# THE HEALING BOUQUET

## EXPLORING
## BACH FLOWER REMEDIES

### VINTON MCCABE

T0273492

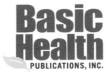

Basic
Health
PUBLICATIONS, INC.

The information contained in this book is based upon the research and personal and professional experiences of the author. It is not intended as a substitute for consulting with your physician or other healthcare provider. Any attempt to diagnose and treat an illness should be done under the direction of a healthcare professional.

The publisher does not advocate the use of any particular healthcare protocol but believes the information in this book should be available to the public. The publisher and author are not responsible for any adverse effects or consequences resulting from the use of the suggestions, preparations, or procedures discussed in this book. Should the reader have any questions concerning the appropriateness of any procedures or preparation mentioned, the author and the publisher strongly suggest consulting a professional healthcare advisor.

Basic Health Publications, Inc.
28812 Top of the World Drive
Laguna Beach, CA 92651
1-800-575-8890 • www.basichealthpub.com


Library of Congress Cataloging-in-Publication Data

McCabe, Vinton.
    The healing bouquet : exploring Bach flower remedies / by Vinton McCabe.
        p. cm.
    Includes bibliographical references and index.
    ISBN-13: 978-1-59120-072-7
    1. Bach, Edward, 1886–1936. 2. Flowers—Therapeutic use. 3. Homeopathy—Materia medica and therapeutics. I. Title.

    RX615.F55M3715      2007
    615'.321—dc22

                                                        2007009682

Editor: Karen Anspach
Typesetting/Book design: Gary A. Rosenberg
Cover design: Mike Stromberg

Printed in the United States of America

10   9   8   7   6   5   4   3   2   1

# Contents

Author's Note, ix

Introduction: Emotional Healing, 1

PART ONE

**Bach's Flower Remedies**

1. The History of the Flower Remedies:
   Healing, Hahnemann, and Bach, 9

2. The Riddle of the Flower Remedies:
   Homeopathy, Allopathy, and Flower Essences, 19

PART TWO

**A Reference Guide to
the Bach Flower Remedies**

3. The Bach Flower Remedies:
   An Introduction, 35

4. Considering the First Mood:
   The Aspects of Fear, 47

REMEDIES FOR THOSE WHO FEAR

Mimulus • Aspen • Red Chestnut
Rock Rose • Cherry Plum

5.  Considering the Second Mood:
    The Degrees of Despair, 85

REMEDIES FOR THOSE WHO DESPAIR

Larch • Elm • Oak • Crab Apple • Willow
Pine • Sweet Chestnut • Star of Bethlehem

6.  Considering the Third Mood:
    The Constraint of Doubt, 139

REMEDIES FOR THOSE WHO DOUBT

Gentian • Hornbeam • Gorse
Scleranthus • Cerato • Wild Oat

7.  Considering the Fourth Mood:
Self Versus Others: Oversensitivity to the World, 185

REMEDIES FOR THOSE WHO ARE OVERLY SENSITIVE

Agrimony • Centaury • Walnut • Holly

8.  Considering the Fifth Mood:
    The Need to Control, 221

REMEDIES FOR THOSE WHO ARE CONTROLLING

Chicory • Beech • Rock Water • Vervain • Vine

9.  Considering the Sixth Mood:
    The Curse of Indifference, 263

REMEDIES FOR THOSE WHO ARE INDIFFERENT

Clematis • Honeysuckle • Mustard • Olive
Wild Rose • White Chestnut • Chestnut Bud

10.  Considering the Seventh Mood:
     The Faces of Loneliness, 321

REMEDIES FOR THOSE WHO ARE LONELY

Water Violet • Heather • Impatiens

PART THREE

# Using the Bach Flower Remedies

11. Taking Cases, 353

12. Combining Remedies, 369

13. Rescue Remedies and Other Blends, 385

14. Using Bach Flower Remedies, 393

# Appendices

Resources, 403

Twelve Healers, Seven Helpers, 409

The Yin and Yang of Bach Remedies, 413

Remedies with Masks, 417

The Ultimate (Baker's) Dozen:
Healers for Your Home Kit, 419

Bach Treatments for Animals, 425

Other Flower Essences, 429

Index, 435

About the Author, 451

## The Bach Flower Remedies Listed Alphabetically

1. Agrimony, 188
2. Aspen, 57
3. Beech, 231
4. Centaury, 195
5. Cerato, 170
6. Cherry Plum, 77
7. Chestnut Bud, 312
8. Chicory, 224
9. Clematis, 267
10. Crab Apple, 106
11. Elm, 93
12. Gentian, 143
13. Gorse, 156
14. Heather, 332
15. Holly, 210
16. Honeysuckle, 275
17. Hornbeam, 150
18. Impatiens, 340
19. Larch, 88
20. Mimulus, 50
21. Mustard, 281
22. Oak, 99
23. Olive, 289
24. Pine, 120
25. Red Chestnut, 65
26. Rock Rose, 71
27. Rock Water, 237
28. Scleranthus, 163
29. Star of Bethlehem, 131
30. Sweet Chestnut, 126
31. Vervain, 246
32. Vine, 254
33. Walnut, 202
34. Water Violet, 324
35. White Chestnut, 302
36. Wild Oat, 176
37. Wild Rose, 294
38. Willow, 113

"Health is our heritage, our right.
It is the complete and full union
between soul, mind and body;
and this is no difficult far-away ideal to attain,
but one so easy and natural
that many of us have overlooked it."

—EDWARD BACH IN *FREE THYSELF*

# Author's Note

I wish to thank Julian Barnard of Healing Herbs, Ltd., for his kind permission to use the quotes taken from Dr. Bach's own writings that have been included throughout this book. Without Mr. Barnard's kind permission to present Edward Bach's core principles in his own words, this book would be a lesser thing. I am deeply indebted to Mr. Barnard, who acted as editor to Dr. Bach in the publication of his collected writings, and to all those who work with him at Healing Herbs, for their guidance and generosity.

All quotations used have been taken from *The Collected Writings of Edward Bach.* For more information on the collected works, and on Healing Herbs, which continues Dr. Bach's works for a new century of practitioners and patients worldwide, please turn to the Resource Guide at the back of this volume.

# Emotional Healing

Like most people, the first time I heard about the Bach Flower Remedies, I heard about Rescue Remedy.

It was about twenty-five years ago, and I had just started to seriously study homeopathy, something about which I was almost equally ignorant.

I was standing backstage at a theatrical rehearsal, rather pompously telling a friend and fellow actor that she should go to see the wonderful new homeopathic practitioner I had just found. Another member of the company happened to overhear me and came over to say that she had been using homeopathy for years. She opened her purse and pulled out a bottle of Rescue Remedy. I had never seen this little bottle before and was unfamiliar with this odd form of medicine that came in liquid form and with the yellow label that has become so familiar to me over the years.

She told me that she always took it if she felt that she had a cold or other form of illness coming on or, as was presently the case, if she was nervous before a performance.

I looked at the bottle, shook it and said, "I don't know what this is, but it isn't homeopathy."

In saying this, I not only let her know (not for the first time, I am sure) how pompous I can be, but I also let her know how little I knew about homeopathy.

And yet there was some truth in my judgmental statement. When you hold Rescue Remedy in your hand, or any other flower essence, for that matter, you are holding a homeopathic medicine. And, at the same time, you are not. You are holding an herbal medicine, which means that you are holding something that must be considered allopathic.[1]

---

1. To readers who may be new to these concepts, "allopathic" medicine is what we think of in the Western world when we think of the word "medicine." Allopathic medicines are given in "material doses," which is to say that they are made from substances, or from chemicals that are created to mimic the physical form and impact of substances. All the medicines you buy in the drugstore and those herbal tinctures that you get in the health food store are allopathic in nature, both because they are actual substances and because of the way they work in your body. Allopathic medicines work by creating "artificial" symptoms that are counter to those your body is experiencing during

In other words, the Bach Flower Remedies can be tricky things, both for those who espouse homeopathy and for those who are dedicated to the practice of allopathic medicine, who tend to try and ignore flower remedies or lump them, with open distain, among those things they rather maddeningly call "alternative medicine." (Alternative to what? To the poisons they are giving? By allowing the use of that word "alternative," those who adhere to more natural forms of medical treatment allow the allopaths to standardize their own treatments—poor though they might be—and marginalize everything else. Don't ever say that word "alternative" to me.). This is especially true of those who, like me, were trained in classical homeopathy. Don't even get me started here—I really hate that word "classical," because it presupposes that treatments that use homeopathic remedies incorrectly, that do not adhere to the principles of homeopathic practice are, in reality, homeopathy, which they are not and will never be. A treatment is either homeopathic or it is not—except for the flower remedies, of course. In the appropriate practice of homeopathic medicine, you can't give remedies incorrectly and then pretend you have "discovered" some new form of homeopathy.

Hard liners, what we call "Hahnemannian" homeopaths, are likely to be very suspicious of the Bach remedies, as I myself was many years ago when I spoke against them with my chest puffed out. They will insist that because the Bach remedies are only slightly diluted and are basically in the same material form they are in when plucked from the soil, they must be considered herbal medicines and not homeopathic. And worse, homeopaths can become alarmed by Bach's theories of treatment, which all but ignore the physical symptoms of the patient and zero in on his or her emotional and spiritual distress.

Again, more on this later, but it is important to note that, from the moment of their creation, Edward Bach's remedies and the thinking process that brought them about were controversial from the very beginning. In his own evolution as a doctor and

your illness. If, for instance, you have a runny nose, you will be given a medicine that causes noses to dry up. This would, in a healthy person, cause a dry nose, but because your nose is running, the thinking is that the medicine will balance things out and return your nose to its "healthy" state.

Homeopathic medicines are different from allopathic medicines in two ways: in the manner in which they are made, and in the way they work in the body. First, they are not given as substances, but are "potentized" into an energy state. And, second, they are not given in opposition to the natural disease, but in a manner that mimics the patient's natural disease as closely as possible. So if you have that runny nose, you are going to be given a remedy that will cause your nose to run more.

That may make no sense right now, but there is a good deal more about this in the pages ahead, especially in the first chapter. For now, just be aware of the words "homeopathy" and "allopathy," and that they are pretty much on opposite ends of the spectrum when it comes to medical treatments.

Bach remedies, however, lurk somewhere in the middle. They are both allopathic and homeopathic, and yet are neither, as we shall see in Chapter Two.

as a healer, Bach more or less cut his ties from both groups of practitioners as he set forth on his mission to bring healing into the life of every man, woman, and child. Even more controversial, Bach placed the responsibility for the healing process and the control of that process in the hands of the patient and not the practitioner, which is something that no doctor of any stripe could ever accept.

Bach was and remains, as we shall see, a truly revolutionary figure in the field of health and healing. His research, his results, and his eloquent writings set him apart from and ahead of nearly every other practitioner of medicine in the Western tradition.

Therefore, I do not think that there can be too many books dedicated to the examination of Bach's work. While his major writings are few enough that they can be gathered in a single volume, and his pharmacy of remedies—only thirty-eight in total not counting Rescue Remedy—is small enough for any family to own and use them all, the impact of his dedication and his discoveries is astounding. As we shall see in the pages ahead, he evolved from allopathic doctor to homeopathically-influenced physician to spiritual healer in his brief lifetime. We see what can be accomplished when passion meets dedication by examining his life, and we uncover subtleties of treatment unknown in any other form of medicine by examining the floral essences that bear his name. His remedies are at once totally safe and amazingly efficacious.

If we can overcome the almost overwhelming prejudice that we all feel in favor of allopathic medicine—a dominance that allows us to accept the niche of "alternative" when we are dealing with anything that the insurance companies don't like—and crawl to a place in which we start thinking of everything that is medicinal simply as "medicine," we can begin untying the Gordian knot that our medical industry has become. And we might find ourselves a good deal healthier a generation or two from now.

> If we can overcome the prejudice that we all feel in favor of allopathic medicine and crawl to a place in which we start thinking of everything that is medicinal simply as "medicine," we can begin untying the Gordian knot that our medical industry has become.

I decided to write this book, not only because I have found again and again over the years that the Bach Remedies offer an avenue to healing that is totally unique among allopathic or homeopathic medicines, but also because I thought it was high time that a book on the Bach Remedies was written by someone schooled in the principles of homeopathy. Every other book I have found was written either by some sort of allopathic practitioner, by an herbalist, or by a therapist trained to work solely in the realm of emotional disturbances. I felt that a book written from the framework of homeopathic thinking could offer insights into the Bach Remedies that no other book to date has offered, because Bach remedies straddle the divide between allopathic and homeopathic medicine, and because Bach's own research was so greatly influenced by the work of Samuel Hahnemann, the father of homeopathic medicine.

There I go, puffing my chest out again, apparently. But I do not mean that I myself have knowledge of homeopathy or of Bach's work that no one else has. I mean that the ways in which the floral essences are used and the results that are obtained are quite different when Bach's work and his pharmacy of medicines are placed within the framework of homeopathy and used in a manner appropriate to that methodology.

The contents of these pages are presented with the intent of giving the reader as complete and thorough a knowledge of Edward Bach's work as possible. It is especially intended that the reader come away with an understanding of what the Bach Remedies truly are and how they became a dynamic and coherent system of therapeutic treatments. In addition, it is my hope that the reader will also receive an education in Bach's remedies themselves, as the majority of the pages in this book are dedicated to the individual remedies. My experience with them tells me that no one book can give a reader a complete understanding of the remedies. But since Bach himself wrote surprisingly little about each of his remedies, writing more about his philosophy of treatment than about his treatments themselves, we must depend upon the writing and research of others to educate ourselves. So, while I hope you will read this book and find it satisfactory, I hope that you will read as much about this small group of remedies as you can. Each book is presented through the filter of its author's bias regarding appropriate medical treatment, as well as through the filters of the author's mind and ego. No book is the last word on this subject for this reason. And all the books in print do not say all that can be said.

In the pages ahead, we shall first explore the history of Edward Bach and his remedies and how they blend the philosophies of allopathic and homeopathic medicine into something unique. Then we shall look at the individual remedies themselves. If you have already glanced at the Contents, you may have noticed that the remedies are grouped differently in these pages than they are in some other books. Many books simply list them in alphabetical order. I have decided to group them in the manner in which Bach himself grouped them. As he polished his new system of treatment, Edward Bach identified seven moods—emotional states that could be positive or negative, acute or chronic ("constitutional" as we say in homeopathic medicine)—and positioned each of his remedies within a group based upon the emotional state common within that group. He identified those groups by a single state: fear, loneliness, and so forth. He identified how each remedy not only stood for a specific and unique emotional state in the group but also how it was a variation on the theme. Therefore, I hope to present the remedies in a way they can most easily be used by grouping them by mood. This way the reader can first identify that he or his patient is described by the fearful group, and then look at the five remedies for fear—each of which approaches the fearful state in a different way and for different reasons—to find the most helpful remedy or remedies. For me anyway, it sure beats having to look through all thirty-eight remedies in alphabetical order before finding the one that is most helpful.

After looking through our potential remedies, we will take a look at how the remedies are used and how they can, singly or in combination, help to balance our emotional states and bring healing to mind, body, and spirit in doing so. You may find that this book differs most from others in this last section, in that, I tend to use the remedies as if they were homeopathic medicines (which is to say, a bit more conservatively than most) because of my background studying, writing about, and teaching homeopathy.

The Resource Guide at the end of the book will give you the best and most up-to-date information I can find on books, pharmacies, organizations, and websites dedicated to floral essences. There is information on other essences that have cropped up in recent years that bring plants indigenous to other parts of the globe to those who share their geography. And, finally, there is a bit of information on the use of floral essences in the treatment of animals. Specific information on the use of each remedy will also be contained in the listing for that remedy.

Throughout all this, I hope to present usable and readable information that will instruct the reader on the safe and effective use of these remedies for self-treatment and for the treatment of the humans and animals we love.

Vinton McCabe
September 2007

# PART ONE

# Bach's Flower Remedies

"Disease is solely and purely corrective;
it is neither vindictive nor cruel,
but it is the means adopted by our own souls
to point out to us our faults,
to prevent our making greater errors,
to hinder us from doing more harm,
and to bring us back to the path of Truth and Light
from which we should never have strayed."

—EDWARD BACH IN HIS COLLECTED WRITINGS

# 1

# The History of the Flower Remedies: Healing, Hahnemann, and Bach

**B**oth the development of the Bach Flower Remedies as a system of therapeutic treatments and the subsequent shift in the goal of treatment from curing specific diseases to encouraging true healing were slow and painstaking processes. They culminated in the work of one physician, Edward Bach, but also involved the efforts of many others over a period of centuries.

Since the time of Hippocrates, medical practitioners realized that they could approach their patients' symptoms in only one of two ways. With one approach, they would try to fight the patient's symptoms by giving him a medicine that would artificially create a new set of symptoms that were in opposition to the symptoms he was experiencing naturally. An example would be giving a sleeping pill to a patient with insomnia—this treatment does not deal with the cause of the sleeplessness, but simply overwhelms the patient's system and irresistibly puts him to sleep.

Or they could do the opposite and work *with* the patient's symptoms. That opposite approach was ultimately named homeopathy in 1896, a word coined by the father of homeopathy, Samuel Hahnemann.

## Samuel Hahnemann (1755–1843)

Samuel Hahnemann was born on April 10, 1755 into the family of Christian Gottfried Hahnemann and his second wife, Johanna Christina Spiess, the daughter of a military captain. His first wife had died years before in childbirth. Christian Hahnemann was a skilled artist, whose work as a painter of Meissen porcelain was particularly respected. He would in later years publish a book on his painting techniques.

Christian Hahnemann's father had also been a painter of some regard and the Hahnemann family had been a prominent one, but they had fallen on hard times during the Seven Years' War. While it had been assumed that young Samuel Hahnemann, who had shown academic aptitude, particularly in foreign languages, would be educated to the highest level, his family lacked the funds to pay for his education.

Hahnemann's teacher and mentor, a Dr. Quarin, introduced the young man to Baron Samuel von Brukenthal, who was the governor of Transylvania. The Baron became Hahnemann's benefactor and offered the young man a job in his personal library. This job would serve two purposes. First, it gave Hahnemann the money that he needed to attend the University of Vienna. Second, it gave Hahnemann access to the many thousands of volumes in the library. Hahnemann read the books as he organized the library, and, in doing so, polished his skill for foreign languages. He was fluent in six languages, including Greek and Latin, by the time he left the Baron's employ. This skill would prove invaluable in the development of what we call homeopathy today.

Samuel Hahnemann received the finest training in medicine available in his day at the University of Vienna. As he studied modern techniques, he also became familiar with those used by past masters, including another graduate of the university, Philippus Theophrastus Bombastus von Hohenheim, or Paracelsus, as he came to be known.

The works of Paracelsus, who was a genius as a medical practitioner (and something of a madman in his personal life, as well as a drug addict, a drunkard, and a wanderer)[1] had great impact upon medical science in the sixteenth century, more than two centuries before Hahnemann. His work was ground-breaking, especially since he bridged the gap between alchemy and chemistry with a passion for both (he likened one to baking and the other to cooking). It is certain that Hahnemann had read Paracelsus' works, although he denied to his dying day that Paracelsus had any impact upon him.

Another aspect of Paracelsus' work, the idea of dilution, is of great importance to homeopathy. In the treatment of the plague, Paracelsus had tested his theory that, if a toxic agent—in this case, the actual excrement of those who were sick with plague—were diluted systematically and to a great enough degree, all toxicity would fall away and what was once poisonous could be used medicinally. He tested his theory in Sterzing and managed to save the village from the disease that was killing half the population of Europe by doing so.

This theory grew in popularity throughout Europe from the time of Paracelsus' experiments. It would, centuries later, become the basis for Edward Jenner's experiments in which he injected a young milkmaid with diluted cowpox and strengthened her system against smallpox. The idea of dilution became the basis for vaccinations as we now know them, and for modern treatments for allergies. It also, as we shall see, became the basis for the creation of all homeopathic remedies.

1. Paracelsus was extremely difficult to deal with. So much so that, in 1532, the citizens of the town of Sterzing, who had only weeks before been so grateful to him for keeping the plague at bay, grew so sick of his antics that they literally drove him out of town. In fact, his wanderings across Europe had as much to do with the fact that populations quickly tired of his drunken brawls as with the fact that Paracelsus traveled to better learn about the medical treatments used in different parts of the world-especially about herbal treatments based upon indigenous plants. Paracelsus would, in fact, die young after one brawl too many. He either fell in a drunken stupor, or was pushed from a second story window and broke his neck. The exact cause of his death remains unknown.

Hahnemann completed his studies and graduated from the University of Vienna. He set up a medical practice in the small village of Hettstedt, a copper-mining town at the foot of the Hartz Mountains. He even married the daughter of a local pharmacist, a marriage that seemed to bode well for all, as it linked an active medical practice with the source of all medicine.

But Hahnemann grew both restless and aggrieved in his practice of medicine. He was repulsed by the practices of bloodletting and leeching, both of which were common medical treatments in his day. Further, he could not help but conclude from his own experience that his patients suffered more as a result of their treatments than they did from their actual diseases.

As Hahnemann began to question the practice of medicine as he had learned it, he also began to put his questions into print. He self-published many small pamphlets that openly criticized both the practice of medicine and those who practiced it. However pure his motivations, his actions were politically unwise. Hahnemann found that he had a harder and harder time making enough money from the practice of medicine to support his growing family.

While he sought a new way of approaching medicine, one that could bring the possibility of health to the sick in a gentle way, Hahnemann was faced with the reality that he had lost the respect that he once enjoyed. Also, the other medical professionals nearby, angered by Hahnemann's publications, were making it difficult for him to practice and even to continue to live in the region. Thus, Hahnemann and his family moved about over the next few years, seeking a place which would accept his new practice of medicine.

Ironically, the same doctors who were unwilling to allow Hahnemann to practice medicine were still quite happy to call upon him for his skill with foreign languages. Hahnemann worked more and more as a translator of medical texts over this period of time rather than as a physician. This work allowed Hahnemann to support his family. More important, it gave him access to the philosophies and methods of medical practice around the globe.

Hahnemann's life changed when he translated the text A *Treatise on Materia Medica*[2] by the Scottish physician William Cullen. In the book, Hahnemann read about a particular bark, Chinchona, which was native to Peru. The bark was known by the natives to be an herbal cure for what was known as intermittent fever. When the European

---

2. The term "Materia Medica" refers to a book that lists all the medicines used within a particular practice of medicine. The term was perhaps first used in the first century A.D., when a naturalist named Pedanius Dioscorides traveled with the Roman army to put together his "De Materia Medica," which described and illustrated in line drawings the plants used in the practice of herbal medicine in Europe and Arabia. This information on all known "materials of medicine" laid the groundwork for the practice of medicine for over sixteen centuries.

explorers came to South America, they suffered from this fever, until they used the herbal treatment. Cullen wrote that the bark, if chewed, would cause symptoms that were similar to the fever itself—chills, aches, and the like.

This small bit of knowledge would literally change Samuel Hahnemann's life.

Could the Chinchona help those who had the fever because it was able to cause the symptoms of fever?

In time, Hahnemann would perform tests with the bark himself and would conclude, "Chinchona bark, which is used as a remedy for intermittent fever, acts because it can produce symptoms similar to those of intermittent fever in healthy people."

This was a whole new way of thinking. And of practicing medicine. It was, in fact, revolutionary, in that it suggested that the manner in which medicine was traditionally practiced in Western culture—indeed, the way in which Hahnemann himself had learned to practice medicine and had practiced it for some years—was, in reality, in direct opposition to the manner in which it should be practiced. Hahnemann changed the nature of medicine with what he would later, after years of research and experimentation, call his "Law of Similars" (stated simply as "like cures like"). In doing so, he learned to practice medicine in accordance with the laws of nature, instead of working against them. Hahnemann established a system of treatment that was both safe and effective through the use of dilution, part of the process by which his remedies were polished from their natural state and made into dilute, non-toxic doses, and the Law of Similars, by which the remedies selected were given to mirror rather than fight the symptoms the patient was experiencing. He added two more Laws of Cure after further years of experimentation. The first of these was Simplex, which insisted that no medicine of any sort should be given in combination with any other, and that all medicines should be given one at a time so their full effect could be weighed and noted. The final Law of Cure was Minimum, which stated that all medicines should be given in the lowest possible effective level of potency and in the fewest number of doses needed. In other words, the patient's system should be troubled as little as possible during the process of reestablishing health.

In time, Hahnemann would name this new system of treatment homeopathy, from two Greek words, *homios*, which means "similar," and *pathos*, which means "suffering." Therefore, the literal meaning of homeopathy is "similar suffering." The name itself reaffirms the core principle of its treatments—that like will always cure like.

Hahnemann also coined a name for the system of treatment he had learned in Vienna that still dominates medicine today. He called it allopathy. Again, it was named from two Greek words, *allos*, which means "different," and *pathos*, which, again, means "suffering." The names define the purpose of the treatments and underline the fact that the two systems of medicine are completely counter to each other.

Hahnemann saw his philosophy and his practice of medical treatment as immutable and inseparable. Only by following all three Laws of Cure could one practice homeopathy. And only by giving remedies that had been fully potentized by following his strict procedure of dilution and *succession* (a method of shaking the diluted substance to better activate their potency) could one administer a homeopathic remedy.[3]

Samuel Hahnemann wrote many more pamphlets about his discoveries. His major work, *The Organon of Medicine*, puts forth his arguments against allopathy and in favor of his new system of treatments. Hahnemann wrote and rewrote the *Organon* over a period of years, taking it through six different editions, each with his increasingly complex vision for the practice of homeopathy. He also developed his own *Materia Medica* of homeopathic remedies. Many of these remedies were created in homeopathic form from the same substances as allopathic medicines, but because they were diluted to the point that none of the molecules of the original toxic substances remained, Hahnemann's remedies were completely safe, while still wonderfully effective in restoring his patients to health.

Throughout the remainder of his life, Samuel Hahnemann saw his reputation grow as his writings found an audience in medical practitioners and patients alike. He lived long enough to see a growing number of practitioners abandon allopathy to practice homeopathy. He saw his philosophy spread from his native Germany through Europe and saw it especially take root in England. From England it would travel to India, where it thrives today, and to America, where it has enjoyed a renaissance in the past thirty years. In the last years of his life, many years after the death of his first wife, Hahnemann married his second wife, Melanie. With Melanie, he moved to Paris, where he taught his methods to a new generation of doctors. He died suddenly of heart failure in the early morning of July 2, 1843. He was eighty-six years old.

Although he had become quite famous as a practitioner of this new sort of medicine, Hahnemann died in poverty. Melanie supported them both in the last years of his life and used her fortune to free him to be able to explore his new methods of practice. She spent all that she had in doing so. Hahnemann was therefore buried in public grave number eight in the Montmartre Cemetery in Paris. When American homeopaths learned of his resting place, they raised the money to give him a proper burial and grave.

Like many others before and after him, Hahnemann proved to be a far better visionary than a businessman. He happily treated all who needed his help, whether they could afford to pay him or not. As a result, the long lines of patients who gathered by his door each morning offered him little in the way of financial reward. Instead, these patients and their cases allowed Hahnemann to codify his practice into a system

---

3. This quick thumbnail of homeopathy will have to suffice for these pages. To learn more about the philosophy and practice of homeopathy turn to the companion volume, *The Healing Enigma: Demystifying Homeopathy*, Basic Health Publication, Inc., 2006.

of treatments that could be taught to practitioners worldwide for these past two hundred years.

## Edward Bach (1886–1936)

It has always seemed odd to me that although Edward Bach was born nearly fifty years after Hahnemann died, and although he lived well into the twentieth century, so much less is commonly known about Bach than is known about Hahnemann. This is particularly true of their personal lives. We know the names of both of Samuel Hahnemann's wives and of all his children, but little is written or discussed about Bach's life.

We know that he was born on September 24, 1886, in a small English village just a few miles outside of Birmingham, and that he was the eldest son. We know that he had a brother and a sister. By all accounts, Edward Bach was something of a sickly child, especially in his early youth, and that, like Hahnemann before him, he seemed from the first to be a natural student. It is said that he could learn anything that he put his mind to.

Bach's family owned a brass foundry. As the eldest son, he went into the family business for a time, but it was determined very quickly that he was not suited for it. Bach noticed the depression and despair that seemed to pervade the workplace, and the negativity of his coworkers affected him. He would remember their sad faces his whole life, and it was in large part for them and for other workers like them that he would develop his system of treatment.

Bach left the foundry to attend Birmingham University, where he studied medicine. He finished his education at the University College Hospital in London and became a licensed doctor in 1912. He developed a particular interest in the subject of immunology early on. Bach became an assistant bacteriologist at a London hospital and worked there throughout World War I.

In 1919, Bach joined the staff of the London Homeopathic Hospital to continue his work in pathology, immunology, and bacteriology. What he saw at the time as a simple step forward in his medical career would prove pivotal in the years ahead.

As Nora Weeks writes about the events that followed in her book *The Medical Discoveries of Edward Bach, Physician*, "Then it was he was given the *Organon* to read, the book written by Hahnemann, the founder of homeopathy.

"This he started to read with doubt in his mind, but the very first page made him reverse his opinion, for he recognized the great genius of Hahnemann, and he sat up the rest of the night and read the book from cover to cover."

Through the act of reading Hahnemann's surprisingly slim volume, the *Organon*, Bach began a process of transformation that would alter the course of his professional life.

As Weeks concludes, "The more he read the more interested he became, for there was a great similarity between Hahnemann's discoveries and his own."

Indeed, Bach had come to question, as Hahnemann had so many years before, both the safety and the efficacy of allopathic medicine. As he stared into his microscope, using technology that Hahnemann could only have guessed at, he marveled at Hahnemann's leaps of logic and vision that identified principles of treatment that only in Bach's time were beginning to be proven with the help of new scientific tools. (Hahnemann's conjectures continue to be proven today, as we refine our methods and improve our technology. Instead of undermining the principles of homeopathy, modern technologies actually support them.)

Central to Hahnemann's vision of homeopathy was the concept of what the practitioner was actually doing when he practiced medicine. And this is perhaps what impressed Bach most as he read the *Organon*. Both Hahnemann and Bach had independently come to the conclusion that the great flaw in allopathic treatment comes from the belief that the doctor is able to treat the patient's disease without treating the patient himself. That toxic substances used in allopathic methods can destroy the patient's disease without harming the patient as a whole being.

> Both Hahnemann and Bach had independently come to the conclusion that the great flaw in allopathic treatment comes from the belief that the doctor is able to treat the patient's disease without treating the patient himself.

As Hahnemann had expressed it, a tenet of homeopathy was that the practitioner treats "the patient, and not the disease." The purpose of homeopathic treatment was to so strengthen the patient's system so that he himself would throw off the illness and return to health.

This approach to medicine insists that the physician see the patient as a whole being in body, mind, and spirit, and always be aware that any treatment affecting any part of this trinity will affect the whole, for better or worse. Homeopathic philosophy further demands that the physician see his patient as a completely unique being, not in any way like or unlike other patients. Each treatment must be geared to the patient himself, and his needs and experiences, not to the idea of eliminating any specific symptom or symptoms.

This makes the practice of homeopathy much more complex than allopathy. The diagnosis of a specific disease immediately suggests a specific course of treatment to the allopath because he is treating the disease and not the patient with the disease. Therefore, his medicines are targeted to the needs of the disease and not to the needs of the patient. That makes them far more likely to injure the patient since his needs are ignored in the treatment.

In treating the patient and not the disease, homeopaths since Hahnemann have insured that the unity of the patient's being will be respected in the treatment, and that the process of curing one part of his being will not take place at the cost of injury to some other part. The patient is respected as a unique individual, so the remedy chosen for his treatment, its potency, and the number of its doses will be chosen for him alone.

This greatly impressed Bach, as it paralleled all he had been discovering in his own work. His reading of the *Organon* changed the course of his life and redefined his work.

Bach soon tried adapting some of Hahnemann's methods of potentization to his own work. The result, over a period of some years, was a group of seven "bowel nosodes." These nosodes—homeopathic remedies made from poisonous or tainted substances—were taken from toxins from the bowels of patients. These toxins were shaped into homeopathic remedies whose actions mirrored those of other, more commonly used remedies. But, as nosodes, the action of Bach's groups of remedies was deeper and more profound than the action of remedies taken from "healthy" substances.[4]

While it might be stretching the point to say that Bach abandoned the practice of allopathic medicine for the practice of homeopathy, it is most certainly true that he increasingly made use of Hahnemann's principles of practice as he searched for his own path in terms of medical treatment.

Unlike Hahnemann's own search for a safer form of treatment, Bach's new approach was not met with anger and criticism. In fact, Bach enjoyed some success as a physician in the years after the development of the bowel nosodes. He opened a practice on Harley Street in London and found a sort of fame as his research was recorded in several medical journals. He even was written about in the *Proceedings of the Royal Society of Medicine*.

Bach's bowel nosodes were used to great success and were, in time, added to the pharmacy of standard homeopathic remedies. They are still in use today.[5]

What would have been the crowning achievement of almost any other physician's career was only a stepping stone for Bach. In time, he turned over his research in the bowel nosodes to his laboratory colleagues. He closed the doors of his practice on Harley Street and set forth, apparently without a specific goal or location in mind. He knew only that he intended to travel through Wales and the English countryside, seeking to learn more about the nature of healing and about the herbal remedies that increasingly fascinated him.

---

4. This is true of all nosodes, and it underlines a principle of homeopathy that states "the stronger the poison, the stronger the cure."

5. Bach had already been working on the idea of using bacteria taken from the bowels to create vaccines when he learned about homeopathic dilutions. Because he believed Hahnemann's methods to be safer, he used his methods for potentizing his nosodes. The bacteria used in the creation of the nosodes were classified by their reactions to four sugars. The nosode's names—Proteus, Dysentery, Morgan Pure, Faecalis Alkaligenes, Coli Mutabile, Gartner and Bacillus #7—reflected their source. Each nosode mirrored some of Hahnemann's other remedies, known as polycrests, in their actions and are commonly used after one or more of Hahnemann's polycrests to complete the cure.

Just what caused Bach to make his move is unknown. In her biography, Nora Weeks tells us that, even before Bach left London once and for all, he had spent some time traveling and had already begun his work developing what would become his flower remedies. He had already created his first three remedies, Impatiens, Mimulus, and Clematis. He had used them enough in his practice to convince him that his new remedies, taken from healthy and benign plants instead of from toxic animal matter, were more capable of bringing about healing than his old remedies.

As Weeks puts it, "So convinced was Edward Bach that he would now be able to replace the bacterial nosodes by the pure and simple herbs of the field that he decided, towards the end of 1929, to give up all other methods of treatment and use these three remedies, the Mimulus, Impatiens and wild Clematis, alone, whilst seeking others to add to their number."

Just what originally inspired Bach's decision to begin work with flowers and make remedies from them is not known. But, in 1929, as he was beginning the last seven years of his life, he did what Paracelsus had also done by choice, and what Hahnemann had been driven to do by adversity. He began to wander. As Hahnemann wandered from town to town in Germany, trying to find a safe harbor, and Paracelsus had wandered before him, learning what he could from herbalists, witch doctors, and tribal healers—indeed, what Dioscorides had done centuries before when traveling with the Roman Legion, Bach set forth on foot to wander through the countryside, looking for what had been overlooked, the flowers of the field.

In the years ahead, Bach would discover a total of thirty-eight remedies, which he would declare to be his complete pharmacy. At that point he began to experiment with combining remedies. The most notable result of this work is Rescue Remedy, which is a combination of five remedies that can be used in all situations involving emotional trauma and/or shock.

Bach would also devise his own system of polishing or "potentizing" his remedies. Bach wrote about this method in his 1932 book, *Free Thyself*:

"Take a thin glass bowl, fill with clear water from a stream or spring for preference, and float enough of the blooms of the plant to cover the surface. Allow this to stand in bright sunshine until the flowers begin to wilt. Very gently pick out the blooms, pour the water into bottles and add an equal quantity of brandy as a preservative.

"One drop alone of this is sufficient to make potent an eight ounce bottle of water, from which doses may be taken by a tea-spoonful as required.

"The dose should be taken as the patient feels necessary: hourly in acute cases; three or four times a day in chronic cases until relief occurs when they can be dispensed with."

By 1932, Bach had discovered the first twelve of his remedies, which he called "The Twelve Healers." With these remedies, he felt that he had identified the twelve archetypes of human behavior and of negative patterns of thought. In time, he would discover seven more remedies, which he called his "Seven Helpers." He felt that these remedies were adjuncts to the original twelve and could be used singly or in combination with those remedies in cases where the first remedies did not create a complete cure.

Bach would refine his remedies and experiment with them during the winter months each year. He used them to treat patients who were not charged for their treatments. In fact, Bach paralleled Hahnemann in his lack of business acumen as he did in so many other ways. Although he had once had a successful medical practice in London, he never considered the acquisition of wealth to be a personal goal. In later years he was often very poor and would be seen wandering the streets in ragged clothes, his pockets filled with vials of his remedies that he offered free to all those in need. It is likely that only his reputation as a physician allowed him to be accepted in spite of his appearance.

In 1934, Bach moved to Mount Vernon in Oxfordshire, where he would remain for the rest of his days. It was here that Bach discovered the nineteen remedies that would complete his pharmacy.

Like Hahnemann, Bach tended to rewrite old works and adapt them to his new discoveries rather than write new titles. An example of this is his work, *Twelve Great Remedies*, which was published in 1933. In 1934, it was expanded into *The Twelve Healers and Seven Helpers*. In the summer of 1936, it was reissued with the same title, although the book now contained Bach's full pharmacy of thirty-eight remedies.

Very little is known of Bach's personal life, partly because he is an obscure enough public figure that no one has yet written an unbiased and journalistically sound biography, and partly because information pertaining to the man and his work is jealously guarded by the foundation that carries on his work today.[6]

What is known is that Bach died at the young age of fifty on the evening of November 27, 1936, after an extended period of ill health.

6. See the Resource section in the Appendix for information on the foundation and a list of titles of books pertaining to Bach, including Nora Weeks' biography.

# 2

---

# The Riddle of the Flower Remedies: Homeopathy, Allopathy, and Flower Essences

A s often as possible in this chapter, I want to present Bach's ideas in his own words. To this end, I want to begin with what I think is an excellent presentation of his core philosophy as presented in his pamphlet *Heal Thyself* [1].

"The main reason for the failure of modern medical science is that it is dealing with results and not causes. For many centuries the real nature of disease has been masked by materialism, and thus disease itself has been given every opportunity of extending its ravages, since it has not been attacked at its origin. The situation is like to an enemy strongly fortified in the hills, continually waging guerilla warfare in the country around, while the people, ignoring the fortified garrison, content themselves with repairing the damaged houses and burying the dead, which are the result of the raids of the marauders. So, generally speaking, is the situation in medicine today; nothing more than the patching up of those attacked and the burying of those who are slain, without a thought being given to the real stronghold.

"Disease will never be cured or eradicated by present materialistic methods, for the simple reason that disease in its origin is not material.[2] What we know as disease is an ultimate result produced in the body, the end product of deep and long acting forces, and even if material treatment alone is apparently successful this is nothing more than a temporary relief unless the real cause is removed. The modern trend of medical science, by misinterpreting the true nature of disease and concentrating it in materialistic terms in the physical body, had enormously increased its power, firstly, by distracting the thoughts of people from its true origin and

---

1. Even the title of the pamphlet is important to understanding Bach and his treatments. In moving away from traditional homeopathy, he sought to simplify Hahnemann's practice of treatment and to offer a method of self-treatment that is both safe and effective.

2. By "material," Bach means that diseases are not the result of germs alone. Certainly, any number of viruses or bacteria associated with disease may be present in the system of a very healthy person and never make him ill. Bach shared Hahnemann's belief that all illness was, at its core, a matter of the disruption of the "vital force," which is the invisible, intangible energy that animates us all and allows our innate healing process to occur.

hence from the effective method of attack, and secondly, by localizing it in the body, thus obscuring true hope of recovery and raising a mighty disease complex of fear, which never should have existed.

"Disease is in essence the result of conflict between Soul and Mind, and will never be eradicated except by spiritual and mental effort. Such efforts, if properly made with understanding, as we shall see later, can cure and prevent disease by removing those basic factors which are its primary cause. No effort directed to the body alone can do more than superficially repair damage, and in this there is no cure, since the cause is still operative and may at any moment again demonstrate its presence in another form. In fact, in many cases apparent recovery is harmful, since it hides from the patient the true cause of his trouble, and in the satisfaction of apparently renewed health the real factor, being unnoticed, may gain in strength. Contrast these cases with that of the patient who knows, or who is by some wise physician instructed in, the nature of the adverse spiritual or mental forces at work, the result of which as precipitated what we call disease in the physical body. If that patient directly attempts to neutralize those forces, health improves as soon as this is successfully begun, and when it is completed the disease will disappear. This is true healing by attacking the stronghold, the very base of the cause of suffering."

In thinking about this quote, it is important to remember its source. Bach is not writing as a religious leader or a tribal healer. He is writing as one of the foremost bacteriologists of his day, and one of the most successful physicians in London. His observations are based upon a lifetime of experience in treating patients, in experiencing successes and failures as a doctor. His conclusions are based upon the empirical evidence he gathered through professional clinical experience. Therefore, his comments were hard earned, and his conclusions were those that stood both the test of time and the test of experience.

In his conclusions concerning the nature of illness and the possibilities for healing, Bach both agrees and disagrees with Hahnemann as to both the nature of disease and the appropriate means of treating those who are sick. In just the same way, he both agrees and disagrees with Hahnemann regarding the creation of his remedies and the manner in which they are used.

## Hahnemann and Bach

In his 1931 pamphlet *Heal Thyself*, Bach identified three men whose work had most influenced his own. He wrote of them: "Such men as Hippocrates with his mighty ideals of healing, Paracelsus with his certainty of the divinity of man, and Hahnemann who realized that disease originated in a plane above the physical—all these knew much of the real nature and remedy of suffering."

From Hippocrates, Bach learned of the body's potential for healing and the boundaries of what is possible in terms of cure. More important, he learned the basic tenet of medical practice: "As to diseases make a habit of two things—to help, or at least, to do no harm."

From Paracelsus, he learned that all innovators must learn to wander, and that they must risk at any moment ridicule, poverty and loss of status if they are willing to fulfill their vision. He also learned the concept of dilution, and the lingering notion of "like curing like" that runs as a slender thread from Hippocrates through to the modern age. Like Hippocrates, Paracelsus knew that the practitioner could only work with a patient's symptoms or against them. Like Hahnemann, Paracelsus concluded that the best, safest, and most effective treatments are those that work with a patient's symptoms.

From Hahnemann, he learned that he must always treat the patient and never the disease, and that he must never allow the disease diagnosis suggest a particular treatment, but must always treat the patient as a whole and unique being.

In a 1931 address that he gave to medical professionals, which has been published under the title *Ye Suffer from Yourselves*, Edward Bach told the audience,

> "The inspiration given to Hahnemann brought a light to humanity in the darkness of materialism, when man had come to consider disease as a purely materialistic problem to be relieved and cured by materialistic means alone.
>
> "He, like Paracelsus, knew that if our spiritual and mental aspects were in harmony, illness could not exist: and he set out to find remedies which would treat our minds, and thus bring us peace and health.
>
> "Hahnemann made a great advance and carried us a long way along the road, but he had only the length of one life in which to work, and it is for us to continue the researches where he left off: to add more to the structure of perfect healing of which he laid the foundation, and so worthily began the building.
>
> "The homeopath has already dispensed with much of the unnecessary and unimportant aspects of orthodox medicine, but he has yet further to go. I know that you wish to look forward, for neither the knowledge of the past nor the present is sufficient for the seeker after truth."

The implication here, of course, is that however good Hahnemann's methods are, they are not, in and of themselves, perfected.

While Bach most certainly embraces Hahnemann, Hippocrates, and Paracelsus and gives them all due credit for the discoveries

While Bach most certainly embraces Hahnemann, Hippocrates, and Paracelsus and gives them all due credit for the discoveries each packed into "the length of one life," he gives himself ample room to make the changes to the homeopathic way of practice that suit his own way of thinking and working.

each packed into "the length of one life," he gives himself ample room to make the changes to the homeopathic way of practice that suit his own way of thinking and working.

Bach continues:

> "Paracelsus and Hahnemann taught us not to pay too much attention to the details of disease, but to treat the personality, the inner man, realizing that if our spiritual and mental natures were in harmony disease disappeared. The great foundation to their edifice is the fundamental teaching which must continue.
>
> "Hahnemann next saw how to bring about this harmony, and he found that among the drugs and the remedies of the old school,[3] and among elements and plants which he himself selected, he could reverse their action by potentization, so that the same substance which gave rise to poisonings and symptoms of disease could—in the minutest quantity—cure those particular symptoms when prepared by his special method.
>
> "Thus he formulated the law of "like cures like": another great fundamental principle of life. And he left us to continue the building of the temple, the earlier plans of which had been disclosed to him.
>
> "And if we follow on this line of thought, the first great realization which comes upon us is the truth that it is disease itself which is "like curing like": because disease is the result of wrong activity. It is the natural consequence of disharmony between our bodies and our Souls: it is "like curing like" because it is the very disease itself which hinders and prevents our carrying our wrong actions too far, and at the same time, is a lesson to teach us to correct our ways, and harmonize our lives with the dictates of our Soul."

We can only wonder what Hahnemann would have made of this. Or if Hahnemann, hearing this, would have given Bach permission to "continue the building of the temple," or if, indeed, he would have thought that he had left the temple unbuilt at the time of his death. Just as Bach felt that, in gathering thirty-eight remedies out of the millions possible, that he had completed and perfected his system of healing, I am quite sure that Hahnemann died believing that he had fully perfected the system of homeopathic practice. I doubt he would have felt the need to turn things over to Bach, or to Schuessler, or, indeed, to Mary Baker Eddy, who borrowed and bastardized much of Hahnemann's philosophy in the creation of her *Science of the Mind*. Just as Eddy capitalizes the "m" in "mind," Bach capitalizes the "s" in "soul" to great impact and great result. Both took the core of Hahnemann's teachings and subtly enlarged upon it in the name of perfecting it.

---

3. The "old school" always refers to allopathic medicine in both the writings of Edward Bach and Samuel Hahnemann.

Bach concludes, "Disease is the result of wrong thinking and wrong doing, and ceases when the act and thought are put in order. When the lesson of pain and suffering and distress are learnt, there is no further purpose in its presence, and it automatically disappears.

"This is what Hahnemann incompletely saw as 'like curing like.'"

Safe to say, Hahnemann would disagree with this. Most certainly, I do not think that Hahnemann felt that his own view of illness or the principle of Similarity ("like curing like") as incomplete.

It is here, in 1931, with the publication of this address, that Bach separates himself from Hahnemann. And it is here that the fundamental differences between homeopathy and Bach treatments become apparent.

While both would agree that man is a whole and unique being, they would disagree as to the nature of disease. Where Bach would say that "disease is the result of wrong activity," Hahnemann would say "yes, it may be in a particular case, but in another case it may not." For Hahnemann—whose view of illness is actually closer to that of the practitioner of Chinese Medicine than anything else—illness is always a block of the Vital Force, that intangible energy that permeates our beings and animates us all as a race of beings. Vital Force is also that which allows us to regenerate and to heal. And when Vital Force is weakened, whether by "wrong actions," toxins in our environment, or exposure to bacteria or viruses, illness results.

For Hahnemann, the fact that he believed his patients to be whole and unique beings meant that every aspect of life, physical, emotional, mental, and spiritual must be taken into account in the case of illness, and the changes in each level of being must be addressed to restore health. This did not mean that he, like Bach or Mary Baker Eddy, was willing to ignore the physical symptoms, although he did consider them to be of lesser import than are the mental or spiritual symptoms. Hahnemann believed in the treatment of the whole man. He believed that only by treating the patient as both a whole and unique being could a treatment be found that could fundamentally improve the patient's health. Hahnemann further believed that each patient was entitled to a medical treatment that brought the rapid, gentle, and permanent restoration of health. It was quite a lofty goal, and remains as much today. Certainly it is in no way incomplete.

Later in his 1931 address, Bach invited his listeners to "come a little further along the road." Speaking now about his own flower remedies, he said, "The action of these remedies is to raise our vibrations and open up our channels for the reception of our Spiritual Self, to flood our natures with the particular virtue we need, and wash out from us the fault which is causing harm. They are able, like beautiful music, or any gloriously uplifting thing which gives us inspiration, to raise our very natures, and bring us nearer to our Souls: and by that very act, to bring us peace, and relieve our sufferings.

"They cure, not by attacking disease, but by flooding our bodies with the beautiful vibrations of our Higher Nature, in the presences of which disease melts as snow in the sunshine."

The purpose of Bach's remedies, then, is to give our minds and hearts an opportunity for change. They can allow us to rewrite our patterns of thought and behavior and make that which was negative become positive. That is a powerful thing, and it certainly has implications for healing as well. As the patient moves to a more positive outlook emotionally, he or she will also surely make changes in lifestyle that can and will support greater health.

In this, Hahnemann and Bach would agree. Just as homeopathic remedies can elicit physical changes in the body, they can also subtly alter patterns of thought and feeling. This is, after all, the reason that homeopaths seek to learn as much as they can about their patient's mind and spirit in the case-taking process. But Bach moves fundamentally away from Hahnemann when he removes all consideration of physical complaints from his healing equation.[4]

He ends *Ye Suffer from Yourselves* with this: "As Hahnemann laid down, all healing which is not from within, is harmful, and apparent cure of the body obtained through materialistic methods, obtained only through the action of others, without self-help, may certainly bring physical relief, but harm to our higher natures, for the lesson remains unlearnt, and the fault has not been eradicated.

"It is terrible today to think of the amount of artificial and superficial cures obtained through money and wrong methods in medicine; wrong methods because they merely suppress symptoms, give apparent relief, without removing the cause."

In this brief passage, Bach brings up two very important concepts, one of which bonds him with Hahnemann, the other of which separates their methods once and for all.

Both would certainly agree (as, for the record, would I) with the idea that there is, in the end, nothing worse you can do for a patient than simply suppress his or her symptoms. This, sadly, is the basis for modern allopathic treatments. Treatments that can, in the long run, offer nothing but continued illness for those who undertake them. Think

---

4. This does not mean that his remedies have no implications in the physical realm. As we shall see in the individual listings for the remedies, many of them have applications for physical symptoms. And, as Bach himself says, all will lead to a state of physical healing over time. I have seen the Bach remedies physically heal patients who found no help in any other form of medicine, allopathic or homeopathic. Remember, Bach removes the physical symptoms in case taking, and tells us to concentrate on the mind and heart of the patient when selecting remedies. He does not say that the remedies cannot work on a physical level—they certainly do. But he does say that that physical level should be ignored, and that it is because doctors have, for centuries, been dwelling only on the physical complaints of their patients that has kept medicine from being truly curative.

about it—when you take a cold medicine or a pain killer does that medicine do anything other than allow you, for a brief time, to pretend that you are not suffering from the illness that you are, in reality, suffering from? An entire industry of supposedly healing pharmaceuticals and practitioners work in collusion to encourage the public to think they are being helped by treatments that actually do nothing at all of a curative nature and, in reality, cause harm.

I sit in amazement when doctors use the word "suppression" as if it could ever be a good thing. Think about what is happening to patients when their symptoms are suppressed. Do they feel stronger and more clear-headed? No, they feel sluggish and dull-witted. Isn't that a sign of something? When a homeopathic remedy is given, the practitioner looks for improvement: an increase of energy, a lifting of the mood, a clearing of the mind, a peaceful sleep. Those are signs of an increase in health. Sluggishness, drugged sleep, and dull-wittedness are all signs of a decrease in health.

When doctors suppress symptoms, they pretend that the body is not a whole unit; that they can shove symptoms down in one part of the body without them appearing anywhere else. This is simply contrary to reality. That which is suppressed must, at some point, rise up again, if not in a repeat of the same symptoms on another day, then in a new symptom in some other part of the body. The allopath, who rejects the idea of wholeness, gets to pretend that the new symptom is a new disease that has nothing to do with his toxic treatments.

And, even worse, when doctors suppress symptoms they are doing nothing at all about the actual disease state (which is why Bach gets so riled up over the idea of disease as a lesson that needs to be learned and that allopathic treatment is a way to avoid learning it). It merely makes the pain go away for a period of time. If the patient is going to get better from these treatments (note the "if"), he is going to have to get better on his own. In fact, suppressive treatments count on the fact that, if you just keep suppressing for long enough, the patient's own immune system will, in time, make him well. Sometimes this actually happens, if the patient's immune system is strong enough. Sometimes it doesn't and the disease recurs, which allows the doctor to suppress it again, like a game of Whack-A-Mole. Sometimes it reappears in another part of the body, which allows the doctor to pretend that it is a whole new disease to be suppressed.

So, Hahnemann and Bach would agree on the toxicity of suppressive treatments and the folly of allopathic philosophy. But they would never agree on a subject that is very important to Bach and his therapies: self-treatment.

For Bach, the whole process of healing is one of self-discovery. Lessons must be learned if illness is to be put aside. While Hahnemann would agree that lessons must be learned in life, and that changes in thought and lifestyle are key to the healing process, he would disagree rather strongly with the idea of self-treatment. While Hahnemann upholds the concept of doctor and patient (although he did have some rather revolutionary ideas on the subject that he writes about in the *Organon*), Bach removes the doctor from the equation as well as the physical symptoms.

For Bach, all truly functional medical treatments must involve the self. And, for him, the self, while taking on the role of the patient, is also perhaps the best choice for the role of the physician. This concept is at once revolutionary and questionable, and it leads us to ask: just what are these Bach Flower Remedies all about, anyway?

## Bach Flower Remedies: FAQs

There are several questions that need to be answered before the more general question posed above can be addressed. Given that these remedies are homeopathic and yet are not, that they are, in some ways, allopathic drugs, in other ways homeopathic, and in some very important ways, something unique and different, they can be something of a mystery to those who are considering using them. Things can get even more confusing when you decide to take them because they are, in some ways, used as if they were homeopathic treatments and, in other ways, used as if they were herbal supplements. So, let's try to answer the most frequently asked questions.

### What Are the Bach Flower Remedies?

Technically, the Bach remedies are what are called "Mother Tinctures." This means that, like homeopathic remedies, they have been diluted in water, in the manner Bach described in the previous chapter. Unlike homeopathic remedies, they have not gone through multiple levels of dilution. They are, therefore, zero potency homeopathic remedies. The Mother Tincture is the substance in liquid state, from which all the other potencies are made.

Therefore, the Bach remedies retain the original substance in a state of simple dilution. Since they retain the material state of the original substance, they cannot be considered true homeopathic remedies—all homeopathics are diluted to the point at which the original substance is greatly diluted or even washed totally away. But since they have been placed in a state of dilution, they cannot be considered truly allopathic (which, in general, all medicines given in material form must be) or herbal.

For me, the Bach remedies represent the perfect balance of homeopathic and herbal medicine. As such, they are unique, an entirely different form of medicine, one that is neither homeopathic nor allopathic and yet, in a way, is both.

Because the Bach remedies are materially different from both homeopathic and allopathic medications and yet retain some portion of the original substance, it was vital to their success as a form of medical therapy that Bach use only the most benign substances for source materials. With his extensive experience in working with toxins (as a pathologist and bacteriologist), he certainly had the working experience to develop a system of treatment that is totally benign in all its uses.

## How Do They Work?

Chemically, that remains a mystery. No medical test known today can prove that the Bach remedies have medical value, just as no machine can show just why the homeopathic remedies have been shown in clinical experience to have empirically proven value.

The impact of the remedies, individually or in combination, however, has been well researched over the last century. It has, for instance, been well established that Mimulus is a remedy that can be very helpful for patients who have specific fears. Many thousands of patients have demonstrated that Mimulus can help those who are afraid to get into elevators, to drive over bridges, or to walk into a dark room.

Bach made a point, when possible, to select flowers as his source materials. It was also important that the flowers from which his remedies were made had no previous track record as herbal medicines. Unlike Hahnemann, Bach did not depend upon the allopathic pharmacy of his day as the source of his own pharmacy of remedies. Instead, Bach went with his instincts and with the empirical evidence of his own clinical experience with the remedies and their actions. As a result, we are dependent upon Bach for the description of their uses when we work with the Bach remedies before we prove the efficacy of the remedies ourselves.

## Is It Okay for Me to Treat Myself with Bach Remedies?

They were created for that purpose. Remember, Bach felt that self-treatment was not only acceptable, but actually the highest form of treatment, because only the self can know the exact nature of the lessons of health that need to be learned.

In *Free Thyself* he writes, "We are all healers, and with love and sympathy in our natures we are also able to help anyone who really desires health."

But remember, because we are all healers, others can be very helpful as we struggle with self-treatment. Those around us, especially our family, can hold a figurative mirror up to our faces so we can see the impact we have on those around us as we begin and continue the healing process.

Trusted friends and family members, even coworkers, can be helpful in measuring our changes. Even more important, those who don't like us and often stand in opposition to us can also be a mirror of sorts. Without necessarily telling them what you are doing to improve yourself, take notice of how the difficult people in your life are apparently changing their attitude to you as you change your behavior. This can give an excellent indication of just how far you've come.

## How Do I Choose the Right Remedy?

Bach has a great answer for this question in his pamphlet *Heal Thyself*. He writes,

"Should any difficulty be found in selecting your own remedy, it will help you to ask yourself which of the virtues you most admire in other people; or which of the failings is, in others, your pet aversion, for any fault of which we may still have left a trace and are especially attempting to eradicate, that is the one we most hate to see in other people. It is the way we are encouraged to wipe it out in ourselves."

Above all else, the selection of the remedy, whether for yourself or for another, involves honesty. It requires a willingness to change and a yearning for health. With those in place, it can be a simple thing.

Bach himself says that we each have within us all thirty-eight of the emotional states described by his remedies, in a mixture of toxicity and creativity. Not all the emotional states need be negative. Where one patient will be fearful, another will have courage. But we each have the *potential* need for any single or combination of the remedies at every moment of our lives. That means that no real mistakes can be made.

In selecting a remedy or remedies, it can be helpful to look at yourself and at others. What, for instance, are your pet peeves when it comes to others? That can tell you a great deal about what you yourself may be doing and thinking without being aware that you are doing it. Think about how you act when you are under the most stress—that can give another strong indication of the needed remedy. We all look pretty good when we are calm and happy.

As Bach concludes, "Seek for the outstanding mental conflict in the patient, give him the remedy that will assist him to overcome that particular fault, and all the encouragement and hope you can, then the healing virtue within him will of itself do all the rest."

### How Do I Decide How Many to Take?

Bach tells us that he believes that the man who has only one negative emotional state or motivation need take only a single remedy to correct that state and free himself from illness. He further states that those who have more than one negative emotional state need to take more than one remedy.

For the sake of clarity and simplicity, Bach grouped his thirty-eight remedies into seven "moods," or categories. It is therefore possible for the physician to first identify the moods from which a patient's negative emotional patterns are coming and then refine the prescription of remedies by identifying which remedy (or, less commonly, remedies) associated with that particular mood best reflects the patient's behavior patterns.

While there is no simple, set answer to just how many remedies one should take, there is a simple rule of thumb: it is always best to take the fewest number of remedies that can create a positive result. If one remedy seems enough to do the job, it should be tried first singly and other remedies should be added if needed.

## How Do I Take Them?

In answering this question in his 1934 book *The Twelve Helpers and Seven Helpers*, Bach writes:

> "To use the remedies, take about a cupful of water and add only three or four drops from the little bottles supplied by the chemist of the needful herb or herb, and stir it up. If it gets stale, throw it away and mix more, or if it is desired to keep it for some time add two teaspoonsful of brandy. It does not matter about being exact, as none of these remedies could do the least harm, even if taken in large quantities, but as little is enough, to make up a small amount saves waste.
>
> "For children, give an egg-spoonful, and for grown-ups a teaspoonful at a time. In very desperate cases doses may be given every quarter of an hour; in severe cases every hour, and in ordinary long-standing illness about every two or three hours spread over the day, or more often if the patient feels it is helping to take it frequently. As the case gets better, the doses will not be required to be given so often.
>
> "If the patient is unconscious, it is sufficient to moisten the lips with the remedy, and if in this case the patient is pale, give Rock Rose and Clematis, or if high-colored, Rock Rose and Vine."

In other words, the rules by which the remedies are given are fluid. Like homeopathic remedies, they are best used "as needed." If a patient feels the need for another dose, by all means allow him one. In acute cases, those that are limited by the nature of the illness itself, like colds or flu, the remedies may be given more often, perhaps every hour or two, until the patient feels that recovery is well underway.

In more chronic cases, I have found that it works best to limit the number of doses per day, allowing only two or three at most, because the remedies are similar to homeopathic remedies. Just as more cases treated homeopathically are ruined by giving too many doses of remedy than by any other mismanagement, I believe that many cases treated with Bach remedies are ruined by giving the remedies too often or by jumping too frequently from remedy to remedy.[5]

## Do I Take the Remedies the Same Way for Acute and Chronic Conditions?

The Bach remedies share Hahnemann's homeopathic viewpoint regarding the goals of treatment in both acute and chronic cases. Both felt that acute situations required acute treatments and that chronic conditions required chronic, or to use Hahnemann's word for it, "constitutional" treatments. Constitutional treatments, commonly, are usually both deeper and longer lasting than acute treatments. They also may be more com-

5. For more information on this and other ways in which the Bach remedies can be used most effectively, turn to Chapter Twelve.

plex, and commonly use a greater number of remedies, in combination or singly, in a greater number of doses over a longer period of time.

An acute emotional state is, by its very nature, temporary and often the result of a particular single cause, stressor, or trauma, so it is expected that fewer remedies in a fewer number of doses are required to return the patient to a state of emotional balance than would be needed to balance a long standing negative pattern of behavior. Constitutional cases have been established over long periods of time and, in terms of either homeopathic or Bach treatments, can often be something like onions. They can have many different layers of illness, often as a result of all sorts of suppressions that need to be peeled away before the patient is returned to a state of health.

### What Will I Feel When I Take These Remedies?

Bach remedies are subtle. Unlike toxic allopathic drugs, they will not impede your ability to drive a car or operate heavy machinery. A patient taking Bach remedies should not feel dullness of mind or heaviness of body. Instead, he should feel a sense of calm, and possibly an increased sense of clarity. Emotional release such as laughter and tears can be common, especially for those taking a remedy for the first time. The patient may have a desire to yawn and take a quiet nap for a few minutes. All of these are signs of a well-selected remedy.

Many who take the remedies, however, will feel no change whatsoever. For this reason, some will think that they are doing nothing at all. In these cases, it may be important to ask the patient to simply be patient and be willing to give the remedies a chance to work. This is especially common in constitutional cases, in which the remedies may have to be used for a period of time before their benefits become noticeable. It may be those around the patient, and not the patient himself, who first notice the improvements that the remedies bring to these cases.

### What Can I Ultimately Expect from the Remedies?

As Bach tells us in *Ye Suffer from Yourselves*, there are four distinct indications that the remedies are working. "First, peace: secondly, hope: thirdly, joy: and fourthly, faith." While this is not an exact answer by any means, it gives an indication of what we can expect from the Bach Flower Remedies.

In my experience, many people use the remedies in the wrong way or for the wrong reasons. And many times it is the person who is giving the remedies that would do well to take them, either along with or even instead of the patient to whom they are being given.

Many times the Bach remedies are given as an act of control over another person, especially by angry spouses or concerned parents. When a patient's flaws are obvious, the loved ones will often decide to intervene with the Bach remedies to "rearrange" the patient's behavior or thoughts in a manner that would be more pleasing to them. This is not what was intended by Dr. Bach in his development of the remedies.

As I will go into more detail in later chapters, I believe that this aspect of self-treatment, that was the very foundation of the remedies in their creation, must always be upheld in all Bach treatments, acute or constitutional: If the patient does not desire to give up his old patterns, indeed, if he does not desire to be healed, then he should never be treated.

So first and foremost, we can never expect that the remedies offer us a method by which we can police the thoughts and control the behaviors of others.

Another thing we cannot expect is that the use of a remedy will eradicate a particular aspect of the patient's personality. This expectation also confuses students of homeopathy. Since homeopathic constitutional remedies, just like constitutional Bach remedies, describe a certain type of person (often down to the details of their dress and skin tone), students often think that if you treat a Sulphur type, for instance, you will end up with a Phosphorus type. In the same way, students of Bach treatments often think that if you treat a Willow type, you will end up with a Clematis. This is not the case.

In homeopathic treatment, if you treat a Sulphur, you will likely end up with a healthy Sulphur. In the same way, Bach treatments of a negative Willow type most often yield a healthy and positive Willow, in whom the negative behaviors of the unhealthy Willow will now be present in their most positive context.

Now, certainly, we often have more than one "type" within us. We are complex beings. But the outcome of a treatment—especially a constitutional treatment—is not easily predicted.

What can more or less be predicted is that, if the remedy or remedies are well selected, and the combination of remedies is allowed to evolve and change as the patient changes with their use, and if the patient's environment also changes, (which is to say that if you treat one person who lives in a toxic environment and do not treat the other aspects of the environment, then you are bound to be disappointed with the results) and especially if others present in that environment support the patient and his healing process, then the results will seem nothing short of miraculous.

Can the Bach remedies, used correctly, elicit a profound emotional change in a patient? Most certainly. They can allow the patient the opportunity to actually change, to rewrite his life, and to let go, once and for all, of old hurts that still remain, becoming the source of his most negative behaviors.

Can the Bach remedies, used correctly, elicit a profound physical change in a given patient? Perhaps surprisingly, the answer to this is yes, most certainly. While the Bach remedies are given on the basis of a patient's emotional needs, they are not limited in any way in the healing they can bring. This is most easily understood in cases of ailments that have a profound emotional aspect or link, like hypertension or headaches. But I have seen these remedies work time and again in cases where the physical ailments seemed on the surface to have no emotional link. And I have seen them have a profound healing impact on every aspect of a patient's life: mental, physical, emotional, and spiritual.

Perhaps it's best to give Bach the last word. In *Ye Suffer from Yourselves*, he writes:

"And so now, in summing up, we can see the mighty part that homeopathy is going to play in the conquest of disease in the future.

"Now that we have come to the understanding that disease itself is 'like curing like': that it is of our own making: for our correction and for our ultimate good: and that we can avoid it, if we will but learn the lessons needed, and correct our faults before the severer lesson of suffering is necessary. This is the natural continuation of Hahnemann's great work; the consequence of that line of thought which was disclosed to him, leading us a step further toward perfect understanding of disease and health, and is the stage to bridge the page between where he left us and the dawn of that day when humanity will have reached that state of advancement when it can receive direct the glory of Divine Healing.

"The understanding physician, selecting well his remedies from the beneficent plants in nature, those Divinely enriched and blessed, will be enabled to assist his patients to open up those channels which allow greater communion between Soul and Body, and thus the development of virtues needed to wipe away the faults. This brings to mankind the hope of real health combined with mental and spiritual advance."

# PART TWO

# A Reference Guide to the Bach Flower Remedies

**An Appeal to My Colleagues of the Medical Profession**

"After very many years of research, I have found that certain Herbs have the most wonderful healing properties; and that with the aid of these, a large number of cases which by orthodox treatment we could only palliate, are now curable.

"Moreover, on-coming disease can be treated and prevented at that stage when people say, 'It is not bad enough to send for a doctor . . .'

"The Herbs mentioned can be used in conjunction with any orthodox treatment, or added to any prescription, and will hasten and assist the treatment in all types of cases, acute or chronic, to be more successful.

"It is a time amongst us when orthodox medicine is not fully coping with a proportion of disease in this country; and it is a time to regain the confidence of the people, and justify our noble Calling.

"The Herbs are simple to every student of human nature to understand, and one of their properties is that they help us to prevent the onset of organic disease when the patient is in that functional state which, in either acute or chronic ailments, so often precedes them."

—EDWARD BACH IN HIS COLLECTED WRITINGS

# 3

# The Bach Flower Remedies:
# An Introduction

As we look at Bach's thirty-eight remedies one at a time, be aware that I have grouped the remedies by Bach's seven "moods."[1] As he lists them, these moods are: Fear, Uncertainty, Insufficient Interest in Present Circumstances, Loneliness, Oversensitivity to Influences and Ideas, Despondency or Despair, and Over-Concern for the Welfare of Others. Note that some of the names for these conditions have been changed slightly in this book. I have also ordered the moods in a manner that, for me at least, makes their study more comprehensible.

Where applicable, I have also noted that a particular remedy is one of Bach's original Twelve Healers, the remedies he saw as archetypes for the ills that plague all mankind. Also, where applicable, I have indicated that a particular remedy may be considered more of a long-term remedy or more often be used only in the short-term. This information can be of particular importance in the individualizing of combined remedies and in giving the Bach practitioner a guidepost for knowing which flower remedies act faster and which work more slowly. In the same way, when administering the remedies, it is helpful to know which are naturally more acute in their actions, and which may be considered to be more or less on the same footing as the polycrests[2] or

1. I have always appreciated that Bach uses the term "moods," in that our moods are transitory things. One day's black mood may melt into a sensation of serenity. While some "moods" may indeed be chronic conditions—depression, for instance may be a deep and long-term condition, and fear may be a life-long crippler—the use of this term reminds us that we have the ability to cast off the conditions that weaken and control us, and repattern ourselves to live freer and healthier lives.

2. In homeopathic medicine, polycrests are the remedies with the widest action. They are those that speak to illness on every level of being—body, mind, and spirit—and are capable of touching every cell in the body with their actions. For this reason, they are the most important medicines in the homeopathic pharmacy. The difference between the terms "polycrest" and "constitutional remedy" have more to do with their use than with their actual action. The term "polycrest" speaks to the actual known action of a given remedy, while the term "constitutional" speaks to a philosophy of treatment—treating the patient in a manner that not only brings an end to the disease state at hand but also, in doing so, strengthens the patient and makes it less likely that the disease, or any other, will recur. Thus, polycrests are commonly used in constitutional treatments in homeopathic medicine.

constitutional remedies in classical homeopathy. (Note that, while all Bach remedies may be used in both acute or chronic cases, some work better acutely, while others are more suited to what homeopaths would call "constitutional" treatments. Such treatments speak to long-term issues or emotional patterns and therefore are used for a longer period of time. Turn to Chapter 12 for more information about the combining of the remedies and their doses.)

For instance, both Rock Rose and Sweet Chestnut are remedies most often used in emergency situations—for those experiencing shock and those who feel pushed past their emotional limits by present circumstances, respectively—while other remedies, like Chestnut Bud and Mustard may require daily doses for months before they complete their work. The person needing Chestnut Bud may need to work with the remedy singly or in combination (it works especially well with Wild Oat) before they can repattern their thinking and get on with their life, and stop making the same mistakes again and again. And the person with feelings of depression that responds to Mustard may need the remedy again and again and again before they feel fully and abundantly alive once more.

Hahnemann's homeopathic remedies are, in my opinion, a "new and improved" version of allopathic medicine. They are created from the same raw materials (originally from the herbal medicines that were part of the medical pharmacy two hundred years ago when Samuel Hahnemann began creating his remedies, and now from the man-made materials in our environment, including allopathic medicines themselves), are based on pretty much the same science, and take the same approach to the notions of medicine and its role in "curing" disease. Bach's remedies, on the other hand, really are something quite different. Bach virtually threw out the rules that had been so fundamental to the doctors before (and after) him. In saying that every patient needs each of the thirty-eight remedies at some point or other in his life, he removed the possibility of making a mistake. Certainly one remedy might be better for a given patient at a given moment in his life than another, but there is no possibility of creating some new burden or new disease through the use of any of Bach's remedies.

Would that this were the case with allopathic medicines—a field of treatment in which the term *iatrogenic* has been created for the diseases that have been actually created through the use of medicines that were prescribed for the original disease.

Even homeopathic remedies, which are commonly thought to be incapable of doing harm, can create deep and dangerous aggravations when used too often or in too high a dosage. These incidents are most certainly not as common or as dangerous as the problems caused by suppressive allopathic treatments. Those tend to consist of layer upon layer of multiple medications, each of which suppress the patient's symptoms, weaken his system as a whole, and expose him to a wide range of dangerous side-effects. Homeopathic aggravations—which are the temporary worsening of the patient's original symptoms brought about either by giving a remedy in too high a potency or giving it too often—can create a great deal of discomfort and mischief in the life of the patient, however. And for patients who are elderly or deeply ill, aggravations can be dangerous things.

Bach's remedies, on the other hand, are even gentler than Hahnemann's in their actions. They are less likely to create an aggravation of any sort, emotional or physical. This does not mean that every patient will find every flower remedy to be completely benign. My experience has taught me that some flower remedies—Crab Apple quickly comes to mind, as does Holly—can be more difficult for patients to adapt to than others. Aggravations are less likely in using Bach remedies than they are with Hahnemann's, but they are not unknown. And just as they are less likely to occur, my experience has taught me that they are less uncomfortable for the patient to withstand when they do occur. But make no mistake, some patients are very sensitive. They will feel some of the more active remedies, like Holly or Vervain, down to the core of their beings. Remember that each of these remedies addresses a way that the patient has become emotionally "stuck." Some circumstance has created a pattern—whether it was just a moment ago, or twenty years ago—and the patient, without some form of help, will continue to replay the pattern until they either digest it, understand it and let it go, or bring the emotional state into the flesh and express it in the form of disease. Therefore, each of these remedies helps us become "unstuck," and that is not always an easy thing. The remedies that speak to our deepest emotional states, our deepest fear or anger, can be uncomfortable things.

I leave it up to each reader to decide how to respond as a practitioner—because that is what we become, a *practitioner*, when we give a Bach remedy to another person or even take it ourselves—to the patient who is having a hard time with a Bach remedy.[3] But as for me, I would never force any patient to continue to take any Bach remedy that causes him an aggravation. Instead, I would seek another remedy or combination of remedies that could help the patient move forward and feel freer and stronger, while still allowing that patient to learn the lessons in life that can bring about a state of healing. I enjoy hearing that a given mixture makes a patient feel happier and lighter; that it allows him to think more clearly and live life more honestly. That, to me, is a successful treatment. The Bach treatment that creates another burden in the patient's already overburdened life is, to me, needlessly and recklessly selected.

3. And let me be very clear about this—the aggravations caused by Bach remedies can, in rare instances, be manifested as physical as well as emotional states. Some will initially cause headaches while others may cause indigestion or a sense of malaise. But most often, the aggravation will be emotional in nature, and the patient will likely feel threatened or shaken by the notion of change.

## Studying the Bach Remedies

When Bach created his remedies, he created something new and rather revolutionary. Just as Martin Luther took the responsibility for spiritual insight out of the hands of the "professionals" when he declared that "each man is his own priest," Bach took the responsibility for healing out of the hands of the professional practitioners and put it firmly and completely in the hands of the patient. Bach sought to create a form of medication that was, by its very nature, simple enough to understand and limited enough in its number of medicines that any person was capable of working with it and, in doing so, could bring about a healing result. Just ask any beginning student of homeopathy how hard it is to get a grasp on the thousands and thousands of homeopathic remedies available, and they will explain to you what I mean.

But to bring about that healing result, we still must have enough knowledge of the remedies to make a choice of the best remedy or remedies to get the job done. Now consider this: since Bach created something truly new in creating his thirty-eight remedies and because he has removed the ability for us to make a real mistake in using them, we have to find some new way of thinking or learning to truly understand them. You see, unlike allopathic or homeopathic medicines, which simply are what they are and do what they do, the Bach remedies (and other forms of flower remedies) are harder to understand. They refuse to be simply what they are and do simply what they do.

> Just as Martin Luther took the responsibility for spiritual insight out of the hands of the "professionals" when he declared that "each man is his own priest," Bach took the responsibility for healing out of the hands of the professional practitioners and put it in the hands of the patient.

When Bach disconnected the physical symptoms of disease from the nature of disease, he did something very, very important. And this makes the understanding and use of his remedies simpler and, at the same time, more difficult than understanding either allopathic or homeopathic medicines.

The reason for this is that, when Bach removed the flesh and blood from the disease state he also removed the physical, natural aspect of his remedies. To put it simply, the Bach remedies are not medicines at all, but are, instead, metaphors. And they must be studied as such.

If you can come to understand the remedies for what they symbolize—what they reflect and what they mask—you will find uses for each remedy that will quite simply amaze you. The uses of these remedies are not limited in their uses by the primary and secondary action of homeopathic medicine or the action and side effects of allopathic medicine. Indeed, they are not limited by their physical actions at all, because they have none. They have only intent—the intent of the physician to put the patient on a path of healing and the intent of the patient to walk that path.

This means that, if each Bach remedy is not limitless in its action, it is, at least, limitless in its possibility. And we are going to have to consider each with a mind that is open to both the metaphor that the remedy represents and how that particular metaphor plays out in the life of a patient.

That's a different way of thinking. And it involves a different way of learning.

And just as making the leap from allopathic medicine to homeopathic medicine requires a change in thinking when giving a medicine, jumping from either allopathic or homeopathic medicine to Bach remedies—which, remember, by their physical nature as Mother Tinctures, are both allopathic (herbal) and homeopathic, and yet, in their use, are neither—requires a leap across a chasm that can be both wide and deep.

Allopathic medicine gives us a mechanistic view of healing. Disease is a matter of parts affected and parts treated, without considering the whole. Always working with material substances as medicines, always working in opposition to the symptoms at hand. Homeopathic medicine gives us wholeness, always moving body, mind, and spirit with a medicine that represents a "magic spark" of energy. Always working with the symptoms, giving a medicine that, in a well person, would create the same symptoms the patient is experiencing.

But in ignoring the physical aspects of illness, Bach makes illness fully and completely a spiritual issue. In doing so, he created a handful of remedies that speak to self, and in learning about these remedies and how best to use them, we are going to have to learn about self. How it is lived and masked and reflected in the eyes of those around us. How it can be lived more freely and honestly, which is the path toward healing.

Therefore, in learning about these remedies, we are going to have to make quite a leap—one that ignores the earache for the sake of the healing. One that begins to wrestle with the notion put forth by Edward Bach that the physical symptoms that we call disease are never the disease itself, but are the symptoms of something deeper—something that is the real disease. And that "something" is always found within the invisible nature of the patient, within the psyche and the soul.

In *Heal Thyself*, Edward Bach writes, "Disease is in essence the result of conflict between Soul and Mind, and will never be eradicated except by spiritual and mental effort . . . No effort directed to the body alone can do more than superficially repair damage, and in this there is no cure, since the cause is still operative and may at any moment again demonstrate its presence in another form."

With such a completely different take on the *nature* of disease and healing, Edward Bach created a system of treatment that requires a different form of understanding and learning. And after more than twenty years of studying and using these remedies, I do believe that grasping their uses fully and completely is a lifetime's work.

# The Language
# of the Remedies

It is important to note the particular language used to express the emotional states of the remedies listed below. In most cases, I refer to patients needing the remedies as being "with" a particular emotional state. In some cases I take things a step further, and say that the patients "are" that state. I do this not only because of the ways language tends to present itself—subconsciously we tend to say exactly what we mean, whether or not we intend to—but also because I want to be quite clear in my own specific meaning. When the phrase contains the word "with" I think that those needing the particular remedy hold that need somewhat apart from themselves and tend to be in an ongoing struggle with the emotional state. But when the word "are" is used, the patient more often has more completely absorbed the emotional state and has taken it on as their norm, sometimes identifying themselves by that specific emotional attribute. Indeed, any of the thirty-eight "moods" can be quite crippling, either as an acute circumstance or as a chronic condition of life. Those that use the word "are" tend to be harder to release, however, as they tend to be more deeply etched upon the persona.

And then there are the remedies I describe as being "in" a particular state. I make this choice of language consciously, also, because I feel that these patients quite literally find themselves located within their emotional state. It is, in their experience, larger than they are, and it contains them.

Finally, we have three remedies that contain the word "obsessive." As the concept of obsession is linked with the chestnut remedies, I have found that those of us needing these remedies (and I admit my own ongoing need for White Chestnut) have perhaps the hardest time of all in learning to release our obsessive habits.

In the list below, I have pulled the remedies into groups that place them not only beside the remedies sharing a common linguistic bond, but also near those sharing their behaviors, whether they are aggressive in their actions, or withdrawn, forceful, or unsure. The groups will help the reader compare and contrast the remedies and select the most appropriate remedies for a given situation or case.

## Remedies for Those "With"

**Agrimony**—for those with false cheer

**Cerato**—for those with self-doubt

**Pine**—for those with guilt

**Mimulus**—for those with fear

**Holly**—for those with anger, hatred and/or jealousy

**Aspen**—for those with anxiety

**Rock Rose**—for those with panic

**Cherry Plum**—for those with hysteria

## Remedies for Those Who "Are"

**Wild Oat**—for those who are unfulfilled

**Clematis**—for those who are vague

**Centaury**—for those who are weak-willed

**Scleranthus**—for those who are indecisive

**Honeysuckle**—for those who are nostalgic

**Larch**—for those who are self-conscious

**Water Violet**—for those who are aloof

**Gentian**—For those who are discouraged

**Hornbeam**—for those who are lethargic

**Olive**—for those who are exhausted

**Wild Rose**—for those who are indifferent

**Gorse**—for those who are without hope

**Elm**—for those who are overwhelmed

**Oak**—for those who are driven

**Heather**—for those who are needy

**Beech**—for those who are intolerant

**Impatiens**—for those who are impatient

**Chicory**—for those who are possessive

**Willow**—for those who are bitter

**Crab Apple**—for those who are perfectionists

**Rock Water**—for those who are rigid

**Vine**—for those who are willful

**Vervain**—for those who are excitable

## Remedies for Those Who Are "In"

**Walnut**—for those who are in upheaval

**Mustard**—for those who are in depression

**Sweet Chestnut**—for those who are in despair

**Star of Bethlehem**—for those who are in shock

## Remedies for Those Who "Have Obsessions"

**White Chestnut**—for those who have obsessive thoughts

**Red Chestnut**—for those who have obsessive concern/worry

**Chestnut Bud**—for those who have obsessive behavior

In this text, I can only give some ideas as to the nature of each of these remedies and the metaphor in which each unfolds. I can only tell you what I know, which, I promise you, is precious little. But I have tried to organize this information in the best way possible, which brings us back to the way the remedies are arranged in this particular book.

I feel that most books on the remedies lose a valuable opportunity for study and comprehension by listing the remedies in simple alphabetical order.[4] By grouping the remedies by the moods that each affects, the reader can easily compare and contrast the action of a given remedy with other remedies in the group. For instance, the reader dealing with a patient who is experiencing fear may well seize upon Aspen as the remedy of best choice simply because it is the first remedy associated with fear listed in most books.

The differences between the remedies and in the way patients need a particular remedy can be subtle. It is important that we understand each remedy within the context of the other remedies that are most similar in action—those that share the same emotional state or mood—to best choose the remedy or remedies that will bring about a state of emotional balance.

I decided to take something of a "kitchen sink" approach to the remedies to do the best job I can in giving complete information. While Bach insists that our physical symptoms are not the disease itself, but only the ways in which it has been made flesh, I include some information about the physical complaints that a person who could be helped by the remedy at hand might be experiencing as a result of his or her deeper spiritual discord. This is not meant to promote the idea that the remedy Crab Apple is good for headaches. Instead, it is included only so that you might consider this as a possible remedy if you are faced with a patient who experiences headaches as part of his or her whole picture. Because, let's face it: Bach's insights notwithstanding, it simply seems to be true that patients with similar mental and spiritual issues often tend to experience similar physical complaints as well. But this information is included as nothing more than a guideline. It is far from complete, and far from conclusive.

I know that this sort of thinking reveals my own strong bias toward homeopathy and the homeopathic philosophy of health and healing, but so be it. In that Hahnemann and Bach were themselves somewhat intertwined philosophically, and I have always felt that my own study of homeopathy informed my use of the Bach remedies.

---

4. I do understand, however, that for simple ease in finding a given remedy most easily and quickly, alphabetical listing is important. For that reason, an alphabetical list of the remedies can be found at the end of the Contents on page v. That way, a reader does not have to be so familiar with the remedies that they know which mood it is associated with to find it in these pages.

And I believe that the homeopathic foundation of this study of the Bach remedies only makes for a richer text.

And, since my training is in the field of homeopathy, I also included the name of the homeopathic remedy that is most equivalent in its action to the Bach remedy. I do this so that the reader can better understand the parallels between homeopathic and Bach treatments, as well as the ways they are similar and the ways they are different. I believe that the more information the reader has about homeopathic remedies the more wisely they can decide the times in life when Bach treatments offer the best course of action, and the times when Hahnemann's more complex treatments can better serve their needs.

While I do this I may, from time to time, also list other Bach remedies that my experience has taught me mix particularly well with the given remedy. Remember, the focus of this section is on the remedies and their actions as individual essences. Since I know that most of us make use of the flower remedies in combination, I am aware that there is a desire for the author to just get on with it and list the best combinations right up front.

I fight this temptation for two reasons. First, I have seen the flower remedies work remarkably well when used singly, and we should never make the ridiculous assumption that more is better. Instead, just as homeopathic medicine teaches us, we should always give the flower essences with the notion that the best healing is the simplest, involving the fewest number in combination and with the fewest number of effective doses.

Second, I present the remedies as I do because I believe that you must first understand the nature of each remedy singly before you can learn to combine them effectively.[5]

This does not mean that there is no place in this book for considering the effective use of the Bach remedies in combination. An exploration of the various methods of mixing and matching these remedies is covered in the following section.

A final word on the remedies themselves and what you should expect from them when they are used medicinally: First, I believe that each of Bach's remedies is a tool for uncovering the truth. They are a mirror we can each of us look into to see the truth of our lives. Just as those who join Alcoholics Anonymous learn that their battle for control of their addiction begins by acknowledging the existence of that addiction, those who take the remedies must first admit the existence of their destructive emotional and behavioral patterns before they can begin to change their thoughts and actions. This is why, I believe, some patients will experience an initial aggravation with the Bach

---

5. I have often advised my students to start out using the remedies singly before they begin to combine them. By seeing what each remedy can do—the broad sweep of its actions—before combining it with others, the Bach practitioner can make the best use of each remedy when they learn to combine it with the others later. I still think this is good advice.

remedies, especially those patients who take some of the remedies that speak to intense emotional states. The shock of the realization of what they are doing and how they are living often causes an initial physical response.

Once the patient sees their emotional block or pattern of thought and behavior they can begin to understand the reasons behind it. Often these patterns date back to childhood, to a message given by someone in authority—a parent or other family member most likely—that the patient has taken to heart. They may have been "told" (perhaps not in words, but by the actions or behaviors of others) they were expected to be perfect, and as a result began to adopt behaviors like those of the archetypal Crab Apple type. Or they may have been "told" that they were just not good enough, and so became a self-conscious Larch.

Or these emotional patterns may be set in place by life's circumstances. The person who has experienced poverty or chronic illness is certainly more likely to adopt the Gorse state of hopelessness than the person raised in a state of health and plenty. For this reason, remedy types may often be generational. Those raised during the Great Depression and World War II have a higher percentage of overly-responsible Oak types than do other generations, because they had to take on more responsibilities in youth than most generations.

Often, our destructive emotional patterns begin in a seemingly positive way. A patient under stress may try a strategy in order to get out of their troubling situation. If that strategy works—if, for example, getting very angry and striking out makes a schoolyard bully walk away—then the patient will likely be very tempted to react in the same manner when other stressful situations arise, and a pattern of aggressive Holly behavior may be chronically set in place. In the same way, our emotional patterns may not be born out of a survival instinct, but from another very powerful instinct: the desire to be liked. The patient who learns at a very young age to give away the toys they love so other children will play with them may set up a lifetime pattern of self-denial for the sake of affection.

No matter the causes of our blocks—traumas that we cannot, without help, move past to get on with our lives—or emotional patterns, the Bach remedies can help us understand ourselves and our real motivations better, and free us to make some decisions. We can look at ourselves with a clear head and decide what we want and need to change. We can see our patterns for what they are—creative or destructive. And we can find the courage to change what we must and move ahead to a life that is freer, one that allows us to inhabit our bodies honestly and live our lives without deceit, being who we truly are.

I see honesty as one of the greatest virtues. Linked with compassion, it is a powerful, creative tool. To me, the Bach remedies give us the great gift of honesty, and, in doing so, offer the pleasure of actual, fundamental change. They allow us to grow up and move on.

Despite this, I have seen many "practitioners" who used the remedies in a somewhat punitive manner. They give the patient the remedies they have selected with the idea that, if the patient would only take these remedies, they would come to see things the way the practitioner wants them to see them, and come to agree that they should live as the practitioner thinks they should. This is most often the case when the person filling the role of the practitioner is a family member, usually a spouse or parent. In these cases, the practitioner usually comes away somewhat disappointed, while the patient is not.

It is certainly true with any form of medicine, allopathic, homeopathic, or any other, that the person giving the remedy can never know what its impact will be on the person taking it. This is certainly true with the Bach remedies. The practitioner cannot know what insights the patient may receive through the remedy. And the practitioner can never predict how the patient will react to those insights. In giving the remedies, the practitioner is offering the patient an opportunity to change—in his own way and his own time. The process of change (that which might, under these circumstances, be called the "healing process") is something that can never be defined, constrained, or timed. It happens how it will and on a timetable that is unknowable.

Therefore, the remedies listed here, whether they are given in a single dose or over a long period of time, or singly or in combination, should always be given in the same way—with a positive hope or a prayer. And the patient must then be allowed to do with that remedy what he or she will, without constraint from the practitioner. Remember, when Bach set about developing this system of remedies, he did so in a manner that set the patient free and allowed the patient, not the doctor, to control the healing process. The practitioner who seeks to establish a traditional allopathic doctor-patient relationship when using the Bach remedies is a practitioner who doesn't know what he is doing.

## 4

# Considering the First Mood:
# The Aspects of Fear

I start with fear because it is an animal emotion. It is perhaps our most basic negative emotional state; certainly it typifies the most basic negative experience of our inner lives and the lives we lead when interplaying with the world around us. Fear lurks around corners, under beds, in small spaces, and in front of large crowds. And we all, at some point in our lives, have clutched our chests in the middle of the night as we realized that we, too, are destined to someday die. We all experience fear many times in our lives, to one degree or another. For some of us, fear is a transitory condition. For others, it is chronic, and it defines and controls their life. It dictates how money is spent, what foods are eaten, even whether the children are allowed to go to a party or school dance.[1] Therefore the remedies in this category—those for patients who fear—are *always* needed, in one way or another, at one time or another, by *every* patient. That is the reason that I list them here first.

The experience of fear may be considered from several different angles and in several different ways, depending upon an individual patient's life experiences and particular stresses.

The most important of these considerations, for me, is the *nature* of the fear itself. Does the patient fear something that he has *actually experienced* at some point in his life, past or present, or is he *conceptualizing* the fear and imaging the worst? Often we will fear a specific thing—a person or a situation—based upon information we have been given by our parents or others who have been in authority positions in our lives, or the experiences of others. These are

> Remember, when selecting an appropriate remedy or remedies for a given case Bach suggests that it can be very helpful to consider the patient not when he is at his best—when he feels safe and confident—but when he is at his *worst*.

---

1. Note that, with some patients, fear can seem to multiply itself from one fear to several to many. A patient's life may narrow continually as fear layers upon fear. The fear of water can lead to a fear of crossing bridges or of any sort of water related travel, which can lead to a fear of travel itself, until the patient withdraws into a very small, unhappy life.

conceptual fears. If a friend of ours is robbed or beaten, we clutch our wallets all the closer. If a friend's loved one is hurt or killed, we hold tighter to those we love, fearing that something will happen to them.

This difference, between the conceptual and experiential fear, can help us determine what remedy from this group will be most helpful in a given case. As we shall see in this chapter, the patient who has experienced being trapped in an elevator or on a bridge and now fears the experience will need a different remedy than the person who is distressed by the idea of being closed in, or the person who, because they have been made to "feel" trapped, now is overly concerned that their child will also be made to feel trapped.

Another way we can consider fear is by how it is *targeted*. Does the patient fear for herself, or does she turn that fear outward, fearing for the sake of others, becoming the Cassandra of their neighborhood, always warning those around her of the dire consequences of life?

As is so often the case when selecting the best possible Bach remedy or remedies, it is a matter of observing and following the flow of energy. In the negative emotional state, does the patient pull energy into himself, or does he direct his energy outward?

In a state of fear, some patients pull inward, and direct their fear to themselves. "Something terrible is going to happen to me." Sometimes that "something terrible" is specific—other times it is vague, an elusive torment. Others who are equally fearful direct that fear outward, perhaps to those they love or to the world in general. Still others leave their fear untargeted. They fear for themselves and for others. This sort of "blanket fear" is a strong indicator of a specific remedy, as we will see.

In considering fear, we must also consider how the patient *uses* the fear that he feels, what his fear causes him to do, how it causes him to act.[2] Does this patient, for instance, mask his fear with anger and lash out when threatened?

Patients may cower when fearful, or strike out and fight back. Some may even take on structured behaviors, like cleaning the house. But remember, as a basic human emotion, fear most often speaks to the issue of fight or flight. Under sufficient stress, a fearful patient will respond from an emotional state that is based on issues pertaining to survival. At this moment their true nature will be revealed.

Remember, when selecting an appropriate remedy or remedies for a given case Bach suggests that it can be very helpful to consider the patient not when he is at his best—when he feels safe and confident—but when he is at his *worst*. Consider the behavior and the emotional patterns expressed by the patient when things seem to be

---

2. I have found over the years that many patients who at first seem to need the remedies associated with aggressive behaviors, such as Holly and Vervain, will not achieve true healing until they are given the remedy for the fear that underlies their behaviors.

as bad as they can be. That will help you select the remedies that can help the patient repattern his thinking and behavior and truly move beyond his fears.

The remedies for those who fear may be used either as long-term or short-term remedies. Patients with deep fear may well need to stay with a remedy or move within the remedies in this group[3] for a period of many months as they release the strictures that fear has placed upon their lives.

Whether the fears are your own or your patient's, whether they are the result of a recent traumatic event, such as a near traffic accident (the old idea of getting right back up on that horse that threw you comes to mind) or fears that have compounded and deepened until they define an entire lifetime, one of the remedies in this chapter will assist in helping the patient understand the nature of that fear and to move beyond it, so that it no longer controls any part of his or her life.

In choosing an appropriate remedy or remedies for those who fear, you begin as you always do, by paying attention to the patient, by observing clearly and actively listening to all you are being told in the process of case taking, and then by following the patient's progress as her heavy load of fear is lightened.

## Fear and the Homeopathic Pharmacy

Of all the emotional states, fear is the most commonly mentioned in the homeopathic *Materia Medica*. Further, the names of more than three hundred remedies are listed under the rubric "fear" in the homeopathic Repertory. These listings confirm that fear accompanies many different other symptoms in our lives. Many disease states, both acute and chronic, carry an aspect of fear with them. But the aspects of fear can play out in many different ways.

For some, such as the typical Arsenicum patient, the fear is directed toward and connected with the disease state itself. The patient will fear their disease, and fear for the worst possible outcome of their disease. Others, like the typical Aconite patient, will fear death.

Some of the fears will be quite specific. The Argentum Nitricum patient will have

---

3. I want to note that, in my opinion, the flower essences work best when they are selected and used individually within each of the seven groups. Therefore, I have found in my years of using the remedies that a more effective combination for a fearful patient can be found by selecting the best of the remedies for those who fear and combining that single remedy with one or more remedies from the *other* groups. Those remedies are, of course, also chosen based upon the mood of the patient, as well as upon his or her actions and, in some cases, physical manifestations of mood. Let me also note that this is not a fixed rule. There are times—most commonly emergency situations—in which remedies from this group can be mixed together with great result. Aspen and Mimulus, for instance may be useful for the patient who experiences both known fears and a general anxiety. And Rock Rose is a remedy that is well combined with any other in a time of true crisis.

fears of heights or closed-in places. The Phosphorus child may specifically fear the dark, or may, instead, have a more amorphous type of fear, dreading many different aspects of the night, from the darkness itself to monsters under the bed.

The depth of the fear is also noted in homeopathic treatment. The fact that a patient is without fear, for instance, contraindicates the remedy Arsenicum, for which fear is the central emotional state.

Remember, however, that in the selection of the remedy used in homeopathic treatment, the mental and emotional state of the patient is just one aspect of the patient's condition considered. Bach, in his system of healing, removes all but the emotional state of the patient, making the understanding of the specific aspects of the patient's fear state all the more important.

While Bach's system of treatment is greatly simplified when compared with Hahnemann's, the five shades of fear listed below demonstrate that Bach realized that fear is one of the great plagues of mankind, and that it could wear many different faces.

## REMEDIES FOR THOSE WHO FEAR

- **Mimulus**—for those with fear
- **Aspen**—for those with anxiety
- **Red Chestnut**—for those who have obsessive concern or worry
- **Rock Rose**—for those with panic
- **Cherry Plum**—for those with hysteria

## MIMULUS · THE REMEDY FOR THOSE WITH FEAR[4]

Bach on Mimulus: "Fear of worldly things, illness, pain, accidents, poverty, of dark, of being alone, of misfortune. The fears of everyday life. These people quietly and secretly bear their dread, they do not freely speak of it to others."

He continues in *Free Thyself*: "Are you one of those who are afraid; afraid of people or of circumstances: Who go bravely on and yet your life is robbed of joy through fear . . . fear of a hundred things?"

---

4. In his book *Free Thyself*, Bach lists his Twelve Healers—the first dozen remedies to become part of his floral pharmacy. Among these he lists Mimulus as the sole remedy for fear. Because of this, and because of the importance of this remedy as I have seen it used over the years, I consider it to be the core remedy of this group. In other words, when fear is present, but you can't get a handle on the situation, try Mimulus. It is almost universal in its impact, as we all have things in our lives that cause us to fear.

- Mimulus is both an acute and a constitutional Bach remedy.
- Mimulus is one of Bach's original remedies, the Twelve Healers.

### Botanical Information

Mimulus (*Mimulus Luteus*) is known as the "common monkeyflower" or the "seep monkeyflower," or even as "Monkey Musk." It is most often an annual, but is known to spread itself (seep) and come back year after year. It is a favorite flower of hummingbirds, but is almost completely deer proof. Mimulus has a profusion of yellow flowers in the spring and can withstand full sun, although it thrives in partial sun. It likes to grow near water and, although it grows in most kinds of soil, it cannot withstand drought. It belongs to the same family as the snapdragon and the figwort. The leaves of the Mimulus plant are edible, and may be consumed raw or cooked.

### Mimulus in General

I recently came upon a quote that speaks to the heart of this remedy.[5] It said that the thing that each of us fears the most is something that has already happened to us, and not something that we have, to this point, avoided. Think for a moment about the truth of this statement. In our hearts, the things we fear the most are always the things we have already experienced, and that have, through the sheer trauma of the experience, in some way limited our lives. Only the person who has been poor—really poor to the point of literally not knowing where their next meal will come from—can truly fear poverty. Only the person who has been abused can truly understand the pain and shame of abuse, and, in understanding it, truly fear it. Just as only the person who has lost someone they loved can truly understand the nature of grief, only the person who has experienced firsthand the specific cause of a given fear can truly understand the ramifications of that fear.

> What can make it so difficult to help Mimulus types confront their fear is that often their fear will seem like a sensible thing. It is rooted in a set of negative experiences that have taught the patient that the safest course of action is avoidance.

These are our deepest fears, the ones that can control us, or, in a more positive aspect, motivate us to change our lives so that they can be lived freely and fearlessly.

Therefore, perhaps the most basic way in which we can select the appropriate remedy for those who have fear is simply to find out if the subject of the fear has ever been

---

5. I am going to attribute this quote to Deepak Chopra. I believe he said it, but it was one of those things that I heard on the fly, and by the time I had stopped thinking about the statement itself, it was too late to be sure just who had said it, or, indeed, where I had heard it or seen it. I apologize if I attribute it to the wrong person.

directly experienced by the patient. Has he been bitten by a dog and now fears dogs? Has she been trapped in an elevator and now fears enclosed places?

For those who suffer from fears of their own imagining, there are other important remedies. But for those who fear specific things, whose lives are limited to the point that they cannot fly, will not cross bridges, or are restricted in other similar ways, there is the remedy Mimulus.

As Bach puts it, "These are the fears of everyday life."

These are also the things, the places, and situations we avoid because we fear them, and, in avoiding them, narrow our worlds and our lives. The fear of these specific things—germs, authority figures, spiders, and snakes—is based within our life experience. Like the child who is badly burned, we learn to avoid the stove. But we do not see the cost of that avoidance, and that, through our fear, we rob ourselves of the freedom to live life to the fullest.

What can make it so difficult to help Mimulus types confront their fear is that often their fear will seem like such a logical and sensible thing. It is rooted in a specific negative experience or a set of negative experiences that have taught the patient that the safest course of action is avoidance.

Now, in many cases, even though the patient *wishes* to avoid a particular place or thing, he or she will choose *not* to avoid it, and will, instead, stoically push the fear aside and get in the elevator, shake the germy hand, or walk past the snake.

Life then becomes a continual choice between continuing onward in the face of fear or avoiding the cause of the fear. Therefore, routes home, foods eaten, animals petted, and many more of the minute aspects of life have to be considered and reconsidered in the mind of the Mimulus. Many Mimulus types will choose never to speak of their fear, and if they are accompanied by others, will choose not to avoid its cause. To those others, the Mimulus looks and acts as if all is well, while, all the while, he or she is in the clutches of fear. Because of the need for the Mimulus to conceal his or her fear, and because of the ongoing struggle between fight and flight, fear is a source of exhaustion for the Mimulus type.

It is the very heart of this remedy and its action that the patient will not only be aware that they are afraid, but will be able to identify the cause of the fear, and, very likely, the reason behind the fear as well.[6]

---

6. This last may not always be the case. Some patients needing Mimulus will not be able to give a reason for a fear. The experience may, on some emotional level, be blocked from their recall, or it may not be a direct, first-hand experience, but one that has been passed down from a parent or other person of great influence, who has impressed upon the patient that this specific fear response is appropriate and sensible. They will, however, still be aware of their fear and have quite specific knowledge of the subject of that fear.

Bach writes that those who need this remedy "go bravely on and yet [their] life is robbed of joy through fear." This is an important aspect of the remedy type. Not only have these patients narrowed their life through the avoidance of things feared, they also have lost the joy of a life freely lived. Their lives are also often robbed of spontaneity because they have to plan the routes of their journeys, select the times during which travel is possible, and base the choice of their destinations in compliance with the rules of life their fear imposes.

In short, their fear is a burdensome thing.

Because of this, Mimulus is a Bach remedy that is often taken for a lengthy period of time. While it is of great help in acute situations—it can help the person who fears public speaking get up and give the speech they have to give, or help the student who fears tests succeed with an exam—it is of its greatest value when taken long term. Then the remedy can help the patient face their fears and move past them, not just get through a momentary crisis. With the help of Mimulus, past traumas can be put aside and the blocks these patients have created that keep them from living in a fearless manner can be removed once and for all.

Mimulus is a remedy that blends very well with other remedies. It can, for instance, be of great value when combined with Gorse. This combination is effective for the patient with a chronic health condition who fears both the pain of his illness and the possibility of a negative outcome and has given up any hope of a cure. It is also an excellent blend with the remedy Holly, for those whose apparent rage contains the underpinnings of fear. And for patients who cannot help but dwell upon their fears, who can think of nothing else, Mimulus combines well with White Chestnut to give them ease of mind and a sense of calm.

In selecting the remedy Mimulus, the depth of the fear is less important than the nature[7] of the fear. As noted above, it can be just as helpful for the patient who fears exams at school as it can for the deeply phobic individual. For both, and for all those who live their lives in the continuum in between, Mimulus offers a method of working through and past fear. As Bach puts it, this is the remedy for those who have fear, but not terror. Instead, Mimulus is helpful for those with "quite calm fear."

## Negative Qualities of the Type

The Mimulus type who is in his or her negative state is too rooted in the world as it is. They see the problems that weigh them down daily and the dangers faced daily just by being alive all too clearly. In time, their vision of fear blocks them from seeing the pos-

---

7. Again, by the nature of the fear, I refer to Mimulus' tendency to be very specific in their fears. These patients know the exact thing or situation that is feared, even if they do not know the reason for the fear. These are not vague fears or uneasy feelings, but concrete, limiting fears.

itive aspects of life, the many situations that, instead of being the basis for fear, should be the basis for joy, for healing, and for harmony. Their fear traps them in an ever-shrinking world of terrors large and small. And as they are drained of their energies more and more by their attempts to avoid all they fear, their lives become smaller and smaller as fear overtakes their world.

The greatest difficulty the Mimulus type has in overcoming his fear is that, to him at least, the fear seems a logical and sensible thing. The situation or thing feared is perceived as being a powerful and threatening thing. It therefore does no good for well-meaning friends and family to try to cajole or tease the Mimulus into abandoning or ignoring his fear. This tends to make the Mimulus less willing to admit or discuss his fear, and does nothing to end it. It may, in fact, make the Mimulus all the more fearful and distrustful, as negative experiences tend to generate a fear and avoidance response. It is important that those who care for any Mimulus type to realize that they have given over a great deal of their own sense of power to the thing that they fear. Only by reclaiming their own sense of power can they see that they have no reason to hold onto fear.

### Positive Qualities of the Type

I find it interesting that when Bach lists the positive quality that presents the other side of Mimulus' fear, that quality is sympathy.[8] This is because those who have coped with Mimulus fears, when they overcome them at last, become natural counselors for others who have had to cope with similar fears. In fact, no other remedy type is as capable of leading others through the minefield of life as Mimulus. They understand the deep fears others feel when confronted with their lives, and they can guide others to learn to deal with those fears with both courage and humor. There is no more sympathetic person than the one who has conquered his or her own fears.

As Mimulus patients begin to deal with their fears, look for several subtle changes to begin to take place. Often, you will find that the first change is the rather delightful restoration of their sense of humor. Where once fear stamped out joy, now joy returns. Often, patients will even begin to find humor in their old fears. As they realize that the

---

8. Obviously, you would expect to find "fearlessness" to reside on the other side of the coin of fear, and, of course, to a great degree this is the case. The Mimulus type who is in a state of health and balance will be able to identify an appropriate response to situations and things that once would have immediately sent them into a state of fear. Now they can honestly evaluate what, if any, response is required of them. Just as the healthy immune system will ignore the presence of bacteria that it does not perceive as a threat while the sickly immune system will create a symptom response when it is not needed, the healthy Mimulus type will no longer fear every stranger, every enclosed space. This frees them to open their awareness to the needs of others. And because they are particularly knowledgeable about all things relating to fear, they can be particularly good at helping others learn to cope with the emotion.

snake that they were so frightened of is trying its best to get away from them, they will feel both freedom and joy.

Next, Mimulus patients who are moving from a negative state to a more balanced and positive one will tend to begin to see the world around them once more. They will take greater interest in that world as well as the people in it. Where they once invested their energy in avoiding the objects of their fear, they now invest it in others, taking interest in the lives and needs of those around them. At this point, their natural sympathy begins to develop. Once locked in prisons of their own fearful making, they now greet the world around them and move freely within their environment.

### The Mimulus Child

These are shy, very timid children. Often, they will be very clingy and will want the reassurance of physical contact with their parents at all times. In cases of particularly clingy children, a combination of Mimulus and Chicory can be very helpful. Look for them to be afraid of people and of things with which they are already familiar. The mother and father will say, "You've met her before. Don't be afraid," and will spend a good deal of time trying to figure out why their child is so timid. These children will blush easily, or may have ears that turn red easily. Look for them also to stammer, and have problems coming up with the right word for what they mean.

### The Mimulus Adult

The riddle here is courage versus fear. Some Mimulus types will be able to reason with themselves to be able to live what appear to be normal lives, although these lives are filled with fear. These Mimulus types will still get on the elevator or still drive their car, although they must talk quietly to themselves the entire time to be able to do so. But, this coping in many ways makes them extremely strong and brave. To do something that you are afraid to do, and to be quietly strong enough to do it and not discuss this fear, is to really be very, very strong. Mimulus adults are also among the most patient people when motivating others to do things that are difficult for them to do. They understand hesitation. They understand fear. They know the methods by which we make ourselves do things that we are afraid to do, since they are afraid of so many things themselves. Mimulus patients of this type, who put so much effort into trying to get through the day and all its many threats, may find help in the combination of Mimulus and Oak, especially if they have reached the point at which they feel they can no longer keep up the appearance of coping with the things they fear.

The Mimulus type who is not coping and reasoning with himself or herself is in a more difficult set of circumstances. This is the person who starts out by being afraid on an elevator, and subsequently never gets on elevators. Over time, escalators are also out of the question, and so on. His or her life becomes more and more controlled by these fears. And over time it becomes very small indeed. This is the person losing the battle for courage, who is surrendering to fear. In this person, look for illnesses to usually begin in the solar plexus area. Often, these conditions will include palpitations and digestive disorders. Like Laura in *The Glass Menagerie*, look for them to get an upset stomach whenever they are called upon to do something that they fear.

Quite often middle-aged patients will need the remedy Mimulus as their lives are taken over by almost innumerable small fears. These middle-aged Mimulus types have lived long enough to know that their lives will not last forever. In the moment they realize that there are fewer years ahead of them than behind them many will become more fear motivated as they seek both safety and long life. As Bach said, these little fears drain the patient's life of all joy, as they trade their sense of freedom in life for an illusionary and elusive sense of safety.

Mimulus is also an important remedy to consider in elderly patients. Quite often, they will move swiftly into a Mimulus state as illness strikes. They can exhibit deep fear of illness and of mortality. Mimulus has helped many patients face the end of their lives with calm dignity.

### The Mimulus Animal

This is one of our most important Bach remedies for domestic animals and pets of all sorts. This remedy works wonderfully for animals afraid of thunderstorms, fireworks, and other loud noises. Use this remedy when animals display distress signals like panting, whining, or pacing. This remedy may be required long term for some animals, while it works best as a simple acute remedy for others. Mimulus, along with Star of Bethlehem (and Rescue Remedy) should always be on hand, especially when a new animal comes into the household.

### Mimulus and the Homeopathic Pharmacy

Many remedies within the homeopathic pharmacy relate in one way or another to the emotion fear. And just as each of the different flower essences in this group relate to a different aspect of the emotion, the different homeopathic remedies also relate to a different aspect of fear, or to different reactions to the presence of the emotion. Argentum Nitricum, for instance, a remedy made from the metal silver, is known for very specific fears that are very similar to those of Mimulus. Commonly, Argentum patients will have a fear of heights, or a fear of crossing bridges. Many will fear flying.

But just as Mimulus is the Bach remedy that speaks to the core issue of fear, the homeopathic remedy taken from arsenic, Arsenicum Album, uses the emotion of fear as a motivating force toward illness. Arsenicum patients also fear specific things—most commonly, they fear death, and especially fear being alone, as they convince themselves that they will die alone. (This fear also suggests the Bach remedy Aspen. The

Arsenicum displays fear as its chief emotional symptom, but this homeopathic type is broad enough in its symptoms to suggest more than one Bach type.) They can experience night terrors and can develop ritual behaviors around their fear. As with Mimulus, Arsenicum types tend to use avoidance behavior for anything and everything they fear. They can become quite rigid in their life patterns, including eating and sleeping habits, all based on their specific fears. Because of this, Arsenicum, among all of Hahnemann's remedies, most closely resembles Mimulus, and should be considered when a patient beset with fears of this sort enters into homeopathic treatment.

Quite often the homeopathic remedy that most closely mirrors Mimulus in the patient's needs and fear and in its action is Calcarea Carbonica, which is made from calcium carbonate. As is often the case with the Mimulus, the fears of the Calcarea patient are slow in growing and develop over a period of years. Rather than having one specific phobia, the Calcarea often has a number of little fears, which he would tend to think of as "dreads." Like the stubborn Mimulus, the Calcarea will often force himself to face his fears daily, and will do everything possible to keep others from seeing that he is afraid. In this way, the Calcarea will continually stress his being, and, as his little fears grow in size and number, look for his physical symptoms to grow in the same way.

### Issues that Suggest Mimulus

Aging; angina; asthma; coma; diarrhea; digestive disorders; dizzy spells; fainting; gas pains; heartburn; insomnia; myopia; overweight; palpitations; stuttering; tonsillitis; ulcers.

### In Conclusion

Mimulus is a constitutional Bach remedy with many acute uses. It is gender neutral and equally effective for both sexes. It is useful for all stages of life, with perhaps a special use for middle-aged and elderly patients. Mimulus works well as a single remedy, and is often very useful as a first remedy for cases in which fear is an important component. It also combines well with many other remedies, especially Chicory, White Chestnut, Holly, Crab Apple (when the fear of germs becomes overwhelming) and Hornbeam (for those who suffer from a fear of failure).

## ASPEN · THE REMEDY FOR THOSE WITH ANXIETY

Of Aspen, Bach writes: "Vague unknown fears, for which there can be no given explanation, no reason. Yet the patient may be terrified of something terrible going to happen, he knows not what."

• **Aspen is both an acute and a constitutional remedy.**

## Botanical Information

The European Aspen tree (*Populus Tremula*) from which this remedy is taken is native to many parts of Northern Africa, Asia, and Europe. Its natural range extends from the Arctic Circle in Scandinavia into England and Scotland, where it is especially common to the Highlands.

The Aspen is a tall, slim tree with naturally gray bark. Its leaves are known to flutter in the slightest wind. The leaves commonly turn yellow, sometimes red, in autumn. The most unusual aspect of the Aspen is that individual trees are either male or female, unlike most trees, which have male and female characteristics on the same tree. The Aspen tree is noted for being a pioneer plant. It will, after a forest fire or other natural disturbance, move swiftly to repopulate the disrupted area.

## Aspen in General

The person for whom Aspen is indicated may be in an acute state of anxiety, perhaps brought on by something as simple as a nightmare (and Aspen is an excellent remedy for anyone who has suffered through a nightmare and wants to get back to a peaceful night's sleep) or perhaps from getting some upsetting news, or just from that vague state of "what happens if . . ." that each of us has played out in our mind in the middle of a sleepless night.[9]

Or the situation may be more chronic in nature, with ongoing vague anxiety. Often, this free-form anxiety is linked with or rooted in a state of sensitivity. The Aspen person is sensitive: to changes in the emotions of self or others, to changes in environment and atmosphere, and perhaps most profoundly, to the state of change that the future represents. Like a handful of other remedies, Impatiens among them, Aspen is a future-focused remedy. Those needing this remedy tend to fixate upon the future, even the near future, and to ignore the circumstances of the present and the past.

Intuition and imagination, along with the aforementioned sensitivity, are keys to understanding the chronic or constitutional Aspen state. Aspen types—especially Aspen children—often have a greatly over-developed imagination. While they fully understand the difference between truth and lies, they do not always understand the difference between imagination and reality. The boundary between what is real and what is imaginative fiction is often paper thin and tissue-fragile.

At the same time, many Aspens have a very strong sense of intuition. They find themselves beset with premonitions and with a vague sense of warning that they can neither fully comprehend nor shake away. Instead, they remain locked in a state of

---

9. For those nights in which your mind keeps racing and the sensation of anxiety is linked with a churning of thoughts, combine Aspen with White Chestnut to restore your sense of mental and emotional balance and return to a peaceful sleep.

vague alarm and heightened sensibility that robs them of their ability to relax, enjoy life or live their life freely and fully.[10]

In the worst case, Aspens enter into a fantasy world that they cannot or will not leave. This world may be a pleasant fantasy or one that is rooted in paranoia and darkness, but, either way, it can become as real to the Aspen as the physical world around them.

All of this might have us believe that the imagination and intuition of the Aspen cannot have any real bearing on the world about him, but this is not the case. Often Aspen types can and will display real skill in what could be called psychic abilities. They can uncover details that they have no way of knowing or foresee events before they occur. They can have an empathy and understanding of other humans and of animals that is well beyond the norm. Even in these cases, however, the Aspen sensitivity can be a mixed blessing, because it comes with an ongoing degree of anxiety unless the Aspen state is recognized and understood and the Aspen type is able to harness and control his or her sensitivity.

Perhaps no other type needs as careful parenting and nurturing as does the young Aspen. And no other type needs to be surrounded by an environment of positive and optimistic values and thought as much as the Aspen. Only when their inherent lack of trust in the future is replaced with an optimistic viewpoint can Aspens release their anxiety.

## Negative Qualities of the Type

The person who remains in a chronic Aspen state lives a life controlled by fear. Aspens are anxious people, whose lives are narrowed by fear. They may be so ensnared by a generalized fear of night, the dark, and their own nightmares that they literally begin to fear sleep itself. For them, darkness and sleep represent situations in which they are at the mercy of things they cannot fully understand or control. Chronic insomnia is common to these Aspen types.

People living in a negative Aspen state seem at the mercy of their own sensitivity, as if they can never be fully comfortable in their own environment and in their own skin. They seek to shield themselves from everything that

> People living in a negative Aspen state seem at the mercy of their own sensitivity, as if they can never be fully comfortable in their own environment and in their own skin. They seek to shield themselves from everything that makes them anxious.

10. In the post 9-11 world, it is perhaps easy to understand the suffering of the Aspen type by thinking of our government's color-coded alarm system. The Aspen lives in a constant state of orange alert, while lacking a reason for that alert. In fact, given that this is the post 9-11 world, perhaps we all have an increased need for this remedy.

makes them anxious. As children, they tend to cling to nightlights and special blankets, and toys to which they can tell their troubles and fears. As adults, they may surround themselves with possessions that make them feel safe, or cling to people whose role it is to help them feel secure, to get them through the night.[11]

Just as they are prisoners of their own fear, Aspens are also prisoners of their own imagination as they conjure the cause of their fears. Their minds—particularly the subconscious mind that is dominant during sleep—resemble those medieval maps of the world divided into known lands and the *terra incognita* that bear the warning, "Here be dragons." The dragons that cause such fear and trembling for Aspens are largely of their own making.

The negative Aspen lacks trust. He does not trust the world that he lives in and often feels alien to it. He also does not trust the future, in that it represents, for him, the true *terra incognita*, the place that none of us can go, that none can see or truly understand. The negative Aspen lives in a world that is divided into what can be known—and, therefore, is not a cause of anxiety—and what is unknown and unknowable —which always causes anxiety.

It should be noted that negative Aspens lack courage because of their fear of anything unknown to them. They tend to adopt the victim's role (if it has not been thrust upon them). Their response to life is overly careful and overly cautious. This can be helpful in identifying the need for Aspen for a particular patient. None of the other fearful types will be so careful of the unknown—from strange dogs to new foods—as will the Aspen. They will tend to shy away from unknown things and people, and their response to those who try to encourage them to simply try something new may well be hysterics.

The negative Aspen, especially the Aspen child or elder, can control the lives of a whole family, because each member, out of love for the Aspen, tries to ensure that he or she is not driven beyond his or her ability to cope. In this way, the entire family can become the prisoner of the Aspen's fears.

The negative Aspen state can resemble the negative Impatiens state in that both are restless and both are future-driven. But the Aspen lacks the irritability that is often linked to the Impatiens restlessness, and the Aspen dreads the future while the Impatiens is driven to it.

It is important to note that not all cases of Aspen relate to anxieties based on imaginary traumas. Soldiers returning from war, victims of violent crime, and those who

---

11. This need for comfort and the ongoing immediate need to "get through the night" often leads the Aspen, particularly the constitutional Aspen type, to turn to alcohol or drugs as a source of comfort. They are people who often easily become addicted to anything—sex, drugs, and alcohol chief among them—that make them feel safe or numb their anxiety. For this reason, Aspen is similar to Agrimony. Just as Agrimony numbs unhappiness with alcohol and drugs, Aspen numbs fear and anxiety.

have suffered mental, verbal, and/or physical abuse may all develop an anxious and hyper-sensitive state of mind that can be treated with Aspen. Those whose trust in the world around them and hope for the future has been wounded by traumatic or terrifying circumstances may need Aspen to bring them into a naturally hopeful and optimistic state of mind. Indeed, very real circumstances of our lives may guide each of us to this remedy, to allow us to lead a life unclouded by anxiety once more.

## Positive Qualities of the Type

When Aspen patients have dealt with their fear, they can become those people who are able to lead us into the unknown, whether that "unknown" is a physical, mental, or emotional state. They are explorers—of mental and emotional worlds as well as our own physical realm. They can be people of great courage combined with their innate keen sensitivity. It is also important to note that, when Aspen types are brought into balance through the use of the remedy, they lose none of their gift for imagination or insight, or their sensitivity to the environment or people around them. But they had better understand both their imagination and their insight if they are to use them as tools to lead better and fuller lives, rather than as hindrances.

Positive Aspens make excellent therapists and natural counselors. They are often gifted in working with animals.

When they are in a positive state Aspens have a well-developed sense of trust. They can gain the courage that allows them to face the future without fear and take charge and help shape that future, both for themselves and for their communities.

## The Aspen Child

This is one of the remedies in which the same issues are revealed in the same way in both the young and the old. Whatever the age of the Aspen patient, the same anxiety, fear, and dread (especially regarding the future and the unknown) will be seen. But in children, look for anxiety to manifest itself in mysterious illnesses, especially stomachaches and vague pains.[12]

Also, all Aspen types are unsure of just what they fear. But, in Aspen children, the issues may seem more like the Mimulus fears—concrete, well-known issues—like visiting the barber or dentist or doctor. You may be tempted to give Mimulus (there is certainly nothing wrong with giving both in combination when in doubt, although a well-selected single remedy will work better), but take a moment to see if the child is sure about what he or she fears, or if the fear is of the unknown that the visit repre-

---

12. Don't be surprised to see some of these pains linked to changes in the weather. Since Aspens are very sensitive to their environment they may, at any stage in life, have acute ailments accompanying these changes. Some may be very sensitive to oncoming storms. Others may have serious rheumatic pains that come and go with each change in the barometer.

sents—if the fear is the fear of a dark future, which is surely the core Aspen issue. Aspen, for both children and adults, is the remedy for apprehension concerning what dire events the future may hold.

Aspen is of great help to children who are "too sensitive for their own good," for children who seem to have been born without a protective layer of skin, and for children who seem as if they were receiving information from other planes of reality. Night after night, they wake alarmed from dreams or nightmares. Think of Aspen for children who do not want to go to bed at night, and who refuse to sleep alone. And especially consider this remedy for children who have hysterics, and those who are uncontrollable in their fear state.

### The Aspen Adult

The central theme of adults needing this remedy is anxiety. Consider this remedy for those who are plagued by vague, gnawing fears. The Aspen person is never sure what they are afraid of—this is the keynote to the remedy. They simply know that something bad is going to happen. The Aspen experiences a sense of anxiety for no apparent reason.

This sense of anxiety can be more objectively apparent in children and the elderly. The Aspen adult, however, who is managing to cope with his or her life in spite of the anxiety, may be harder to spot. It may take a good degree of honesty on the part of the Aspen or a keen eye on the part of the practitioner for the need for this remedy to be uncovered.

Aspen people can be almost supernaturally sensitive. As well as feeling anxious, they may see ghosts, auras, and be guided by hunches and feelings. Like the Aspen child, the Aspen adult has to deal daily with insights and impressions that seem to be coming to them invisibly from other dimensions. They are also people who are very interested in fairy tales, fantasy fiction, and other writings that, like Aspens, seem to be aware of invisible places. As if they are radios able to receive far more stations than most, Aspens are sensitive to many impressions the rest of us simply miss.

While the Aspen child usually feels the anxiety in the stomach, the adult will usually feel it on the skin, with goose bumps and tingles of all sorts. The stomach's "butter-flies" may remain in adulthood, however, and will usually become chronic nausea and digestive disorders.

Aspen is considered by many to be a "mood"[13] remedy, best used in acute situa-

---

13. There are two ways of expressing this idea: Those of us with a background in homeopathic medicine consider remedies to be basically "acute" or "constitutional" in nature, determined by the length of their impact as required by the nature of the conditions that they are called upon to treat. Those of a strict Bach background call these two types of remedies "mood" remedies, which are used to treat the more fleeting acute conditions, and "type" remedies, which work for those of a specific constitutional type.

tions. Certainly all of us experience the Aspen state to some degree or another almost every day of our lives. We are experiencing Aspen each time a particular stressor pushes us into a state of anxiety or vague fear. The near-miss traffic accident that causes some of us to have a fear of a particular road where the accident almost took place, or a particular time of day or weather condition that we believe was responsible for the near miss can lead to the need for Mimulus, but if that same near miss leads to a vague sense that all is not well, that we may not miss the other car again in the future, then Aspen is needed to set things right.

However, those who think of Aspen only in the acute context rob it of its ability to assist in cases of deeper need. I have known it to work wonders in chronic or constitutional situations. Aspen combines well with Rock Rose for panic attacks, and it also is often a key remedy in working with phobias of all types. It will often be called for in a mixture with Crab Apple for people with eating disorders as well as other illnesses involving a feeling of helplessness and/or loss of control, in which it combines well with Cherry Plum. When dealing with a situation in which a patient is in a state of anxiety that seems all too harsh, or too real, consider combining Aspen with Star of Bethlehem for a treatment that soothes, calms, centers, and encourages healing.

Aspen is also of great help to people who have worn their egos thin through the use of drugs because it can calm and balance the hysterical trauma caused by drug use. Often these people will feel unsafe at all times and in all places. They see the world as a chaotic, frightening place.

In all things, look for Aspen to increase strength and confidence. Look for it to bring the ego back into balance, and to give the person a sense of well-being and safety.

### The Aspen Animal

Aspen is an excellent remedy for animals (especially dogs) that whimper, quiver, cower, pant, or show any other signs of anxiety or fear without apparent cause. It is effective for horses that spook easily. It also is helpful for pets that urinate in the house due to stress or fear. Consider this remedy for animals that are rescued from shelters and have unknown backgrounds. Consider mixing Aspen with Rescue Remedy and/or Walnut for animals that are failing to adapt after they are brought into the home.

### Aspen and the Homeopathic Pharmacy

Aspen can resemble the homeopathic remedy Arsenicum Album, which is made from the poison arsenic. Both are used for patients who are victims of anxiety, who seek to control their environment and life in an attempt to cope with this overwhelming fear state.

But perhaps the remedy most similar to Aspen is Phosphorus. Both help patients who tend toward vague fears, such as the dark, or even the oncoming dusk, where Arsenicum's fears often are very concrete, in that they fear death, poverty, or being alone. This last major fear of Arsenicum's is very Aspen-like, in that this fear of being alone is vague and nagging and tied to the concept that, if he or she is alone, "something bad will happen." Therefore, it is this fear that most links Arsenicum with Aspen.

Like Aspen, Phosphorus is often considered an excellent remedy for children, especially young and sensitive children. And Aspen and Phosphorus patients share a powerful sensitivity. They are acutely sensitive to their environment, both their emotional and physical environment. They also are sensitive to changes in the weather, and will often have fears linked to those changes such as fears of oncoming storms and other weather-related catastrophes.

### Issues that Suggest Aspen

Addictions of all sorts; cardiac weakness; digestive issues such as abdominal cramps, heartburn, acid reflux, nausea and/or ulcers, eating disorders; headache; hormone imbalances; hyperactivity; hyperventilation; hysteria; insecurity; insomnia; myopia; nervous conditions; overweight (mostly in adults) or underweight (in children); paranoia; palpitations; physical, emotional, or sexual abuse; travel sickness.

### In Conclusion

While the patient who experiences the full weight of Aspen anxiety and distrust may be somewhat rare, this sensation of oversensitivity and anxiety is common to us all. Each of us has moments when we fear for the future, both for ourselves and for the whole of the human race. Each of us knows the sensation of the quickening of the pulse as we feel the hollow dread that accompanies anxiety. And as the world becomes ever more dangerous a place in which to live, our need for the remedy Aspen grows. As our television screens nightly bring us images of war, of terrorism, and of dangers real and imagined, our need for the remedy Aspen grows. Perhaps there was a time when this remedy was not needed in every home, but was only needed in homes with a sensitive child or a fearful elder, but today the home without Aspen is a home that is, in a very real sense, unprotected. For the moments after the nightmare, for the moments of pure dread before facing the coming day, and for the "mortality" moments in the still of the night when death seems to come all too near, there is no better remedy than Aspen.

One final note: it is important that, while under treatment, Aspen patients avoid anything that overwhelms them and sends them into anxiety. Alcohol and drugs must be avoided—even coffee or too much sunlight may interfere. They must seek calm and quiet. This is one of the Bach remedies that, while it may do some good immediately, truly needs some time to work, and the patient some time to recover. Anything that brings the patient into a state of calm and security should be allowed, and anything that is disruptive should be avoided.

## RED CHESTNUT · THE REMEDY FOR THOSE WHO HAVE OBSESSIVE CONCERN/WORRY

Bach writes: Red Chestnut is "for those who find it difficult not to be anxious for other people. Often they have ceased to worry about themselves, but for those of whom they are fond they may suffer much, frequently anticipating that some unfortunate thing may happen to them."

• **Red Chestnut is both an acute and a constitutional remedy.**

### Botanical Information

The Red Chestnut tree (*Aesculus Carnea*) is, outside of Bach circles, best known as the "red flowered horse chestnut." It was created as a hybrid between the Red Buckeye (*Aesculus Pavia*) and the Horse Chestnut (*Aesculus Hippocastanum*). It is a drought-tolerant tree, with pink to bright red bell-shaped flowers. The red chestnut tree is small, rounded and slow-growing.

### Red Chestnut in General

The Red Chestnut fear state can be difficult to target because, in many cases, it comes disguised as a virtue. After all, on the surface, what can be more natural and loving than concern for those we love?

The problem, when it reveals itself, is multifold. First, the concern for others that motivates the Red Chestnut type is constant, and can never be resolved. Therefore, the Red Chestnut type can never relax and go on with his or her life, and the loved one can never be released from the chains of the Red Chestnut's concern. In this way, Red Chestnuts take on the role of the parent who cannot be pleased. But instead of being dissatisfied with their loved ones' choices in life, and thinking they do not measure up, Red Chestnuts are constantly concerned that these choices (unless a choice happens to coincide with what they think is best) will put the loved one in danger.

Now, while it is most common for the loved one to be the actual child of the Red Chestnut, it certainly does not have to be the case. The loved one can be anyone (human or animal) that the Red Chestnut has chosen to obsess over. Which brings into play the second aspect of the problem of the Red Chestnut's concern: it is obsessive in nature. Because the Red Chestnut is obsessed with the loved one, the love he or she feels and expresses is smothering and controlling in nature, not nurturing and freeing. This can make the Red Chestnut's love something of a noose for the recipients.[14]

---

14. Don't think that the Red Chestnut can't be obsessively worried about more than one person—they certainly can. Constitutional Red Chestnut types can have an entire family of people and pets on very short leashes. Their phones will ring almost constantly as each member of their "circle of concern" checks in with nearly hourly reports.

Many believe that Red Chestnut is a "mood" remedy, rather than a "type" remedy, because no one can live at the level of anxiety that Red Chestnuts constantly feel for those they love. These people never met my mother. While the Red Chestnut state is indeed often fleeting—the result of a snowy evening and a child who is out driving and is late getting home—it is certainly possible in many cases for the Red Chestnut state to become more or less permanent, and for the Red Chestnut patient to be in a chronic state of alert and worry. Just as the Aspen type can remain in a more or less constant state of upset and anxiety, the Red Chestnut patient can and will worry about the object of his or her concern on a sunny, warm afternoon nearly as much as on that snowy night.

It is indeed possible for negative Red Chestnuts to feel fear for those they love during every moment of their lives and for these people to constantly need to know that all is well and everyone is safe. This is a way to keep from having to deal with the issues of their own lives—to live in denial of self and the issues of self, and if possible, heap their fears onto those they love instead.

This is the final aspect of the problem this emotional state can bring. Not only does this obsessive overconcern for the loved one damage the relationship between the Red Chestnut and the loved one, it also impairs the Red Chestnut's ability to live his or her own life fully. Red Chestnuts choose—without being asked—to deny their own needs in order to ride herd over the needs of those they love.

In some cases, the Red Chestnut's apparent love and concern can seem so noble, even saintly, that anyone would be hard-pressed to consider it negative in any way. In these cases it is important to look at the loved one—the one who seems to be so cherished—to see if the apparent love is bringing about a positive or negative result.[15]

Perhaps it is best to understand Red Chestnut by considering two other Chestnut remedies: White Chestnut and Chestnut Bud. Each of these remedies is taken from a related plant, and each of the Bach remedies taken from these plants shares the emotional attribute of obsession. Each remedy type targets a specific aspect of life and clings to it. White Chestnut patients are given to obsessive thoughts. They lock onto a particular idea and will not, cannot let it go. This can be anything from the acute thought of what they should have said to their boss when he criticized them in that meeting—a thought that keeps them up that night instead of sleeping peacefully—to a deep chronic obsession, a plan for revenge, or a work or creative goal that literally takes over their life and shapes their future. The Chestnut Bud type shares the characteristic of

15. Keep this in mind when dealing with a Red Chestnut: the fact that they are worried doesn't mean that they are *right* to be worried. The Red Chestnut's obsession has warped their ability to distinguish between times when any reasonable person would be worried about those they love and times when their obsession is simply blinding them.

obsession, but places it in action rather than thought. These are the people (nearly all of us, to some degree) who take a behavior that once worked for them and lock onto it as a way of life. This can be embodied in bad habits, like smoking or overeating, which the Chestnut Bud knows is bad for him, but over which he has no power. Or it can be embodied in a string of bad marriages or failed jobs, in which the Chestnut Bud continues to make the same bad decisions and do and say the same foolish things over and over again, long after she is aware she is doing and saying something foolish.

Red Chestnuts are obsessive in the same way, but they have turned their obsession outward. They target one or more loved ones and direct their life energy onto them, simultaneously depleting their own life energy and smothering their love object.

The intermixed love and worry of the Red Chestnut comes at a high cost for both the Red Chestnut and the love object. For the Red Chestnut, the worry takes a physical as well as a mental and emotional toll. Red Chestnuts' ceaseless worry and hand wringing leads them into illness in the same way that Aspens weaken themselves into illnesses with their constant anxiety (like a car that is idling too roughly, they can never simply relax). Family members have often gathered over the casket of a Red Chestnut to extol his or her virtues and loving nature.

There is a cost to the loved ones as well. Those who are loved by the Red Chestnut must bear the burden of that love, as well as a sensation of always being watched and always being fussed over. They have taken on the weight of that love as if the energy pouring from the Red Chestnut (their own life's energy turned outward) were a physical thing. The loved ones will feel this energy not so much as a sensation of love, but as a method of control. If they do not constantly make choices that set the Red Chestnut's mind at ease, they bring the Chestnut to even higher states of alarm in which—within the context of love and concern—the Chestnut becomes even more demanding of assurances that "all is well," and that the loved ones are wearing their boots, carrying an umbrella, doing well at work, keeping a clean house, staying away from alcohol and bad influences, and on and on and on.

## Negative Qualities of the Type

For a remedy type that, on first glance, is often viewed as benign and loving, the negative qualities of the type are actually many and varied.

First, Red Chestnut types—either in an acute or constitutional context—place their focus on the worst-case scenario in every situation. They assume that their loved one is dead in a ditch although there is no evidence at all that this is the case. This places Red Chestnut alongside Gorse as one of the most pessimistic of all Bach types. Red Chestnuts will never believe that their loved one is well and happy. And the fact that their pessimism comes wrapped in what is supposedly a blanket of warm, cozy love makes matters all the worse.

Because the Red Chestnut and, often with these cases, those around him accept the belief that the obsessive concern is actually an aspect of healthy love, the overwhelming pessimism is often not only accepted but encouraged as being "loving." This allows the obsessive thoughts to fester and, in time, grow, both for the Red Chestnut and for the loved one. The Red Chestnut state—either as an acute or a chronic condition—is poisonous for both the "loving" Red Chestnut and for the loved ones.

The second negative is the nature of the worry itself. Along with the Red Chestnut's message of worry and concern comes a warning. This warning says, "Don't." It tells the loved one not to go there, not to do that, not to stay out late, not to drive. In time, it cripples the loved one, and it depletes the Red Chestnut in the process.

The natural concern we all feel for those we love must have some boundaries. We should be concerned for our own lives, just as we are for those we love. Some balance is needed, and some boundaries. What we should want for those we love is a life lived fully and freely—to be in a healthy and happy place in their own life. We should also want to be healthy and happy ourselves. The Red Chestnut type takes this natural flow of mutual love and (when it is called for) mutual concern, and warps it into a destructive thing—no matter how it is sugar-coated.

## Positive Qualities of the Type

No other type can match Red Chestnuts in their ability to love those they choose to love. Their devotion is complete. And, when they are in a positive state, no other type can match them for their ability to create positive situations for those that they love. When Red Chestnut types move into a positive state, they do not lose their ability to truly love. Instead, they lose their pessimism. Instead of always seeing some terrible catastrophe involving those they love playing out in their minds, they see their loved ones as happy and complete. They trust that their lives can be long and their achievements many. They trust that they have, in their loved one, someone who has the wisdom to walk a good path in life and the ability to work through the issues that life can bring.

Positive Red Chestnuts stand ready to help when called upon, but are busy with their own lives and focused on their own accomplishments.

## The Red Chestnut Child

Don't make the mistake of thinking that Red Chestnut types are usually middle-aged or elderly adults. It is likely true that the majority of those who enter into the Red Chestnut mindset at a chronic level are adults, but children can and do share this mindset. The child in a Red Chestnut state worries about the welfare of his or her parents. In simple cases, this can result in a form of separation anxiety on the part of the child; in more chronic cases it makes for a relationship in which the usual roles are reversed.

The child who takes on the constitutional Red Chestnut role will tend to take control of the household. This child will usually seem older than his actual age, and the aspects of his fear will also tend to be far more adult than his actual age. Like the Red Chestnut adult, he will curtail his natural interest in PlayStations and television and will, instead, worry over airplane safety and terrorists. The safety of all those for whom he cares, including the family pets, will be the chief concern of this child and the ongoing topic of his conversation. Worry will cause the Red Chestnut child much anxiety, and this anxiety will be a terrible burden upon the whole family.

### The Red Chestnut Adult

The constitutional Red Chestnut has taken a great virtue—true love for another being—and turned it into a negative mental and emotional state. This state can cause great harm for both the Red Chestnut and his or her loved one. The Red Chestnut has taken on the role of parent to the loved one, whether the object of this love is an actual child, a mate, or even a cherished pet. Whether it is appropriate or not. Whether it is desired by the loved one or not. Remember, one of the aspects of this remedy type that makes it so negative is that the loved one is not given any choice about being the love object and being so worried over. He or she is, in reality, an object of obsession, not love. In extreme cases, the loved one may not share any feelings for the Red Chestnut and may, indeed, be doing everything in his or her power to get free.

When the Red Chestnut and the loved one are unrelated and adults, the relationship is often a sexual one, in which the over-concern masks deep longing for the loved one. The desire to control the loved one's action is concealed by the message of concern. In this situation the power of each individual is equal, in that each person has the freedoms associated with adulthood.

When, however, the loved one is a dependent child or a pet, they are all but completely controlled by the obsessive worry of the Red Chestnut. The loved one will be weighed down by the constant concern and the restrictions to his or her lifestyle and movements. In cases like this, the Red Chestnut becomes "the loving tyrant."

### The Red Chestnut Animal

This is not a remedy that adapts easily to use with animals, but it does have one particular use that may be very helpful. Consider this remedy for the animal that works itself up while waiting for its owner to come home. The anxiety usually begins about an hour before it is time for the owner to arrive. The animal gets nearer and nearer to the door or to a window from which it can watch the arrival. Before the owner arrives, the animal has worked itself into a near frenzy, upsetting the entire household. And when the owner at last arrives, he or she must pay a great deal of attention to the animal—even more than to the others in the family. For this situation, Red Chestnut is a wonderful remedy.

### Red Chestnut and the Homeopathic Pharmacy

In that this remedy presents an ongoing riddle of selflessness versus selfishness, it in many ways is most similar to the homeopathic remedy Natrum Muriaticum, the polycrest remedy made from table salt. Like Natrum Mur patients, Red Chestnuts will tend to push all their will outward to those they love: they will sacrifice anything for their children. The problem is that Red Chestnuts pay no heed to their own needs. Instead, they focus on the lives of those they love, often creating situations born of their fears for them. They can be overly protective, and have problems with over attachment and lack of appropriate emotional boundaries. Red Chestnut also mirrors the Bach remedy Heather in this respect. Both will impose inappropriately, both will pry, and both will stand too close and intrude too much.

### Issues that Suggest Red Chestnut

Addictions; anorexia and other eating disorders; belching; breasts: lumps and cysts; excessive appetite; far-sightedness; foot problems; insomnia; obsessive behavior; pregnancy; sterility.

### In Conclusion

Each of us is perhaps more vulnerable when it comes to those we love than we are even when our own life is on the line. None of us can bear to think that harm will come to those we love, to whom we have opened our hearts. And this is as it should be.

The Red Chestnut state takes this natural vulnerability and perverts it into a negative emotional state, in which natural concern for others becomes targeted and obsessive, and the natural concern for self withers as a result.

The Red Chestnut state is hard enough to deal with as a momentary mood. There are, after all, snowy nights when our loved ones are out on the roads and we have reason for concern. But, as every parent knows all too well, we have to turn them over to whatever gods we know in these circumstances. We have to hope for the best as we prepare for the worst. And we sit long into the night, keeping the dinner warm and the house well lit.

In these times, Red Chestnut can help balance and calm. It can help us believe the best and not yield to irrational thoughts.

When the Red Chestnut mindset becomes chronic, it can be very difficult to bring back into balance. First because Red Chestnut (and all the Chestnuts, really), like Willow, will tend to deny that there is anything wrong. What we see as obsessive and irrational they perceive as loving and natural and, therefore, they are quite likely to refuse to even consider treatment.

Even if the Red Chestnut patient agrees to try the remedy, you should be prepared for the second reason this is a particularly tough mindset to balance: Red Chestnut is a remedy that does not work quickly or easily. The Red Chestnut state is a particularly tight knot to untie. It takes time and patience on the part of all concerned.

Finally, it is important to note that the needs of the loved one must also be attended to when treating the constitutional Red Chestnut. Often you will find that they have been beaten down into a Cerato state, in which they are now rather timid, and have become quite used to the domination they have experienced. Others will carry deep grudges and need Holly as an aid to let go of the anger they have long carried.

## ROCK ROSE · THE REMEDY FOR THOSE WITH PANIC

Before he developed the mixture that would take the name, Bach considered Rock Rose to be "*the* rescue remedy[16]." And when this first concept of rescue remedy was superseded by Bach's five-remedy mixture, Rock Rose became a component of the new version.

Of Rock Rose Bach writes: "The remedy of emergency for cases where there even appears no hope. In accident or sudden illness, or when the patient is very frightened or terrified, or if the condition is serious enough to cause great fear to those around. If the patient is not conscious the lips may be moistened with the remedy. Other remedies in addition may also be required, as, for example, if there is unconsciousness, which is a deep, sleepy state, Clematis; if there is torture, Agrimony, and so on."

In other words, it is important to note when beginning our study of this remedy that Rock Rose is very seldom considered a constitutional or "type" remedy, because very few people could exist for long at the emotional pitch the remedy suggests. It is, instead, one of our most important remedies for acute crisis situations.

- Most often, Rock Rose is used in acute situations.
- Rock Rose is a component of Rescue Remedy.
- Rock Rose is one of Bach's original remedies, the Twelve Healers.

### Botanical Information

While Rock Rose (*Helianthemum Nummalarium*) is native to Southern Europe, it is grown throughout Northern Europe and North America. It is particularly prized in England, but the English climate makes the plant's survival questionable as a perennial. It is a sun-loving and beautiful shrub, known for its brightly colored flowers, which may appear in a range of colors but are most commonly bright yellow.

16. See Chapter 13 for information on the history and uses of the Bach mixture known as Rescue Remedy, if you're not already familiar with it. For now, just know that it is a mixture of five Bach remedies: Cherry Plum, Clematis, Star of Bethlehem, Impatiens, and the remedy we are now considering, Rock Rose.

## Rock Rose in General

It is possible to witness the emotional state objectively when dealing with a patient who is experiencing a feeling of true terror. The patient's body may be literally frozen in fear, like the proverbial deer in the headlights. The patient's body becomes rigid. The heart pounds, so that it seems it will explode, or simply stop once and for all. These symptoms can remain for seconds, minutes, or days after the event that triggers them— or for much longer. The cause of the terror and panic can be any number of things, from the near miss on the turnpike to violent crime or abuse to a shocking natural occurrence such as a tornado or an earthquake. In dealing with the patient in a Rock Rose state, we are dealing with someone whose life has likely been put into jeopardy, someone who has experienced the deepest sensation of fear possible. We are dealing with the full expression of shock, terror and panic, or with its aftermath.

Although the specific reactions of individuals may vary from person to person while they are in a state of panic, some aspects of its cause tend to be similar from person to person and case to case.

First, the cause of the fear and panic is usually sudden. It comes seemingly from nowhere when a dog attacks, or a car swerves into your lane. Any existing plans for life and its living are quite literally thrown out the window, and you are placed in a situation for which you have no plan, no strategy. These are moments that we can only hope we will never experience, or that, if we do, some divine hand will guide us in our actions.

Second, the cause of the Rock Rose state is almost always external. Something happens *to* you that is not caused by you or in any way planned by you. Again, this means that the person experiencing such a crisis is working outside of his own thoughts and his own plans and is usually acting on equal parts instinct and adrenalin.

These two aspects of the catalyst to fear mean that the person is faced with a loss of control, which is a trigger to fear for almost all of us. An ice patch on a dark road can make our car skid, so we can no longer control the speed and actions of the two thousand pounds of steel to which we have strapped ourselves. The loss of control triggers the fear; the situation into which we have been thrust and our understanding of just how dire it is leads us to respond emotionally as well.

No two of us will react in the same way to the same set of circumstances. To put it in Bach terms, the quick-witted Impatiens may react to the icy patch swiftly enough to put things right and experience little shock, while the Clematis, who has been abruptly dragged back to reality from his usual dream-state, may be slower to react and therefore experiences a higher chance of fatality and a deeper shock. The Vervain may see the whole thing as a challenge, while an already anxious Aspen may experience deep trauma and may add winter nights to his list of things that are better avoided.

So it has to be remembered that when each of us is thrust into unknown and threatening circumstances, we go into those circumstances with a different set of strengths and weaknesses. Therefore, not everyone dealing with the same threat will respond with a Rock Rose reaction of panic and shock. Therefore, it is always necessary for the Bach practitioner to witness the patient and his emotional state. Too often this remedy (along with Cherry Plum, which follows next) is given based on the circumstances of the threat to the individual instead of on the individual's response to the threat itself. And while giving Rock Rose or any other Bach remedy in error will not threaten the patient's health and well-being further, it will not help the patient as much as the correctly chosen remedy. In the interests of understanding the Bach remedies and using them in the best way possible, it is always important to select a remedy based upon the patient's response to a given situation or mood, and not because of the situation or mood itself.[17]

Many sloppy homeopaths automatically give the remedy Arnica for every patient who has a bruise, often missing a better-selected remedy like Bellis Perennis. In making assumptions when they should be paying attention to their patient, they deny that patient a remedy that truly could have helped him. In the same way, Bach practitioners sometimes give a remedy based on the circumstances surrounding the patient and not on that individual patient's specific reactions to that situation. Worse, all too often the flawed Bach practitioner will give the remedy based upon *what he or she would need in the same situation*, which likely will offer no help at all to the patient. We can do no good at all with these wonderful remedies if we cannot remove ourselves from our own needs and our own heads and pay attention to the patient in front of us.

In dealing with the patient, it is important to realize that, when placed in a traumatic situation, the patient will experience the trauma not only while the circumstances causing the trauma are occurring. The trauma will continue to be experienced after the circumstances have ended. Indeed, the patient will not be able to move ahead without fear until he or she is able to fully digest all that has happened and has reached a point of understanding the full impact of the experience.

That's what the Bach remedies can help the patient do—digest what has happened (whether it is of the patient's own causing or has been forced upon him), learn from it, and move ahead freely and without fear.

In the case specific to Rock Rose, you are truly administering first aid when you give this remedy. It will restore a patient lost to trauma and panic to his right mind and

---

17. This is easily proven when working with animals. Many aggressive dogs, even those who growl and snap at their owners, can be helped with the fear remedy Mimulus. Those looking only at the current circumstances would likely give Vervain and Vine in combination for the dog's excitement and aggression. But those who pay attention to the dog itself will see the fear underlying the aggressive behavior.

a clear head. When the bottom has fallen out of life, when all that was once planned and safe and sunny now seems dark and threatening, this is the remedy that will set things right.

> In the case specific to Rock Rose, you are truly administering first aid when you give this remedy. It will restore a patient lost to trauma and panic to his right mind and a clear head.

As I have noted above, Rock Rose is almost always an acute remedy. Few of us could survive living in such terror. So Rock Rose is used fleetingly. The need for the remedy ends as the patient begins to return to himself, as his panic fades and his rational mind returns.

But that does not mean that the need for Bach treatment ends. Just as Arnica is often given homeopathically to begin healing and then is followed by other remedies to complete the cure, so, too, the fleeting Rock Rose, having served its purpose, is followed by other remedies in Bach treatments. It is often followed by Star of Bethlehem (or combined with it from the beginning) in cases in which the trauma has left an emotional wound.[18] Rock Rose also combines well with or precedes two other fear remedies, Aspen and Mimulus, depending upon the fear state of the individual. Rock Rose is also often combined with or precedes Scleranthus for patients who are unable to function at all due to their state of shock and fear.

Having written at some length about the dire circumstances that can lead to the appropriate use of Rock Rose, it is, in closing, important to note that the cause of panic is not always life threatening. Studies have shown that many people fear public speaking more than they do death itself. For some, the fact that they are going to have to face a stage or a podium is reason enough to panic. Rock Rose can help these people. The same may be said for those who panic when taking tests (especially driving tests, when the panic can have dire results). And this remedy can help all those people who tend to "lose their minds" just a little when facing any of life's little emergencies, like a trip to the emergency room with a child who is injured, or a trip to the dentist. It is, after all, a part of the Rescue Remedy blend because it brings us back to our right minds when we have lost them, even a little—no matter the cause.

One final note: Rock Rose should be considered in cases in which the shocking circumstances have to do with medical emergencies as well. It can calm a patient who is having a heart attack or stroke, and also assist those caring for him to remain clear

---

18. These two remedies are often very useful for those who have been traumatized in war and for those who—as the term was first coined after World War I—are "shell shocked." The two remedies can be given in combination or in sequence, as the case suggests. In such cases of post-traumatic stress, the patient may need to use or revisit the remedy Rock Rose more often than most other people needing the remedy for other causes, other reasons.

headed. While the use of any Bach remedy should not keep you from performing appropriate first aid or from calling 911, it can be used to help fill the gap of time until that help arrives, and it can be of great value to all concerned.

## Negative Qualities of the Type

The negative Rock Rose state is one in which we are incapable of clear action because we have entered into a state of deep fear, panic, and shock. The problem with this state is that it is the same whether the situation is one of true danger, or one in which the Rock Rose is incapable of effectively reacting to that danger.

It is this aspect of the remedy that is useful in constitutional Bach treatments. Those who have entered into a chronic negative Rock Rose are always in a state of alarm, always ready to flee any perceived danger. They have lost the ability to know what circumstances are truly life threatening and which are not. The chronic negative Rock Rose sees life as a series of acute situations and traumatic events. Each of these events brings about the same response: panic. The patient's well-being disappears; his or her clear headedness disappears and is replaced by a panic response: shortness of breath, pounding heart, wild eyes and flailing limbs. Rock Rose can help set things right when used in combination with other remedies. Note, however, that when Rock Rose is used as part of a combination of remedies, it will have to be taken for a longer period of time than it would if used singly as an acute remedy.

The patient in a negative Rock Rose state, whether it is acute or chronic in nature, should be considered to have a contagious disease. By this I mean that, when someone near you (especially someone emotionally close to you) is in a Rock Rose panic, they will tend to project this emotional state onto those around them. When circumstances require Rock Rose it is best that everyone take the remedy, so *all* can remain clear headed and take whatever action is needed.

## Positive Qualities of the Type

Since Rock Rose is most often an acute remedy given in the short-term, it does not offer the fully-felt transformations that more constitutional remedies enjoy. But that does not mean that Rock Rose does not bring about almost operatic results when it is well used. In many cases, the patient's improvement will become obvious in just a matter of seconds after the first dose of the remedy. You will be able to watch as the patient returns to himself and regains his ability to cope. Those who have been given Rock Rose in a time of need are those who will be able to take action when all others have lost their heads to fear. They are those who are rational when others have become irrational.

## The Rock Rose Child

Just as with adult patients, children who need Rock Rose most often need it in the short term as an acute treatment. And the reasons why the remedy is needed remain the same in children and adults. Very few children chronically live in a Rock Rose state, and those that do are most often in truly threatening situations—children of war and of violence. These children are motivated by their panic and their terror. They have nightmares and awaken suddenly in a panic state. They also start at every noise, and overreact to the dangers at hand.

### The Rock Rose Adult

Because we are dealing with true emergencies when we consider the circumstances that create and shape a Rock Rose state, there is little difference between the needs and actions of the Rock Rose adult and the Rock Rose child. Indeed, true emergencies often reduce the strongest of us to the state of helpless and fearful children. What Rock Rose offers is the possibility of returning the adult to an adult state, with his or her fully rational mind, knowledge of experiences, and capabilities.

### The Rock Rose Animal

Since Rock Rose is a component in Rescue Remedy, I suggest that you have that mixture on hand in your home at all times. It can be used in any emergency situation, and I suggest that you use that remedy in place of Rock Rose. And I suggest that, if members of your family need Rescue Remedy, you give it to your animals as well. Use it any time any domestic animal or pet displays "escape behaviors," which is to say any time they try to scratch their way out the door or bite through the fence. Consider it in cases of physical trauma as well because it will calm the animal and help it cope with physical pain.

### Rock Rose and the Homeopathic Pharmacy

Because this state comes on suddenly and shockingly, it relates most strongly with the homeopathic remedy Aconite, taken from the plant Monkshood, with which it shares the suddenness of symptoms and the shock that the situation at hand creates. Both remedy types share the feeling of an "ill wind" suddenly blowing upon them. Both feel the shock in the solar plexus, and usually feel a physical symptom of chilliness in their body.

In the homeopathic *Materia Medica*, Rock Rose can also suggest the remedy Arnica, which can be used for the treatment of those in shock, who have been physically or mentally traumatized and need help in beginning to heal. In homeopathic treatment, we often use the alternating remedies Aconite and Arnica for what might be considered a Rock Rose state in Bach treatments, as in the case of the child who awakens in panic from a nightmare or an entire family who has survived a house fire or violent crime.

### Issues that Suggest Rock Rose

Anxiety attacks; auto accidents; death and dying; heart attack; hysteria; nightmares; panic attacks; physical trauma; shock; stroke.

### In Conclusion

If the remedy Aspen dreads the future and is convinced that it will not go well, the remedy Rock Rose is, as Bach wrote, "terrified as to what will happen." The patient needing Rock Rose is both unsure as to whether or not there will be a future and whether or not he wants there to be a future. This is a person whose perception of life has been shocked into the exact second in which he finds himself. Most of us, in our daily lives, blend memories of the past and past experiences with hopes and plans for the future in our moment-to-moment lives. The person who has been forced—and that is the word, as no one chooses the Rock Rose state—into a Rock Rose state of mind has shaken away the past, except for yearning for it, and is terrified of the future, even the next instant. Where most of us live in terms of days or weeks, the Rock Rose lives in the instant, not knowing what to do in the next moment, or even if it will occur.

I like the way Bach himself concluded his section on Rock Rose in *Free Thyself*, and can think of no better way to conclude here: "You are learning to be brave against great odds, and fighting for your freedom, and the beautiful little yellow Rock Rose, which grows so abundantly on our hilly pastures, will give you the courage to win through."

## CHERRY PLUM · THE REMEDY FOR THOSE WITH HYSTERIA

Bach has important words about Cherry Plum: "Fear of the mind being over-strained, of reason giving away, of doing fearful and dreadful things, not wished and known wrong, yet there comes the thought and the impulse to do them."

Of this remedy, the *Flower Essence Repertory*[19] states, "The circumstances of life oppress and condense the soul, so that it literally feels that it cannot take any more pressure or stress. There is the fear that one will lose control and become erratic, destructive, or even suicidal or insane. The soul tries to protect against this fear of losing control by tightening its grip, which leads to more pressure and stress. At these extreme times, Cherry Plum is indicated . . . Cherry Plum flower essence brings strength and encouragement, helping the soul to overcome its extreme tension and fear."

---

19. The *Flower Essence Repertory* is the product of the Flower Essence Society, an American organization dedicated to education on the subject of the Bach Flower Essences, as well as those created by the Society. The organization has published an excellent repertory that contains information on all its essences and Bach's as well.

• Most often, Cherry Plum is used as an acute Bach remedy, although it can be very valuable as a constitutional or "type" remedy.

• Cherry Plum is a component of Rescue Remedy.

### Botanical Information

The flowers of the Cherry Plum (*Prunus Cerasifera*) open in the early spring, from February until April, and are pure white in color. The shoots of the tree are thorn free, and the plant itself is shrublike, growing to a little over four feet in height.

Cherry plum is most often planted in rows to fence property and to act as a windbreak.

### Cherry Plum in General

Cherry Plum shares the general emotion fear with the others in this group. However, in the case of Cherry Plum, the fear is fixated on the loss of control.

Cherry Plum is often considered to be solely a "mood" remedy, called for only in acute situations. And it certainly is a valuable remedy for sudden stresses and traumas that lead to an intense state of fear in which the patient feels that he or she is no longer in control of his thoughts or actions. But Cherry Plum, as we shall see, is also an excellent remedy for constitutional or long-term use, and can help those with chronic destructive impulses that can cripple a lifetime. Indeed, it is the remedy for impulsiveness.

To begin with the acute uses for the remedy, the typical Cherry Plum state is one in which patients feel driven up against a wall emotionally. They feel that something has pushed them until they can stand no more, take no more. Cherry Plums feel that they may literally lose their reason and all control of their thoughts and actions at any moment. It is important to note that while the Cherry Plum feels driven to emotional extremes, in all reality the cause of their distress may well be of their own making. Where the Rock Rose, for instance, is always driven to emotional distress by external forces, the Cherry Plum may choose to believe that he has been driven to extremes by something outside himself, while, in truth, his distress may be only in his mind. Those nearby may be as shocked by the Cherry Plum's hysterical behavior as the Cherry Plum is shocked by the perceived threat.

But no matter how the Cherry Plum got there, the Cherry Plum is in a state of hysteria, and, in that state, feels as if he or she will soon be unable to control his or her behavior. This torrent of emotion may build slowly, or it may appear explosively—it may also, as we shall see, be a long-term situation—but once it has built, it needs to be taken very seriously. Even the acute Cherry Plum state of hysteria can reach levels of thought and behavior that can threaten the patient's mental health. And it can most certainly threaten the Cherry Plum's relationships, as he or she may say or do things to loved ones in the moment of explosion that are not easily taken back or forgiven after the explosion has passed. In a Cherry Plum state, a patient is capable of suicide, or totally irrational or even psychotic behavior. In a chronic or constitutional Cherry Plum state, a patient is also capable of obsessive behaviors that can include paranoia, revenge fantasies, and stalking.

Of course, not all Cherry Plum states, acute or chronic, are so threatening. Most often, the remedy is used in acute cases in which the patient has worn down their emotional defenses through extraordinary stresses or deep illnesses. When a final catalyst appears or is perceived, the patient begins to fear that they can take no more and hysteria results. A dose or two of Cherry Plum can restore the patient's sense of calm and clarity.

In acute situations, consider this remedy in combination with Elm for the patient who has been worn down to a state of exhaustion leading to hysteria, or with Sweet Chestnut for the patient whose hysteria threatens even more extreme actions, such a suicide. The three remedies combine beautifully for those patients who have worn themselves down in caring for a critically ill loved one. It is of especial help if that loved one has lost their struggle and their life, leaving the caretaker in a state of exhausted grief that leads to hysteria.

In considering the constitutional Cherry Plum, I am reminded of a medical diagnosis that was often made in the beginning of the last century—*neurasthenia.*

That diagnosis, coined in 1869 by George Miller Beard, referred to a state in which the central nervous system was totally depleted and the patient was in a state of nervous exhaustion. It was a disease of the upper classes, especially in British society, during the period of urbanization, in which the stresses of everyday life increased to the point of destroying the patient's ability to enjoy his or her life. It was a diagnosis that was more often than not applied to female patients, most notably Virginia Woolf. The neurasthenic patient was considered to be sensitive and high-strung; an emotional, as opposed to a logical, thinker, given to bouts of fainting, crying, and hysteria, all without cause.

Although the diagnosis of neurasthenia has fallen into disuse today, doctors today still tend to consider those patients given the diagnosis of chronic fatigue syndrome or fibromyalgia the same way that neurasthenics were considered a century ago. Those who are prone to hysteria today are often quieted with antidepressants or antipsychotic medications and left to cope as best they can.

Constitutional Cherry Plums find themselves in a state of constant imbalance. Their constant fear is that they will fall victim to their stresses, to the things that threaten to overwhelm them, and that they will lose all reason as a result. They fear they may lose control of themselves at any moment, and this fear causes them to behave in an erratic and hysterical manner. Because the catalyst to this hysteria may or may not be objective and known or witnessed by anyone other than the Cherry Plum, those close to the patient likewise find themselves in a state of unbalance, and they cannot be sure whether anything they might say or do will bring on a hysterical outburst.

Like the acute Cherry Plum state, the chronic state may also contain moments of extreme emotional outbursts and dangerous behaviors. Cherry Plums fear they may lose all reason, and the resulting irrational behavior based upon that fear causes a "chicken or the egg" situation. Is the fear of losing control based upon a past history of actually losing control? Or is the actual loss of control based upon the ongoing drumbeat of fear and stress that wears the Cherry Plum down into such a state of emotional exhaustion that they can no longer stay in control? It is impossible to know. But one thing is sure: the Cherry Plum state, especially when it becomes chronic, can be a dangerous thing for all concerned.

> Cherry Plums find themselves in a state of constant imbalance. They fear they may lose control of themselves at any moment, and this fear causes them to behave in an erratic and hysterical manner.

Often there is a valid reason that a given patient has moved into a chronic Cherry Plum state. One major cause is abuse—child abuse, physical abuse, verbal abuse, or, especially, sexual abuse. These patients are and have been abused for some time and, as a result, have lost all trust, first in their abuser and then, as the abuse continues over time, in the world around them that fails to protect them. Finally, as they are driven downward and their coping mechanisms fail, they lose trust in themselves. At that point the explosive emotionalism of the Cherry Plum type comes to the fore.

The cause of the condition is not always easily knowable, however, nor is it always external. Many of those in the Cherry Plum state are, in all reality, not threatened in any way, but they perceive a threat, and, as a result, end up in the same Cherry Plum emotional pattern.

The patient in a chronic Cherry Plum state will tend to go from outburst to outburst, with periods of relative calm in between. The outburst itself can often seem to calm the patient, drain him of his pent-up hysteria and/or anger. But since no one, including the Cherry Plum himself, can know exactly when the next outburst will occur, life with a Cherry Plum and for the Cherry Plum himself is a journey through a minefield.

The remedy Star of Bethlehem combines well with Cherry Plum for those in a Cherry Plum state due to abuse. For those who have worn themselves down into a Cherry Plum state through overwork, also consider combining the remedy Oak. For those who have become obsessive in their brooding thoughts, which can drift into paranoia, blend White Chestnut with Cherry Plum.

## Negative Qualities of the Type

When dealing with a patient who is in a constitutional Cherry Plum state, you are dealing with a person who is choosing between rational and irrational behavior and between clear reason and total abandon in every moment of their life. The Cherry Plum is seen by others as a chaotic person who cannot be fully trusted or depended upon, because it is impossible to predict when he or she may become hysterical. Family members and other loved ones tend to walk on eggshells around a Cherry Plum, as they can never be sure just what will set that person off into an emotional outburst. The Cherry Plum himself is equally aware of the onus of his condition and lives in a continual state of fear that he will soon lose control. In truth, the Cherry Plum has no more idea as to just what it is that will set him or her off than anyone else does.

This ongoing fear of loss of control is the key to understanding the Cherry Plum's plight. Just as Aspen's state of chronic anxiety and Red Chestnut's constant worry exact physical and emotional tolls, so, too, does Cherry Plum's ongoing struggle to stay in control of his or her mind and emotions.

The Cherry Plum type is high-strung, usually more sensitive and intelligent than the average person and usually, like Water Violet, somewhat refined in nature. They will, like Aspen, seek to surround themselves with "safe" and "comfortable" things, possessions that can be depended upon in a way that living things cannot. But where Aspens may turn to alcohol or drugs to numb their anxiety, Cherry Plums will most often totally avoid anything (or any place or any person) that makes them feel as if they might lose control. So alcohol and drugs (with the possible exception of tranquilizers) are something that they often tend to avoid.

Like Aspen, the Cherry Plum type lacks trust. But Aspen suspects the world of evil intentions, does not trust his environment, and suspects the future of all sorts of evil possibilities. The Cherry Plum has, instead, lost trust with himself or herself, and this loss of trust sets up an ongoing inner dynamic that mixes tension with fear.

The Cherry Plum state is usually progressive. It starts mildly, but becomes more and more crippling as the weight of tension and fear continues and actually grows as fear leads to more fear and still more fear.

As their emotional state worsens, the Cherry Plum can resemble the Water Violet in that he or she will tend to retire from life as much as possible. They will also tend to become sensitive to more and more catalysts, such as specific foods, smells, and colors, and to light and sound. Left untreated, their lives can become very difficult and very small.

## Positive Qualities of the Type

The Cherry Plum type who has learned to deal with his fears and to accept and trust himself can open himself to those around him, fully able to live in peace and harmony.

The key to the Cherry Plum type who is in a positive state is that they are completely clear minded. Their natural insight and intellect is still in place, and they make discerning and sensitive counselors for all in need.

Equally important, they can rest assured that they are able to meet each stress or crisis with the amount of emotional energy it requires, and no more. No longer does the Cherry Plum have to expend energy straightjacketing himself with the fear of loss of control, or, worse, with the actual loss of rational thoughts and actions.

### The Cherry Plum Child

Cherry Plum is usually considered to be an acute remedy for children. It is most useful at moments in which a child is hysterical. It is also used when a child is very ill, such as when he becomes delirious with high fever. Another common illness associated with Cherry Plum is toothache.

When a child is in a Cherry Plum state, their parents will tend to be shocked by his or her behavior, as it strongly deviates from the norm. They will experience a sudden outburst of temper from a usually calm child, or a child who has become hysterical for no apparent reason. When the child is in a Cherry Plum state, he or she will tend to overreact to every stimulus and will be uncontrollable with no apparent cause.

For the rare child who seems to be a constitutional Cherry Plum, the remedy combines especially well with Holly (for cases that combine hysteria with rage) and Impatiens (for hysterical hyperactivity). Consider combining Cherry Plum with Aspen for the child who is highly sensitive and hysterical.

### The Cherry Plum Adult

This remedy is useful for those moments when life does not seem worth living. When a wife loses her husband of many years and no longer wants to live, or when a person has been driven to the brink of a nervous breakdown. For such people, Cherry Plum is an acute remedy that will help them move forward and release the self-destructive impulses in a safe manner.

But for millions of others, this remedy may be needed day-to-day. A friend of mine adopted a young child who was born into poverty and warfare in a third-world nation. As the child grew, he proved to be far more wounded than could have been guessed. He was virtually uncontrollable. The schools did not know what to do with him, and, over time, neither did his adoptive mother.

While that child was successfully treated with homeopathic remedies and was able, in time, to be both happy and healthy in his new environment, it was Cherry Plum that got his adoptive mother through the many months in which she was pushed past her ability to cope with this child's behavior.[20]

And that's the key to Cherry Plum. The thought that: "I've been pushed past my limits and now I just don't know what I'll do." Or: "I'm mad as hell and I'm not going to take it anymore." It is for the moments in which, as Raymond Chandler writes, wives are looking at the back of their husband's necks and fingering knives.

Whether used acutely or constitutionally, look to Cherry Plum to guide the patient through a process of transformation. Look for an increased ability to cope. Most important, look for a more unified sense of self. The positive, adult Cherry Plum is a person in whom the conscious and unconscious are in direct and complete communication.

The Cherry Plum then knows what is and is not appropriate behavior. They know the consequences of their actions. They are able to cope with the stress of life and (to paraphrase Kipling) keep their heads when all those around them are losing theirs.

### The Cherry Plum Animal

This is not a remedy commonly needed by animals. However, it may be of value to you if you have an animal that is highly strung, with behavior you cannot predict or trust. Consider this remedy particularly if the animal displays destructive behaviors based in hysterics. If the animal has moments of being totally out of control, consider Cherry Plum. It can be very helpful for animals that panic and may do damage both to themselves and their surroundings when they are left alone.

### Cherry Plum and the Homeopathic Pharmacy

Staphysagria is the homeopathic remedy most similar to Cherry Plum in behavior. Both patient types most deeply fear loss of control, and both are victims of situations that have pushed them beyond their ability to cope. Both feel they have been treated unfairly and that external forces have forced their hand.

The other remedy type that closely mirrors Cherry Plum is Ignatia Amara, which is often a remedy for those who feel that they have been betrayed. Ignatia shares the sensitivities of Cherry Plum, particularly to smells, sound, and light. More important, the Ignatia patient will often explode in displays of high emotion for apparently no reason, suddenly running out of the room crying and leaving their family in a state of confusion as to the reason for the outburst. As with Ignatia, the Cherry Plum state can come on as a result of the loss of a loved one, either through death or divorce—a loss that has been interpreted as a betrayal of sorts.

### Issues that Suggest Cherry Plum

Allergies; bedwetting; child abuse; compulsive behaviors; destructive behavior; eating

---

20. Parents or others who love some of the "tougher" personality types, such as Vervain or Vine constitutional types may also need a few doses of Cherry Plum from time to time to help them stay calm in the face of myriad difficulties.

disorders; headaches, especially migraines; hyperactivity; nervous conditions; physical or verbal abuse.

## In Conclusion

For a small number of patients, Cherry Plum is the most important and valuable remedy. It can restore a life that has been lost to fear and to hysteria.

For most of us, however, Cherry Plum is a remedy that is called upon only from time to time, when we have been worn down or pushed to the limits of our emotional strength. At these times, Cherry Plum can restore order from chaos.

I find that some people, men especially, tend to avoid this remedy and do not even consider taking it, since they perceive it to be a remedy for the weak, for the feminine. This bias blocks Cherry Plum from fulfilling its full potential. The hysteria associated with Cherry Plum is an unpleasant thing, to be sure. But worse, when a large man is in a Cherry Plum state and yielding to his own hysterical impulses, it is often coupled with rage (blend in the Holly—but don't count on Holly alone to do the job) it can be a terrifying thing for all concerned. The man who is wise enough to recognize his limits—especially when he is dealing with children who are crying or dogs who won't behave—and can take Cherry Plum before his emotions build can help create a safe and harmonious environment for all those he loves.

5

---

# Considering the Second Mood:
# The Degrees of Despair

Henry David Thoreau wrote that most "men live lives of quiet desperation," and, in writing it, revealed his knowledge of the human condition. How many of us have let go of joy in our day-to-day lives and replaced it with the dull sensation of depression or the ache of despair?

Simple depression may well control the lives and actions of more people than any other emotional state. The remedies in this group relate to the many millions who have lost touch with excitement and joy in life, whose lives are largely defined by a daily to-do list of responsibilities and chores that have long since ceased to challenge or interest them. In the same way, life's relationships, which once caused the greatest excitement possible, now seem to involve only thoughtless gestures and evenings lit by the light of the television screen.

Therefore, the remedies listed in this section can be very helpful for a wide range of emotional states. They can help us rediscover who we are and our natural passions when we find ourselves in a rut. Or they can help us through times of deep despair, when the weight of the world is on our shoulders. As with the other Bach remedies, those gathered together around the range of emotions in Bach's category of despair fall into two camps—acute and constitutional. Two remedies in this group—Sweet Chestnut and Star of Bethlehem—are often thought of as "mood" remedies, best used in acute situations and rather fleeting in their actions. The other six are typically considered to be "type" remedies, and are given for a longer period of time to help the patient change an ingrained emotional pattern. As always, however, it is best to remember that all Bach remedies can be used in acute situations. All are equally valuable in the short-term and even remedies, like Sweet Chestnut, that are most often only needed to help a patient cope with a moment of crisis, may be of value over a longer period of time. Therefore, it is best to understand the nature of a remedy and the issues to which it speaks without trying to lock in the specific uses of a given remedy. Once we come to understand the remedies to the point that we can see them acted out in actual human behavior, we can be free to use them as they are really needed.[1]

I have found in past experience that, with the possible exception of Sweet Chestnut and Star of Bethlehem, those persons who need the remedies in this group are among the most difficult to treat. Many are completely unaware of the fact that they have a problem. The driven Oak or the perfect Crab Apple will tend to feel that the world would be a better place if more people were like them, and the insecure Larch often cannot bear to look at his own issues. So you should not expect a great degree of objective self-awareness or even a desire to change when dealing with those who are gathered here.

Perhaps the most difficult aspect of dealing with patients in this mood state is that they often feel there is an aspect of nobility in living their lives in despair—that they are enduring all that life throws at them. They tend to feel that they are coping rather nicely with their lives, even if the weight of their responsibilities is nearly overwhelming. They also tend not to notice the impact their particular emotional pattern is having on those around them. Willows will not see the cost of their negativity; not only to them, but also to those they love. Crab Apples will only see their organized and clean environment and not the unhappy looks on their children's faces.

This makes them hard to treat, especially if, like me, you don't believe it is ever appropriate to simply slip the remedy into their morning coffee, no matter how tempting that might be.

Often the solution to this issue presents itself because the patient will ask for help with other issues. Their sense of "quiet despair" may be accompanied by anxiety or exhaustion. The case can therefore be opened with other remedies and the appropriate remedy for despair can be introduced in combination with the other remedy or remedies. In time, the patient may be willing to discuss his sense of despair—or may not—but the result is the same: he will feel a lifting of the weight he had been carrying, and a wonderful sensation of freedom and possibility.

For that is what is lacking in these patients: a feeling of possibility—the possibility that something wonderful might happen to them or they might accomplish something truly wonderful with their lives. It is as if their visual sense of color has, over time, narrowed and narrowed until all they perceive are shades of gray. With the help of these remedies, their eyes are opened once more to the full spectrum of colors around them. Imagine the joy that such a shift in perception would bring.

---

1. In other words, while it is important to understand that some Bach remedies are best used in acute situations and others are more typically needed in the long term for constitutional treatments, don't lock yourself in by rigid rules when actually using the remedies. While the nature of a given remedy—"mood" or "type"—may help guide you in choosing and/or using a remedy, don't let that simple categorization block you from using any remedy as needed. A solid constitutional remedy like Crab Apple, that usually takes quite some time to have an effect, may act in a single dose, while Sweet Chestnut, commonly thought of as an acute remedy, may be needed by a particular patient for months. Let the case, not the rulebook, guide you.

Those needing the remedies listed here must be reminded that we are meant to explore this lifetime like an unknown mountaintop. Those who merely accept despair are like those who bury their talents, risking nothing, and then wonder why their behavior is not honored by those who creatively risk and grow.

## Despair and the Homeopathic Pharmacy

The concept of despair can be difficult to treat homeopathically, as it can be expressed in myriad ways that are not easily defined in "rubrics" (the individual symptom listings in the homeopathic Repertory). If you were to look under the mental symptom of despair, you would find a complex rubric containing many dozens of remedies, prominent among them the remedy Lycopodium. Lycopodium is known as a remedy that feels very stressed easily and is deeply challenged by any sort of change in their thinking, their methodology, or their relationships. These are people of strict demeanor, rigid rules, and issues of self-confidence. As such, they relate to most of the remedies in this category. Other remedies are likely to fall prey to feelings related to despair: both Arsenicum and Veratrum Album can be perfectionists whose perfectionism covers deep chasms of doubt; Calcarea Carbonica can quietly despair of their life choices and situation; and Ignatia Amara can experience moments of deep, terrifying despair.

In the Repertory, the concept of despair can seep into other mental/emotional states as well. It can be expressed as discontent, or dissatisfaction, as with the remedy Natrum Muriaticum, who often feels very disappointed with those he loves. Or the patient may feel discouraged, which again suggests Lycopodium, or the remedy Lachesis, which, when needed, suggest a patient who, for all his apparent bluster, feels deeply that he will never achieve his goals in life. Mental dullness may also be an aspect of despair, as with the remedy type Sulphur, whose mind drifts into confusion and discord as a means of not dealing with the underlying deep despair.

In a very real way, the Bach remedies can offer much more to those wrestling with despair and its allied emotional states than Hahnemann's pharmacy. The Bach remedies can assist the patient who knows despair, both in the moment of acute crisis, and with the lifelong patterns that are formed in response to the emotional state.

## REMEDIES FOR THOSE WHO DESPAIR

- **Larch**—for those who are self-conscious
- **Elm**—for those who are overwhelmed
- **Oak**—for those who are overly-responsible
- **Crab Apple**—for those who are perfectionists

- **Willow**—for those who are bitter
- **Pine**—for those with guilt
- **Sweet Chestnut**—for those who are in despair
- **Star of Bethlehem**—for those who are in shock

## LARCH · THE REMEDY FOR THOSE WHO ARE SELF-CONSCIOUS

Bach says that Larch is the remedy "for those who do not consider themselves as good or capable as those around them, who expect failure, who feel that they will never be a success, and so do not venture or make a strong enough attempt to succeed."

- **While Larch may be a very useful acute remedy, its greater strength is in constitutional use, especially in young people.**

### Botanical Information

Larch (*Larix Decidua*) is an unusual tree, because, although it is a conifer, it is also deciduous. Most conifers are evergreen, but the larch loses its needles in the winter. And the needles themselves are patterned differently from other conifers. The cones of the larch are small, from one to two inches long. There are only ten species of larch in the world. It grows throughout the colder northern regions of Europe and North America. The larch is also known as the "tamarack."

### Larch in General

The Larch type—and this is, most frequently, a "type" or constitutional remedy that will need to be taken for a lengthy period of time and/or combined with other Bach remedies to bring about a change—has locked into a sense of self that is very negative. The Larch tends to be, like Heather or Chicory, overly self-aware, and, like the Willow or Water Violet, judgmental. But the Larch reserves this critical attitude for himself. He tends to observe himself at all times, judging his own words, the sound of his own voice, his own appearance, and finding them all lacking. This is a shy person, a timid person, because he considers himself to be inferior to others.

This sense of inferiority would push another patient to attempt accomplishments by which he could attain a sense of achievement and self-worth. But, for the Larch, this sense of inadequacy undermines every attempt at any goal. The Larch is convinced that anything he attempts is destined to fail, simply because it is he who is attempting it. And so you will find the Larch abruptly giving up on his work, his vision, and his goals in life again and again, apparently for no good reason. But to the Larch, any sort of difficulty or resistance to his work or ideas from any quarter is reason enough for him to abandon his project. Because the Larch goes into the project convinced that it will fail, he interprets the slightest problem as a sign of worse things ahead—a sign that failure is imminent. And so he simply drops the project and collapses back into himself, perceiving the "failure" as reinforcement of his own inadequacy. As proof that he is as big a failure as he thought he was to begin with.

This is the cycle of the Larch's life, or, better put, the downward spiral. With each turn of the wheel and each new failure that was, in truth, an unnecessary abandonment of his cause, the Larch becomes more and more convinced that he is doomed to failure and more and more likely to fail again in the future.

In truth, the issue with Larch is a matter of proportion. They fail to understand that each of us lives a life that is a mixture of failure and success, and that this is an acceptable part of life for most of us. Most of us try to learn from our failures, and, more important, develop a sense over time of when a project is worth continuing and when it is not. The Larch lacks this ability. They cannot step back from themselves for a moment to objectively judge the amount of work required against the possible reward, and then decide whether or not to continue a project that involves some difficulty.

Because he lacks a sense of proportion and perceives every sort of difficulty—great or small—as the same (which is to say enormous and unsolvable), and because he is stuck in a place of self-consciousness that will not allow for objectivity, the Larch perceives no other way to resolve issues than to quit and run away. In the ongoing battle between fight and flight that controls much of our lives, Larch is locked into the "flight" option. Others, perceiving the Larch as weak, shy, and easily intimidated and put upon, then reinforce his emotional pattern by treating him as if he is indeed inferior and not worthy of respect. And so the cycle continues and is strengthened, both by Larch's own assumptions concerning himself and by the subsequent treatment he receives from others.

This, of course, is the worst case Larch scenario. In most cases, even the constitutional Larch is seen by others as being a very pleasant, friendly, and emotionally open person. They seem, on the surface, to be as capable and able to achieve as anyone else. Indeed, their pleasant demeanor often makes them very popular. Others tend to see them as having not a problem in the world.

This does not mean, however, that this sort of Larch is not beset internally with feelings of self-doubt. While it may not be readily apparent, they are thoroughly convinced that they are just not as good as others. Even Larch types that function well in society must constantly wrestle with feelings of shyness, of fear of what others think of them.

All of us need Larch from time to time in an acute context. This is the remedy to turn to when you are having a moment of self-doubt, when you feel that you cannot possibly succeed with the tasks at hand, when you are called upon to speak in public and feel all but crippled with worry about how you will be perceived. Larch can help with all these issues, and with the times of transition in our lives in which we come, for a time, to doubt ourselves and our abilities. Larch can help each of us judge our own weaknesses and strengths fairly and truthfully and assess our abilities honestly. Further, it can work miracles for those times when we fall prey to self-judgment and self-consciousness. It helps us get out of our own heads and change a subjective viewpoint of the world into an objective one.

I find that Larch, because it is a remedy with a very "fixed" viewpoint, blends particularly well with two of our chestnut remedies: Chestnut Bud and White Chestnut. White Chestnut can help the Larch who is at the point of perceived failure to quit running the struggles of the day through his mind. It can release his obsessive thoughts and help him clear his mind to tackle the real work in an objective manner. Chestnut Bud—which is, in my opinion a greatly underused remedy—is an excellent blend with Larch, particularly for those who, in middle age, find themselves at a dead end in their career, and who must reinvent themselves in terms of their skills and work persona to find a new career path or succeed in their current path.

Larch also combines well with Wild Oat for those patients who tend to collapse inward in times of perceived failure. They tend to have no idea at all of where to go from here when they feel they have failed. Instead, they want to hide, to curl up on the couch and watch TV. Wild Oat will help the patient discover his path and passion while Larch helps him develop the inner strength to move forward with his life.

Finally, consider Walnut to mix with Larch for patients who combine self-consciousness with a willingness to listen to or follow anyone. These patients are quite willing to set aside any sort of goal or vision of their own for one supplied by others.

### Negative Qualities of the Type

Since the Larch trapped in a negative state expects that whatever they attempt will surely fail, they create that reality within their lives. And fail they do. And, having in their own eyes failed often enough, they stop attempting any new thing.

But that is not the end of the story. No matter how many times he has failed, the Larch yearns to accomplish something, to live a life that contains adventure; that attempts what is surprising and new. Although they seem passive in nature, in their core they are yearning to attempt new things, to find ways in which they can come to respect themselves. This creates an uncomfortable dynamic for the patient. The negative Larch has deep and uncomfortable feelings of helplessness and impotence that are coupled with equally deep yearnings for accomplishment. They struggle to overcome their shyness and their negative emotional state, but because they cannot jump the hurdle of the stresses of accomplishment, because they cannot perceive what lies beyond the mountain of difficulty before them, they give up again and again, and fall back into failure.

It is not that the Larch is unintelligent or untalented. It is simply that he is locked into a prison of self-consciousness that blocks him from the accomplishments he craves.

Thus the Larch must be considered as self-defeating, in that he has not been dealt any more challenges than the rest of us. But because the Larch perceives himself as inferior, he also considers his efforts as second-rate at best and abandons them when faced with challenges.

The Larch must first open his eyes to the world around him and the other people in it. He must come to see that he has been dealt a hand that mixes strength and weakness, success and failure, just like the rest of us, and that he is no better or worse than anyone else. And then he must fight his way through one series of challenges toward one set of goals. In winning one race, he can learn to pace himself for the rest.

## Positive Qualities of the Type

Positive Larches are the world's leading realists. They have a true understanding of who they are and where their talents lie. They know what they can and cannot do. Further, they have a realistic notion of what can be accomplished by an organization, society, or culture. They teach the valuable lesson of perseverance and show that, if you never give up, you can accomplish great things. We need those with a positive Larch outlook in our society to help us understand the realistic possibilities of our present time as well as our future.

On a personal level, the Larch's innate shyness becomes true modesty when it is placed within a positive emotional state. This is the person that others can turn to for support and wise counsel when they themselves are not sure whether or not they are up to the tasks at hand. The positive Larch is never one to overstate or to boast. Instead, he will give clear-sighted opinions about the path ahead, both for himself and for others. The once timid Larch who has moved from the negative to the positive emotional state will be amazed to find that he is perceived as a tower of strength by others.

## The Larch Child

This is one of the remedy types that tend to develop in early childhood. Therefore, you will find many young people needing this remedy. Young people who have somehow, early on, taken in a message that they are not good enough, smart enough, strong enough, or pretty enough. This message has been taken to heart and it motivates the actions—or, more correctly, the lack of actions—on the part of the young Larch.

This is the child who may have done his homework, yet will not raise his hand in class because he feels he risks humiliation by giving what he is sure will be a wrong answer. As a result, he tries to make himself invisible in the classroom. Sports, public speaking, and, especially, any form of public competition—are all a form of torture for the Larch child. They tend to see gym class as what Jerry Seinfeld once called a "Lord of the Flies" experience. They take any parental encouragement to attempt competition as a form of punishment, because they feel as if their parents are exposing them to failure and humiliation.

In young people, Larch combines especially well with two of our fear remedies: Mimulus and Aspen. The Larch/Mimulus is a great combination for children whose fears and limitations are known by all—fear of sports, for instance, or tests in school. The Larch/Aspen child is one who experiences anxiety along with his lack of self confidence, who may have panic attacks the night before tests or other public activities.

### The Larch Adult

The Larch adult needs to learn the lesson that there is no shame in failure, and that we stand to learn more from our failures than from our successes. Also, that failure is most often an individual concept. That when we set our standards too high, we can never see ourselves as successful. And what we ourselves may perceive as a failure others may see as a qualified or complete success. The fact that Larch locks in on certain failure often makes him overlook the good that has actually come out of his struggle.

The Larch needs to confront his very real feelings of inferiority and, with the help of this remedy, work through them to a more balanced view. They usually need other forms of support, from public speaking classes to therapy, to assist them on their way.

### The Larch Animal

While it is impossible to know whether your dog or cat has an inferiority complex, it is still possible to use the remedy Larch with some success for an animal patient. There are, after all, shy and/or timid animals—the dogs that have to be coaxed to come, the cats that hide behind the couch. Larch can work wonders for shy animals, and blends particularly well with Aspen for the animal that seems ill at ease, especially in a new home. The remedy is also useful for show animals that seem ill at ease in public.

### Larch and the Homeopathic Pharmacy

In terms of homeopathic remedies, it is easy to find the parallel to Larch. The remedy Lycopodium most closely resembles Larch's psychological situation. Like Larch, Lycopodium feels inferior and is beset with issues of self-confidence. Lycopodium patients may also collapse into an inert state, convinced that whatever they attempt is doomed to fail. But they are more likely to use their inferior state and their feelings of overcompensation to fuel their way to success. With each success, Lycopodium patients can, for a moment, forget their feelings of inferiority, only to have them return soon. Like Larch, Lycopodium's life is a balancing act between the desired result and the tendency to quit when times get rough. Both have deep feelings of inadequacy, and both use these feelings to color and control their experience of life.

### Issues that Suggest Larch

Acne; allergies; athlete's foot; arthritis; bleeding gums; career issues; digestive problems; father issues; fatigue; procrastination; rejection; sexual dysfunction and sexual shame; shyness; spine malformations and pain.

### In Conclusion

Bach wrote that all of his remedies were universal, which is to say that all of us will need every remedy at one time or another in our lives. And while the true Larch type, who is locked in a state of self-consciousness and failure, is somewhat rare, each of us will have a need for this remedy in our lives from time to time. Indeed, I consider it to be one of the most important remedies for the crisis of middle age—for the moment in life when we realize that we are not likely to win an Academy Award or a Nobel Prize and we wrestle with feelings of failure and question whether all our struggles have been worth it. For this and other moments of crisis in self-confidence, we should turn to Larch, which gives us a clear head and clear eyes to see our lives and ourselves as we really are. Larch lets us accept and even possibly rejoice in what we are and with what we *have* accomplished.

## ELM · THE REMEDY FOR THOSE WHO ARE OVERWHELMED

Bach writes that the Elm type are "those who are doing good work, are following the calling of their life and who hope to do something of importance, and this often for the benefit of humanity. At times there may be periods of depression when they feel that the task they have undertaken is too difficult, and not within the power of a human being."

• **While Elm can be helpful in acute situations, it is far more useful as a constitutional remedy.**

### Botanical Information

The remedy Elm (*Ulmus Procera*) is taken from the English Elm tree, which is known for its shady cover. It can grow to more than 100 feet tall. There are nearly forty different species of Elm and the tree is known for its easy hybridization. It is grown throughout all the temperate regions of the Northern Hemisphere.

It should be noted that more than twelve million elm trees have died since 1967, the year in which Dutch elm disease reached Great Britain. This same disease has devastated nearly all the species of the Elm and has killed millions of trees worldwide.

### Elm in General

On the surface, Elm would seem to be perhaps the only Bach remedy that can be discussed in terms of its positive traits. After all, Elm people are fair. They are hard workers. They are the salt of the earth. They are the people to whom others bring their troubles and depend on for support. And that's fine with the Elm. They like to be depended upon, to be thought of as "go to" people. Elm likes to be needed and is happy to help out.

But the story does not stop there.

Typically, the Elm type is motivated by two driving forces: responsibility and ambition. For some Elms, one force may dominate over the other, but all Elms have some blend of each. And although this remedy may be of use for most of us from time to time when our responsibilities become too much for us and we get overwhelmed, Elm is predominately a "type" or constitutional remedy that speaks to a behavioral pattern or personality trait that is deeply engrained and not quickly or easily brought back into balance.

The Elm takes all the responsibilities that life has given him very seriously. If the Elm is married and has children, he or she will become even more determined that they will see to it personally that every member of his or her family is well provided for—even if he or she has to sacrifice the relationship with those loved ones in working to raise the money for that purpose.

But Elm is also ambitious. It is common to the type that Elms suffer from too much ambition, a drive not only to achieve, but also to acquire. They tend to be people for whom the riddle of what they want to do in life has already been answered. They know their life's work, and are already busy doing it and doing it well. They tend to be decisive, capable, and successful. The problem is that they all too often become victims of their own success.

The Elm type often works himself into exhaustion, and, once exhausted, into a state of depression and despair. Sometimes this exhaustion and despair is the result of some sort of downturn in business or other setback at work. The Elm, as a response, redoubles his efforts at work, dedicating his time and energy to the task at hand. In time, his energy depleted, the Elm falls into a pattern of exhaustion and depression.

When the situation becomes too much for the Elm to handle, he breaks down. Physical illness is the result, along with a temporary lack of interest in his work and responsibilities.[2] This temporary lack of interest may be seen and treated as an acute state.

---

2. Often this exhaustion and depression will bring about a withdrawal of sorts. The Elm will tend to pull into himself and to pull back from everything that adds stress to his life, including the sources of his sense of responsibility—his loved ones.

And this is important: the exhaustion and depression of the Elm are always temporary things, an acute state. The pattern of moving in and out of this state may be a constitutional issue, when you have a workaholic who reaches the point of driving himself or herself into illness through overwork and exhaustion again and again, but the state itself is self-limiting and temporary. This characteristic allows us to differentiate between Elm and some other allied remedies.

Elm can, at times, be rather like Hornbeam, as each tends to feel exhausted. However, Hornbeam's exhaustion is emotional—they have wearied of work they once loved, or they have reached a temporary block in their work—while Elm's exhaustion is not just emotional but physical as well. They have physically worked themselves into exhaustion, and have emotionally reached the point at which they feel they simply cannot continue and are ready to give up.

This physical component is important to understanding the type, and because of it, Elm can be very similar to Olive. Olive is also exhausted, worn out. They, too, are physically depleted. But, remember, Elm's exhaustion is temporary. They are just in a moment in which they feel overwhelmed and overburdened by responsibilities they usually enjoy, that they themselves have selected for their life. Olive, on the other hand, is truly and completely exhausted. They have fully depleted their life energy and need to not only recharge, but fully recover. Theirs is not an acute state, a momentary weakness, but a life-defining change if left untreated.

Finally, it is important to differentiate between Oak and Elm. Both of these types tend toward over-responsibility. But, remember, this is a state that is usually harmonious for the Elm. They like their responsibilities and have a great deal of natural ambition that drives them forward. Therefore, the Elm is motivated from within. They choose to work hard, choose their life's work, and choose to push forward as best they can. The Oak, on the other hand, adds tremendous will into the mix, and takes on external responsibilities to mix with his own. What you have with an Oak, if you will, is an Elm who has moved up and on to the next level of unhealthy behavior. The Oak has become rigid in his thoughts and actions, incapable of changing his methods or goals once they are locked in place. As a result, the price he pays for his work ethic is even greater than the Elm's. The Elm finds himself on the edge of illness through stress and overwork, but the Oak goes over that edge and still pushes onward.

> It is important for the Elm to understand that, unless he actually learns to balance the needs of self with the needs of others, he will come to the point of breakdown again and again.

So the difference here is often one of degree, and of age. Elm is the remedy of the young buck, the up-and-coming worker. Oak is the remedy of the older, driven worker: the one who, if left untreated, will work until his heart stops from his efforts.

It is important for the Elm to understand that, unless he or she actually learns to balance the needs of self with the needs of others, they will come to the point of break-down again and again. And, in time, he may well move into other negative states—typically Willow, which blends negativity, bitterness, and despair, or Oak, which breaks where the Elm bends low.

Most of us need the remedy Elm only in passing, during those moments of life in which everything just seems too much to bear, when we are overwhelmed by every-thing that needs to get done by Friday. A dose or two of the remedy and we feel ready to get up in the morning and work a bit harder and a bit smarter to put things right once more.

But the person who has become an Elm type has lost sight of the fact that they don't have to keep repeating the pattern of success and near failure over and over again if they get enough sleep, if they are a bit more creative, or if they know when to say that they can't meet a particular deadline. They also tend to lose sight of the cost of their behavior on those they love. Often the Elm is very puzzled to find that his wife and children are actually hostile to him because he works nights and weekends when they would prefer to spend time with him. And the Elm has also, of course, lost sight of the physical and emotional cost of his pattern of actions to himself. Elm must learn to pace himself, to reward himself with rest, with proper food breaks, and with a reasonable workday. Many Elms, as they get older, are shocked to learn one day that their bodies simply cannot withstand the treatment they have received over the years, and that they have actually done physical damage by neglecting their own physical and emo-tional needs.

Where other remedy types may seem to be forever young and childlike, or prema-turely elderly, the Elm seems locked into a mindset of young adulthood. Thus many forty-year-old Elms carry with them the idea that they are twenty-five and capable of missing a night's sleep or an evening meal. They are shocked when they, usually during a health crisis brought on through overwork, suddenly have to deal with the physical reality of their lives.

### Negative Qualities of the Type

So many other types have such easily apparent negative qualities. Some are bossy, telling everyone what to do and how to do it. Others are bitter and evil. And others are filled with rage. But look at an Elm and what do you see? Someone who takes his life's work and life's responsibilities seriously. Someone who works hard. Someone who cares about the quality of his work and achievements.

So, on the surface, it would appear that Elm has no negative qualities. But you have to look a little deeper than the surface to understand the negatives that underlie the praiseworthy positives.

Elm types do not take enough time for themselves. They do not bother to tend to their own needs or wants, as they put their responsibilities in the place of their needs. And they must learn the lesson that, if they work too hard and never balance the stresses of work with everything else that life provides, they will, in time, stop working altogether. It is better to balance life with work and rest and work for a lifetime, than to work without ceasing until undone by exhaustion and then not work at all.

The negative Elm seemingly cannot control himself. His ambition pushes him to try a bit harder, risk a bit more. And the more he risks, the more stress he places upon himself. And, let's be honest, in moments of stress the Elm can be very difficult to be around. In their time of despair, they tend to act out, to be overly blunt to the point of cruelty. Worst of all, the negative Elm tends to expect all those around him to be able to read his mind and realize that his present behavior is a result of stress and that "he's not himself."

As the Elm pushes himself right to the edge of the cliff again and again only to act out his exhaustion drama and "not be himself" each time, he will find that those around him become increasingly weary of acting as support systems and mind readers and less and less willing to supply him with excuses.

After all, unlike the Oak, the Elm has no intention of going over the cliff. (This is not to say that some don't accidentally fall over, to their own great surprise.) But they have a drive that impels them to go right up to the edge and to push themselves to the limit. This remedy can help change that pattern. It can help the Elm learn that he or she actually will accomplish so much more by working for the long term and not, as they are accustomed, from crisis to crisis.

## Positive Qualities of the Type

There's almost nothing but positive qualities about Elm. Elm types are those we want for our parents and our children, for our wives and our husbands, and, perhaps most especially, for our bosses. They are fair, honest, and hard working.

What more could you want?

In treating an Elm, we are really just trying to tweak their behavior patterns a bit. To get them to rein themselves in just a bit. To help them learn their limits and their strengths. In treating an Elm, you are trying to turn a sprinter into a long-distance runner.

When an Elm is in a positive emotional state, no one is more capable, more balanced, and more direct in his or her efforts. The positive Elm mixes passion and compassion, love for others and love for self. They learn to balance that which once caused them a great deal of stress: the needs of those they love and the needs of the workplace. In learning this, their ambition turns to the best possible result, as shaping the lives of their children becomes as important as empire building.

### The Elm Child

Many parents dream of such a child. They keep their room clean, and they are willing to do their part for you as well: doing the laundry, setting the table.

Further, these are confident children, solid and strong. But they can lose confidence and strength through overwork, through taking on too much. Parents must resist the teacher's idea that they be moved to a higher class or take part in too many activities. Parents would do well to praise such a child and teach them that they need not accomplish all things to earn love.

While other children may need their parent's help to find and prepare for their path in life, the Elm child comes with this software already loaded. They will, at a very young age, determine the sort of work that they want to do and begin training for it. In these cases, it becomes the parents work to help train the child to develop talents in all aspects of life—the social as well as the career aspects. It is also important that the child learn how to go about accomplishing their desires in a way that does not involve an ongoing series of crises revolving around the attaining and conquering of goals.

### The Elm Adult

A healthy Elm wishes good things for everyone and is willing to work to bring these things about. They are strong enough people to be true servants of humanity. But, when Elm begins to move into a negative state, they can become perfectionists, taking on more and more, trying to accomplish much more than they need to or are reasonably able to. They become overwhelmed and despondent, and must rest to recharge their energy. As their negative state increases, they must spend more and more time recharging. In this way, they move from the Elm pattern into the deeper Oak or Willow patterns, which carry with them the same despair as Elm, but in a far more long-lasting manner.

### The Elm Animal

While this remedy is not often used in the treatment of animals, consider it when an animal has been ill for a long time and is struggling through a slow recovery. In this situation, blend Elm with Gorse for best results.

### Elm and the Homeopathic Pharmacy

The homeopathic remedy most similar to Elm is Calcarea Carbonica. The Calcarea type is the worker bee. They come to work early and work late. They take responsibility for their own work, and are only too willing to help others as well. Like Elm, Calcarea types can threaten their own health through overwork.

### Issues that Suggest Elm

Anxiety attacks; co-dependent behavior; chronic fatigue syndrome; depression; exhaustion; midlife crisis; nervous collapse; stress and stress-related illness; sudden acute illnesses of all sorts.

### In Conclusion

Elm types, with their respect for work and responsibility, would likely distain gambling. And yet they tend to gamble continually with their own strength and energy. Instead of working within the limits imposed upon them by life and working for long-term achievement, they seize upon a short-term result and turn it into a crisis that requires all their strength and wit—to say nothing of their family's patience—to resolve. And the Elm type repeats this cycle again and again, feeling the strain of the crisis and the wonderful release of its successful skin-of-your-teeth resolution.

We all have experienced Elm's state of being over stressed and overwhelmed in our own lives. When the desk's a mess and the work's piled up and there seems no way that things can come out right. For these moments, Elm is the remedy that can bring things back into balance.

## OAK · THE REMEDY FOR THOSE WHO ARE DRIVEN

Bach writes, "Oak is for those who are struggling and fighting strongly to get well, or in connection with the affairs of their daily life. They will go on trying one thing after another, though their case may seem hopeless. They will fight on. They are discontented with themselves if illness interferes with their duties or helping others. They are brave people, fighting against great difficulties, without loss of hope or effort."

• **Oak is very seldom an acute remedy. Its great strength in the Bach pharmacy is as a constitutional or "type" remedy.**

### Botanical Information

The "Common Oak" (*Quercus Robur*) or "British Oak" can live for an astonishing 1,000 years or more. It can live in virtually any kind of soil, even thriving next to the sea in soil that is saturated with salt. Oaks are among the most common trees on Earth, and are often found in mixed woodlands. They are native to the Northern Hemisphere including England and Ireland and can be found throughout Western Europe and Asia Minor.

### Oak in General

When dealing with the Oak type, you are dealing with a person who can be described in a few words: rigid, willful, uncompromising, and, perhaps, obsessive. Because of this, Oak is similar to a handful of other remedies, all of which strictly adhere to a specific approach to life. There is Crab Apple, who demands perfection, both from himself and from all those around him. There is Rock Water, who shares the Oak sense of responsibility, but who has become martyred in her lifestyle and joyless in her approach to life. And there is Elm, who shares much of the Oak drive and ambition, but who instills life with more drama than does the Oak, and who still enjoys periods of rest between crises. All of these remedies, as well as bitter Willow, compulsive Vervain, and the bullying Vine have themes that are somewhat similar to Oak's, and all blend well with this remedy.

What these remedies all share is "yang" energy. Each is willful, using the force of their will to exert influence upon others. Each, therefore, might be said to have an overabundance of male energy, and all need to learn to balance their dominance with a sense of calm.

On to Oak.

Like Elm (and I suggest you read both of these remedies to make the best choice between them), Oak may be discussed in terms of some very positive traits. These are, after all, the people in our communities about whom we might say, "This is the one person we can rely on!" Like oak trees, Oak people stand tall and strong, with roots running deep into the community. Like Elm, they are strong silent types, doing their work with a minimum of fuss and a maximum of care. They seem almost regal in their bearing, with good manners and strong "family values." They are the people we pattern ourselves after, or the ones we take for granted, who pay our bills without acknowledgment or thanks.

Oak and Elm are alike in that both are work centered. Both have a need to be needed and a great desire to accomplish something in the world. Both like to be noticed for their work and expect to receive the rewards due them.

Oak is unlike Elm, however, in that Elm feels that their work is their calling, and any exhaustion they might feel is only temporary. Oaks see work as duty, and are quite willing to keep working even if their work brings them no joy and precious few results. Exhaustion and a sense of being overwhelmed is a momentary thing for Elm, part of their crisis-to-crisis life cycle. Exhaustion is chronic in the Oak. And Oaks reveal their compulsive nature in their willingness to work to the point of exhaustion and beyond.

Oak is the remedy for those who are truly driven. It is needed for those who have reached a negative emotional state in which they have quite literally perverted their natural positive traits of strong will, clear vision, and willingness to work into a state in which these positives have become warped and negative. The Oak is rigid in his demands, both of those around him and, especially, of himself. This is the man who will be the first to arrive at the office every day and the last to leave at night, and who, in all honesty, does not understand why others expect to be able to leave in time to have dinner with their children. To the Oak, this sort of behavior reveals a lack of dedication to the task at hand.

Another thing that the Oak cannot abide is a complainer. Oak is a stoic. He will plod along, working, working, working, but he will never complain. The aches and pains of the body, the inconveniences of letting your family and friends down as you dedicate yourself to work, are part and parcel of achievement to the Oak. They should be expected and accepted without complaint. The coworker or family member who complains reveals himself or herself as not being a team player.

Oak, again like Rock Water, Willow, and Crab Apple, tends to be humorless, joyless. For him, there are rules about how work should be done and how the workplace should be inhabited.

This brings up another point about Oak: like Honeysuckle, Oaks tend to be past-oriented. While the goal of their work may point them to the present and the future, Oaks tend to lock onto a mode of grooming and a code of ethics that traps them in the past. They want the twenty-year-old of today to act like a twenty-year-old did in their day. Further, Oaks tend to lock on to a particular way of dressing or wearing their hair from a time of their youth—usually in their early thirties—in which they think they looked particularly well, and to hang onto that look for as many years as possible.

More than other remedy types, it is possible to compare the person needing the remedy Oak with the oak tree itself. Like the oak tree, Oaks are towering, powerful things. Oak trees are, after all, known to be able to thrive in soils and climates in which other trees cannot. In the same way, the Oak's will gives him incredible endurance, and the ability to apparently thrive in situations in which others would collapse.

But, again like the tree, Oaks are rigid creatures. And while the oak is huge and powerful, it is not a tree that bends in the wind. It also can have surprisingly shallow roots given its size. Oak types break and fall in the same way when challenged beyond their capacity because they will not bend.

Because Oak is compulsive in his behavior, he will not even consider bringing balance into his life. The usual outcome of his negative emotional state is that he wears down his health through his willful refusal to consider that he might, at any moment, be unable to keep pushing ahead with his life. The best hope for forestalling an outcome that includes chronic pain or a heart attack is for the Oak to be told in no uncertain terms by a person in authority—and a person he respects—that he must change his ways. A doctor in a white lab coat who tells the Oak he must change his diet, take a vacation, stop smoking, or whatever else is specifically needed in the way of lifestyle modification, might well get the Oak to modify his habits. But it is usually the first heart attack that finally does the trick and gets the Oak to reconsider his life's choices.

The waiting rooms of the world are filled with Oaks, middle-aged and beyond, most of whom—having survived what they will take to calling their "wake-up call"—are finally willing to listen to reason. The golf courses of the world are filled with Oaks who feel that they have been unnecessarily put out to pasture and who still yearn for the years behind their desks.

A better solution is for the Oak to learn his lesson earlier, and realize that yoga is not a silly and unnecessary thing and that humor isn't just a waste of time without having to survive a health crisis first. The remedy Oak can help bring a patient into balance. But, as Oak is almost always a constitutional remedy, it most often needs to be taken in the long term. And it likely will not only need to be blended with other remedies (most often from the list of those mentioned above) but also with other modifiers, such as yoga[3] and other exercises that stretch the Oak out of his natural rigidity.

Unlike most other Bach remedies, Oak has few acute applications. Certainly, it might be helpful in cases where a student is working on a term paper and becomes obsessed with the paper to the exclusion of the rest of his life. But even the "acute" circumstances that Oak speaks to are in reality all rather long term. It is a remedy that can definitely help in times when we are being called upon to work extra hard, to dedicate ourselves to a task. It can help with the stresses of work and help keep us in balance as we see our task to completion. But Oak is not a "momentary" remedy. There is no shocking event that creates an instantaneous Oak result. Instead, Oak is a remedy that slowly reveals itself: it is a life path we settle into, as we surrender the joy and recklessness of youth to the predictable, conservative grind that is Oak.

## Negative Qualities of the Type

Oaks' greatest negative qualities are that they take some very positive traits and make them negative. That they suck all the air out of any room they are in.

Oaks are overly responsible and do not know when to stop. They are plodders, who tend to work slowly and steadily and who cannot be stopped once they have begun a project. They are out of touch with themselves and their own emotional wants and needs. They fear showing any sort of weakness, and, for this reason, they will never complain, never seek help, even after they have reached past the point at which any reasonable person would have stopped, rested, or sought medical treatment.

---

3. Like all well-written television shows, *King of the Hill* gives us a wonderful portrait of an Oak type in the title character Hank Hill. Hank is a middle-aged man who has worked his way up to manager of a propane company through hard work and dogged loyalty, not only to the company but to "Lady Propane" herself. In one episode, Hank is suffering from intense low back pain, a typical Oak complaint, and, after medicine fails him, has to take yoga classes to get help. After much resistance, he finds that not only does he enjoy yoga, but that it also actually helps with his pain. As soon as the pain is gone, however, he quickly (and typically for an Oak) puts the yoga behind him and returns to his old ways.

Oaks' compulsive need to push forward despite the odds may cause them to quite literally work themselves to death. Among the ailments that commonly beset the constitutional Oak type are heart disease, hypertension, and chronic joint pain.

## Positive Qualities of the Type

Oaks see themselves as living the American dream in a strictly American way: with endurance, reliability, steadfastness, strength, honesty, and good old-fashioned common sense. All the things we were taught were good traits, especially in men. And, in truth, Oak has all these qualities. Added to these, Oak is self-sacrificing, even to a fault. He is also responsible and trustworthy. A secret told to an Oak is a secret taken to the grave.

In other words, Oak makes for a very good friend and an even a better neighbor. They may not be the most entertaining or delightful company, but they make for a neighbor who can be trusted, and who likely is very good with his backyard grill.

Oaks make excellent coworkers as well, and even better employees. What boss does not want a worker who is up for any task and who never complains?

In some ways, they are also good spouses. They may be rather demanding when it comes to a clean house and dinner on the table, and they may be rather plodding in relationships, often less than creative when it comes to gifts and romance, but they can be trusted, and their actions can be predicted in most situations.

## The Oak Child

Plainly put, Oak is not a natural state of children. This is a remedy type that tends to be formed over time and is a remedy most commonly needed in middle age. Therefore, the child who needs Oak has been prematurely forced into this state, often as a result of terrible stress. Something has thrown the child's life and its natural rhythms out of balance. This can be a family trauma, like the death or serious illness of a parent, which threatens not only the child's emotional state, but also the financial health of the family. Or it can be a national or global emergency, such as war. The children who lived through our nation's Great Depression were often driven into a premature obsession with security that led into a chronic Oak state.

Oak children tend to be solid children who are seldom sick. When they are sick they ignore the illness to the point of denying it, and just keep on going. In the classroom, they are diligent students who do their homework on time, but with little creative flair. Other children come to depend upon the Oak child, bringing their fears and troubles to him. This child will appear to be positive in his outlook, but needs to learn to be in touch with his needs and emotions early and to have solid boundaries of what is and is not his responsibility. An Oak's parents must guard against feeding into the notion that the child is in many ways capable of parenting his own parents.

### The Oak Adult

I feel that the remedy Oak comes into its full glory in adults. It is especially valuable to those who have lived some life and have experienced ups and downs, wins and losses. Therefore, it is one of our great remedies for middle age and beyond.

The middle-aged Oak is in his or her glory years. As life changes around them, as their children grow up and leave, as their own bodies age and change, Oaks fixate even more on the tasks at hand, ignoring all else. This is the time of life when they are still young enough to ignore their aches and pains, and old enough to have a track record of successes and an ingrained sense of how things should be done. The fact that their children have moved on only allows them one less distraction as they concentrate on their work.

Because of this, the middle-aged Oak is also in his or her danger years. They have reached the time of life when they begin to reap what they have sown in terms of wear and tear on their bodies. This is the time of life when hypertension begins to make its impact on the body. When the joints ache and the teeth crack. Oak will want to ignore it all, of course, and see it as only one more inconvenience, another block in his or her path to be mowed down. And this can have terrible consequences to the Oak.

Remember that Oak is listed among the remedies for Despair. I haven't discussed this aspect of Oak yet, but it is important to understand. Oak can be an excellent remedy for midlife crisis, especially if the crisis is linked with, or brought on by, a health scare. The midlife crisis for the Oak involves two things. First, it involves that terrible moment (and you know it if you have experienced it; if you haven't experienced it yet, you will) when you realize that you yourself are mortal. It usually happens in the middle of the night. It may be brought on by a health crisis or a near-death experience. But the result is the same: while you have witnessed the deaths of others you loved, it somehow hadn't registered that you yourself would one day die, and that you haven't a clue as to what that really means or what happens afterward. Despite any religious beliefs you might have, this moment shakes you to your core.

The second aspect of the crisis is a reexamination of your life so far. This leads to an examination of all your failures: in work, in relationships, in your home, and of all the many mistakes you have made along the way.

The Oak who is moving through these two phases may plunge into a deep depression, into a state of chronic despair. And what is true physically for the Oak is also true emotionally. Because of their rigid nature, they will not bend in a storm; they will, instead, break. So when the Oak moves into midlife crisis, they break, and fall into deep despair.

The remedy Oak can be of great help, of course. It can help moderate this despair, help the Oak come to terms with his life and begin to live his remaining years in a more valuable way. It can help establish flexibility in the place of rigidity.

Oak is also an excellent remedy for the elderly. It can be an excellent aid for those at the point of retirement and for those who have retired. It can help them rethink their life strategies and live at peace with their quieter pace. It can also help elderly patients who feel exhausted, who feel that they have been worn down by life. It can help reignite a spark of life for those who prematurely feel that their life is done.

Two remedies that Oak blends with wonderfully well for those who are in a state of exhaustion and depression are Mustard, our best remedy for those who are depressed, and Olive, which is very helpful for those who are physically and emotionally exhausted. The three remedies together can be a powerful aid to those in need.

## The Oak Animal

This is not a remedy often needed for animals, and therefore it is not necessary in the average household. It can be very useful, however, in a specific set of circumstances. Use Oak for older animals, especially animals that once had a specific work or task central to their lives. Oak can be a valuable tool for animals that are worn down, especially animals that are lame or have arthritis or any other form of joint pain. Oak and Olive make an excellent blend for animals that have reached the last stage of life and are exhausted and when getting through the day has become a burden.

## Oak and the Homeopathic Pharmacy

The homeopathic remedy most similar to Oak is Kali Carbonica, a remedy well known for its conservative values and strong work ethic. Both Kali Carbs and Oaks will literally work themselves into an early grave because they will not, like Elms, take the time to rest, but will keep right on working even when exhausted.

Oak also parallels the remedy Aurum Metallicum, which is made from the metal gold. Both types are work driven, and both are given to deep depression, even suicidal thoughts.

## Issues that Suggest Oak

Anemia; apathy; arthritis; bleeding gums; chronic pain: joint pain, rheumatoid arthritis, or gout; constipation; deafness; fatigue; heart disease; Hodgkin's disease; hypertension; hypoglycemia; kidney problems; neck and/or back pain; pneumonia.

## In Conclusion

Because Oak either involves a negative emotional state that develops slowly over a period of time or is forced upon a patient prematurely by incredible stress, the need for this remedy is never a sudden thing, and it is seldom needed in the short term. The evolution of the Oak type from a negative to a positive emotional state is a slow process as well. Oak blends well with other remedies and I find that it seldom is used on its own.

Most often it is blended with Mustard or Olive in the patient who has been broken by the demands of his life's path, or with Willow, Crab Apple, Elm, Vine, or Vervain, for the Oak who is still in all his majestic glory and is still compulsively pushing ahead through his will and pigheadedness alone.

## CRAB APPLE · THE REMEDY FOR THOSE WHO ARE PERFECTIONISTS

Bach writes, "This is the remedy of cleansing. For those who feel as if they had something not quite clean about themselves. Often it is something of apparently little importance: in others there may be more serious disease which is almost disregarded compared to the one thing on which they concentrate. In both types they are anxious to be free from the one particular thing which is greatest in their minds and which seems so essential to them that it should be cured. They become despondent if treatment fails. Being a cleanser, this remedy purifies wounds if the patient has reason to believe that some poison has entered which must be drawn out."

• **Crab Apple is both an excellent acute remedy and a constitutional remedy of the first order.**

### Botanical Information

The crab apple (*Malus Pumila,* although it may also be referred to as *Malus Sylvestris*) tree is a small or medium-sized deciduous tree that is perhaps the most common fruit tree on Earth. It is thought to be native to Southeastern Europe and Western Asia, although it grows in temperate climates around the globe. Crab apples may be cultivated or grow wild in thickets and woodlands. They have flowers that are pink on the outside and white inside.

### Crab Apples in General

There are two things I want to note about Crab Apple right up front.

First, Crab Apple is different from the other Bach remedies, in that it has a specific use outside the realm of the emotions. As the quote from Bach suggests, Crab Apple also has a purely physical application. It can be used to cleanse the body, just as it can be valuable in balancing compulsive emotional behaviors. Impurity is the key to understanding the action of Crab Apple, and it can be used to purify either the body or the spirit.

This gives Crab Apple an almost allopathic use. Especially in cases of allergies, or with any sort of food poisoning, even for hangovers, Crab Apple acts as a "specific," which is an old homeopathic term for a medicine that can always be used in a given specific situation.

This gives us a knee-jerk use for Crab Apple: it can be used whenever toxins of any sort are suspected, and it can be quite effective. This represents sort of a bastardization of Bach treatments, however, because it totally ignores the all-important emotional state of the patient and simply treats on the physical sphere instead.

In many cases, the physical need for Crab Apple will be mirrored in the emotional sphere as well, and the patient will have those feelings of being unclean and impure that are core issues of the type. I leave it in your hands to decide how best you can use the remedy, and whether you look to the mood of the patient as you would with any other Bach treatment, or consider it to be the hangover cure you have looked for all these many years.

The second important fact about Crab Apple is that, of all the Bach remedies, it is the one I have found again and again that simply cannot be tolerated by everyone (Holly being another, to a lesser degree).

The Bach remedies are, as a group, remarkably benign. They can be given to anyone, taken with or without food or drink, used in combination with virtually any other therapy[4] without aggravation, and certainly without harm.

Crab Apple is the exception to this. I have found that it can create aggravations in some people, especially in highly sensitive people or people with many allergies. Crab Apple can be a very hard remedy for them, one that stirs up a great deal and aggravates the situation at hand. For this reason, I always suggest that you try Crab Apple on its own for a day or two before blending it with other remedies. That way, you can be sure of the impact of Crab Apple first, and not be left wondering why your blend of remedies created such a negative result.

Purity—the search for perfect purity—is the central issue for all Crab Apples. This can be manifested in several ways.

Most commonly, Crab Apples tend to attempt to find purity through either cleanliness or organization. On a physical level, they seek perfection by being sure that both they and their environment are completely clean. This usually includes being sure that they are pure in their personal habits as well. Most Crab Apples are careful eaters. Most avoid alcohol and other toxins, like drugs, both because they disapprove of anything

---

4. Let me be very clear about this: In my opinion, Bach remedies can be given safely to anyone who is taking an allopathic medicine or any herbal remedy or supplement. This does not mean that, as medicinal substances, they should be taken without the knowledge of your physician. They should not. You should always discuss taking any form of medicine, over the counter or not, with your physician before taking it. Also, while Bach remedies are perfectly safe to take with most forms of allopathic medicine, they do not blend well with "energy medicines." Therefore, I would never mix Bach remedies with homeopathic medicines or cell salts. Nor would I mix Bach remedies with acupuncture. Since Bach remedies are, in a way, a form of energy medicine, in that they are homeopathic in their nature, they do not blend well with these treatments.

that is less than pure, and because their systems tend to be more sensitive to toxic substances.

So the first movement for Crab Apples is toward cleanliness. Once things are clean, they also want all elements of their environment—personal and professional—to be completely organized. Crab Apples have an actual emotional need for order. Things that are well organized are perceived as beautiful to them.

Crab Apples also yearn for purity on an emotional and metaphorical level. This means they seek to clean and organize not only their physical and personal environment, but their spiritual environment and being as well. Crab Apples seek to be moral in all things. They will try to organize their own thoughts and emotions to guard against any taint of thought or action.

Crab Apple's ongoing struggle toward perfection creates havoc for him, both within his own being and within his work and home environment.

Few other remedy types—and, here again, we are dealing with a remedy that is far more often needed in constitutional cases than in simple acute circumstances—have as much difficulty in dealing with or working with others as do Crab Apples. Like Rock Waters, Crab Apples tend to be locked into their way of thinking and performing tasks. They tend to become convinced that their way is not only the best way, but is also the only way to proceed. This creates friction between Crab Apples and others, especially others for whom perfection is not a constant goal.

This friction can be very uncomfortable for Crab Apples, as they tend to be rather passive types. They want to please, because any discord with others is perceived, once more, as less-than-perfect behavior on their part, and, therefore, as a personal failure. The Crab Apple negative emotional state is most often shaped in childhood, when the child of overbearing parents receives a message that he or she can never be good enough, perfect enough. Once this state is established it can last a lifetime, as the Crab Apple constantly attempts to attain a state of perfection that can never be reached.

Because Crab Apples tend to judge themselves far more harshly than they do others, they tend to have difficulty expressing the judgment that they feel for others—especially for those for whom chaos and filth are the natural shape of things. Crab Apples, therefore, can best be described as having a devil on one shoulder and an angel on the other. Try as they might to ignore or remove the devil, he stays on their shoulder, whispering in their ear. The Crab Apples' continual struggle is toward perfection, away from their own flawed human natures.

The ongoing problem is that Crab Apples display compulsive behavior patterns. They feel unclean and disgusted with themselves. They feel they are not and can never be good enough or clean enough. They cannot bear their face in the mirror, and so they look only at their nose, or lips, or eyes—again focusing on details when the whole is too difficult to bear. This becomes their pattern in life: never seeing the whole picture, always focusing on the details alone. Thus their lives become more and more controlled by details and by obsessive patterns of dealing with the details.

In a negative state, Crab Apples can develop rituals by which they accomplish the tasks of their days. They may count things—steps, the number of digits in a phone number, words in a sentence. They may lock in on the idea that specific tasks must always be performed in a specific order. These are Crab Apples at their most compulsive. Left untreated, Crab Apples' lives can be taken over by ritualized behaviors.

This negative state can also lead Crab Apples to become obsessed with cleanliness and an ongoing war on filth. They can become constant cleaners and the fussiest of people. They can be terrors as customers, in that they demand the same perfection from employees and service providers that they do of themselves. Pity the poor waiter who brings a dirty knife to a Crab Apple.

Crab Apples may also typically focus on their own personal health as part of their obsession with perfection. Even if they are in a state of good health, Crab Apples will exhaust a good bit of energy in staying healthy. And, if they feel that their health is threatened in any way—and this may be a core fear for many Crab Apples—they will take extreme action to restore and maintain health. And as they do with other service providers, Crab Apples will expect much from their medical personnel, and may attempt to control the nature and pattern of their health care.

In the acute sphere, Crab Apple can be a helpful remedy for situations in which physical cleansing is needed. It will detoxify the body and can be particularly helpful for all sorts of skin conditions and infections. It can be very helpful for cases of chronic inflammation.

Emotionally, consider this remedy when you are feeling a bit fussy, when you feel displeased with yourself and with everyone else. When there seems no pleasing you. In these moments, Crab Apple will set things right.

## Negative Qualities of the Type

Crab Apple, when in a negative state, will be controlled by small things: details, germs, dust motes. And because they themselves are controlled by minutiae they will seek to control all aspects of their environment. They micromanage their own lives and the lives of all around them. They will seek to control the small things because they feel their life overall is out of control. So you will see them cleaning, straightening, and controlling, all in an attempt to feel better about themselves.

Crab Apples in a negative state will be equally controlling in the emotional context. They feel they are sinful, dirty, ugly, or unclean. Some may feel as if they have committed some sin for which they can never be forgiven, no matter how hard they struggle. They may turn to religion and seek redemption from God, or may humanize the struggle within themselves.

This is not to say that Crab Apple's dilemma is not a universal one, that we don't all wish to improve ourselves, or even wish to be forgiven or perfected. But Crab Apple's move toward perfection is done in denial of self, and his or her real, human needs. Instead of the natural evolutionary process that we all, hopefully, experience as we live our lives, learn our lessons, and grow older, Crab Apple's reach toward perfection is punishing—a controlling and humorless thing. It is done in denial of the reality of self and life and thus becomes meaningless. That is the great irony of the Crab Apple struggle. Although the Crab Apple attempts, through personal struggle, to become perfect, the rituals that he uses to move him toward perfection are utterly devoid of meaning and therefore can get him nowhere. Remember, the Crab Apple's need for perfection and order is not a noble quest. It is, instead, a compulsion that controls his life and keeps him from truly living.

Three remedies commonly combine with Crab Apple. The first is Rock Water. Since both of these remedy types tend to be very rigid in their behaviors and locked in to their mindsets, the combination of the two can be a powerful tool in cases where the patient combines the strict discipline of the Rock Water with the perfectionism of Crab Apple.

For patients tormented by thoughts of their many failures, or tortured by the notion that they are tainted and can never be forgiven, mix White Chestnut with Crab Apple.

Finally, for the patient who, as a response to his need for perfection, totally withdraws either emotionally or physically from others, combine Water Violet with Crab Apple. People who are germ phobic can be helped by this mixture.

### Positive Qualities of the Type

When Crab Apple is in its positive state, it has the wonderful ability to improve all things, to see the flaws in the details and help organize and change them for the better without emotional turmoil or upset. Positive Crab Apple is able to balance the detail with the overall picture, and is able to deal with the fact that the world is not perfect with calm understanding.

### The Crab Apple Child

Children who move into Crab Apple behaviors have been wounded. They have taken a message from someone they respected or feared deeply to heart. They have been told they are not good enough, and that message motivates all their behaviors.

Crab Apple children are little adults. They are children who are careful not to make too much noise, not to do anything that may, to most of us, be equated with the actions of a normal child. They are careful not to dirty or stain things. Careful never to break anything. They tend to be excellent students and to excel scholastically.

It is important to note that the Crab Apple's parents have failed in two ways, in giving their child the message that he or she must struggle daily for perfection.

First, they have established a pattern of neurotic and even compulsive behavior that will, if left untreated, hamper their child's ability to live life in a truly free and healthy manner.

Second, they have created a child who will tend not to think for himself or herself. The Crab Apple child has been taught not to question authority, not to struggle against his or her elders, especially teachers and parents. In doing this, they have drained the child of his or her natural will, and his or her ability to make decisions for himself or herself. They have created a person who will not question authority[5] and who will seek to please others above all else.

Parents need to be careful not to instill the idea in children that they are not good enough or cannot satisfy their parents, no matter how hard they try. Children must learn to develop their own expectations, their own goals, and their own moral compass.

One final note: consider Crab Apple for teenagers struggling with feelings of inadequacy, especially for teenaged girls moving toward eating disorders as a means of attaining perfection and controlling one aspect of a life that feels out of control. In these cases, the remedy Larch may blend well with Crab Apple to help establish a sense of self. Or the remedy Rock Water may be called for, when rigid rules of behavior—specifically, eating and dietary behaviors—become compulsive.

### The Crab Apple Adult

If the Crab Apple person has not dealt with their issues by adulthood, look for many physical issues to have risen in response to the emotional state: anorexia and other eating disorders, acne, and allergies are all common, as are migraines and psychosomatic illnesses.

While we as a culture tend to consider the Crab Apple state to be a funny thing, and fill our literature and movies with fussy people and hypochondriacs, the struggle of the Crab Apple is far from funny. These are people who, as they grow older, remove themselves more and more from the realities of life, and replace those realities with rituals that are at once controlling and meaningless.

---

5. This is true in all circumstances, save one. As the Crab Apple moral code is all-important to him, the Crab Apple will need to be able to bring his respect for authority into balance with his own unquestioned moral code. Should his government, for instance, pass a law supporting something that is against the Crab Apple's moral code—a law legalizing abortion, for example—then the Crab Apple will have to wrestle with the issue within himself. Often, the Crab Apple will choose his own moral compass over the authority of his government. This is done, however, with great discomfort and after a period of soul-searching.

## The Crab Apple Animal

I have never found a use for Crab Apple that involves the emotional state of animals. Perhaps a sensitive owner of a cat can see the need for the remedy in a tabby that is struggling toward perfection, but that is beyond my own abilities.

Instead, I suggest that you keep this remedy on hand to use on a purely physical level. It can be very helpful for an animal with diarrhea or any other sort of intestinal disorder. It can also be a great deal of help to animals with chronic or acute skin problems of all sorts, from dandruff to mange to eczema. It is helpful as a cleanser for animals with worms. And it can be very helpful if you have an animal—a dog especially—that seems to attract ticks and fleas.

## Crab Apple and the Homeopathic Pharmacy

No one remedy truly parallels Crab Apple. Arsenicum, in its obsessive patterning, comes close, as does Causticum, with its demands of personal perfection. But the remedy I choose as being closest would be Calendula. Used as a topical remedy, Calendula, made from the Marigold, is a detoxifying remedy and a natural antibiotic. It takes whatever is unclean and purifies it.

## Issues that Suggest Crab Apple

Acne; adolescence; allergies; asthma; cancer; eating disorders; emergencies; immune dysfunction; hay fever; food allergies; menopause; migraines; poisonings, especially food poison; sexual dysfunction.

## In Conclusion

Little has been left unsaid about the Crab Apple, but in closing, it is perhaps important to note again that, like so many other remedies, Crab Apple takes an aspect of human nature. In this case, it is the positive wish to become better than we are, more perfect than we have been, that is perverted into a negative state. Crab Apples are not seeking to become better; they are, instead, demanding that they themselves and others around them become perfect. And that they become perfect right now.

Their method of attaining perfection involves control. Control of thoughts, actions, behaviors, desires. And, especially, control of the details of life. These methods are often expressed in ritual behaviors that are devoid of meaning.

Finally, remember that Bach considered Crab Apple to be a remedy for despair. In their forced march toward perfection, Crab Apples are miserable. And their misery and sense of despair only grows deeper as they continue their march, without rest and without result.

## WILLOW · THE REMEDY FOR THOSE WHO ARE BITTER

According to Bach, Willow is "for those who have suffered adversity or misfortune and find these difficult to accept, without complaint or resentment, as they judge life much by the success it brings. They feel they did not deserve so great a trial; that it was unjust, and they become embittered. They often take less interest and less activity in those things of life which they had previously enjoyed."

- **Willow is both an acute and a constitutional remedy.**

### Botanical Information

The white willow (*Salix Vitellina*, also called *Salix Alba*) grows as male or female trees, both of which produce yellow flowers in May. This particular willow is unique in that its branches turn a bright yellow-orange in the winter, making it particularly appealing in the bleak winter landscape. For this reason, it is often called the "coral embers willow." It is a small tree, one that prefers full sun or light shade to thrive. It needs a great amount of water to do well. The white willow is native to Europe and grows in temperate climates worldwide.

### Willow in General

A heavy weight of negativity lies in the core of the Willow personality. And an air of dissatisfaction, no matter what life brings them. Willows are a heavy burden, both to themselves and to their community. It is not enough for the Willow to have others admit that he or she—the Willow—has been greatly punished by fate. To satisfy the Willow, others must also be willing to give up their own happiness in life. Bitterness is the keyword of the Willow type, and the bitterness and despair of Willow always demands a sacrifice, and the sacrifice must be made by another for the sake of the Willow.

In my opinion, the Willow state is the hardest of all to treat. First, it tends to be a deeply engrained emotional pattern. Second, and more important, I have never yet met a Willow who was willing to admit that his or her negative emotional state was a problem, or who sought any help in moving away from bitterness.

Like Miss Havisham in Dickens' *Great Expectations*, the Willow has, at some point in her life, been injured. She has been betrayed or wronged in some way that has left her

> A key to understanding the Willow state is that they hold themselves blameless in whatever event triggered their bitterness. And as they move forward with their lives, they continue to hold themselves blameless while they blame everyone around them for everything.

scarred. Because of this moment of perceived betrayal,[6] the Willow is first shocked, and then, as time unfolds, moves into an emotional state in which she blames the world, or some specific aspects of it, for her plight.

What can make the Willow especially difficult to deal with is the fact that his injury is, on some level, quite real. The state may have been created in a childhood in which the Willow was physically or emotionally abused, or in an abusive marriage. Something has actually happened to the Willow for which he was blameless, and that event now colors every aspect of the Willow's life. And, if the Willow is permitted, it will color the lives of everyone around him.

A key to understanding the Willow state is that these people hold themselves blameless in whatever event triggered their bitterness or thirst for revenge. And as they move forward with their lives, they continue to hold themselves blameless while they blame everyone around them for anything and everything that happens. In essence, they hold everyone in their lives hostage, forcing them to apologize on a continual basis for everything that goes wrong in the Willow's life.

Willow tends to be an active and "yang" type. They send their life energy out and crowd out other people's own energy and personal space with their own. They tend to have rather mean mouths, and are quite capable of saying hurtful, even vengeful things on a regular basis. In the same way, they are quite capable of taking action specifically intended to bring harm to another. When they injure another, as they believe that they themselves have been injured, you will often see a look on their faces that expresses a simple thought: "Now you know how it feels."

Given all this, it is obviously difficult to have to deal with or treat Willows. They tend to fight change and to be totally unwilling to give up their "red badge of courage," the emotional wound that is the source of their personal power and their despair. Because Willows are powerful, everyone tends to yield to their wants and needs, simply because it is far easier than risking an outburst of anger or an act of "getting even."

But, sadly, as is so often the case, Willows undermine their own happiness with the emotional state that was developed with the hope of creating happiness. After all, Willows yearn for happiness above all else. They want to return to the moment before the betrayal, to the time of trust, pleasure, and hope. But their drive toward happiness has been warped by bitterness. So they continue to hope for and seek happiness, all the

---

6. The key idea is that the Willow has experienced a "perceived" betrayal. The emotional wound may not have been an actual or intentional betrayal—it may, for example involve the death of a loved one that has left the Willow feeling deserted, even as he or she realizes on a rational level that the loved one did not want or intend to leave. The emotional wound, irrational as it may be, still festers. In other cases, like poor old Miss Havisham, the Willow has been humiliated, injured, or wounded in some way by someone they loved, respected, or trusted. This wound keeps them from trusting again, and, quite often, becomes the wellspring of destructive or petty behavior.

while acting in a manner that all but guarantees that no one, least of all themselves, will be allowed even the briefest glimmer of joy.

Along with happiness, Willow also seeks justice. In the mind of the Willow, it is very simple. Something happened—some setback, some failure, some betrayal—that has taken the scales of justice and thrown them out of balance. In his own mind, the Willow is just trying to bring the scales back into balance. The problem is that nothing ever quite manages to do this. The Willow takes action, he speaks up, and yet the scales never seem to move. Ultimately, the Willow will come to understand that it will take a lifetime of work to set the scales in balance. In the meantime everything else will fall by the wayside: relationships, career, amusements or joy of all sorts.

Some Willows will take up a specific cause, often a political or religious cause, and focus laserlike upon it as the means by which the scales can be balanced. They will work tirelessly for their cause and will perceive every small setback as another betrayal, as another log on the fire of their rage.

Just as Willows tend to find themselves blameless in all things and to blame others, they also tend to find themselves right on all occasions and to assume that others are, therefore, wrong. Willows cannot bear to have others disagree with them, especially in public. And worse, they cannot bear to have anyone else point out their faults, even though they spend a good deal of their time telling everyone else their myriad failings.

As is common to the remedies in the "Despair" mood, Willow is emotionally rigid, and this rigidity masks an underlying fragility. Willows perceive themselves as being rather weak, as just barely able to work through their day, but others tend to see them as gigantic, as a powerhouse of negative energy, and certainly as people who should never be crossed. But to feel compassion for Willow—who is in what is really the most negative and difficult of all emotional states—we must remember that this is a remedy for Despair. And Willows do feel terrible sorrow and despair, no matter how they act. Inside them is the memory of that calm and vulnerable person they once were. And Willow wishes nothing more than to be that person once more.

Obviously, Willow is a deep constitutional remedy needed in many doses to help the patient back into a state of emotional balance. It is also a remedy that will likely have to be used in combination with several others over time. Willow tends to be what I think of as a "tent pole" remedy. Those who need this remedy may always need it to keep from falling back into their old patterns. While the other remedies in their personal mixture may change over time, Willow—like the obsessive Chestnut remedies—will be needed in the long term.

In cases that involve a Willow type who obsesses over his or her injuries, combine Willow with White Chestnut to create a wonderful result. It also is very commonly combined with Mustard for cases in which the Willow negativity leads to deep depression. And consider Willow mixed with Water Violet when the bitter Willow withdraws from the world and from relationships, or for cases in which the Willow negativity is a result of physical illness that restricts freedom of movement and the patient's ability to carry on a normal life.

Willow does have some acute uses as well. Think of this remedy for any little slight that seems to have grown in your imagination or memory. For those disappointments and setbacks that loom large. Willow will help you absorb the harm on the emotional plane and release it to move on with your life. Again, combine Willow with White Chestnut for those nights when you toss and turn and think about "What I should have said," after you have been humiliated or wronged. The two remedies will help you put your mind on the future and to release the injury before it festers.

## Negative Qualities of the Type

This most destructive of types is known first and foremost for bitterness. They take every kind thought and action and twist it into something negative and damaging. At their worst, they can be emotional black holes, taking whatever they can from anyone wishing to help them, giving nothing in return. And this is an important note: Willow projects a powerful persona, but like a black hole, they pull everything into themselves. They may dominate every conversation in which they take part, and may seem at times to be issuing lightning bolts from their fingertips, but, at the same time, they drain others of energy, and of any other resource they can get their hands on. They will take advantage of any perceived weakness in others to benefit themselves. Like any injured person, Willows want to be paid attention to, and waited upon. In this way, they tend to "use up" relationships. Others find themselves exhausted by any contact with the Willow. And they will, eventually, begin to wonder why they feel guilty for things they haven't done, or why they have to do penance for another's crimes. In time, those others will want to have less and less to do with the Willow, even if that Willow is their own mother. Having had to tread lightly for so many years, the others will, one day, tend to sneak away once and for all.

And Willows, who are very sensitive to the issue of betrayal, will sense the withdrawal and add it to their overwhelming weight of sorrow and negativity, and will move further into despair and grief. Once more, the happiness yearned for has been denied and the Willow is, once more, alone.

In short, in their negative state, Willows refuse to see their own negativity or to take responsibility for the unhappiness they create. Worse, they may even take perverse pleasure in the unhappiness they cause and the damage they leave in their wake.

## Positive Qualities of the Type

It seems impossible that we could consider the positive qualities of this most negative of remedy types, but, once transformation takes place, Willows become able to take responsibility for the fact that they and they alone have created their situation in life, even if they were blameless for the original betrayal that set up their emotional dynamic. At this point, they can begin to create a new life for themselves. In other words, Willow will cease to be a victim of fate and will instead be the creator of his or her own life.

At this point, the Willow can actually demonstrate some wonderful positive attributes.

The positive Willow understands that life has ups and downs for all of us, that everyone receives emotional wounds along the way, that we have all blamelessly received injury along the way. They are, when in a positive emotional state, not only able to balance the ups and downs, but to help others do so as well.

And when in balance, Willows can, at long last, achieve the happiness they long sought. They are finally able to let go of old hurts, not to return to an emotionally naïve state, but to move on to a state of wisdom that understands the negative, but stresses the positive.

It is a riddle of the Bach remedies that those who are at first trapped in deeply destructive emotional states, like Willow, Holly, or Vine, can and do become the strongest positive forces in our communities once they have worked through their emotional issues. While Willows make for difficult patients, they become tremendous sources of light once they are healed.

### The Willow Child

Any child who is beginning to display the patterns of Willow behavior, such as any form of acting out or blaming others in their family for their own unhappiness, must be given strong parental messages as well as the concept of personal responsibility and an acceptance of reality. Willow children are chronically dissatisfied with their environment as it is. They tend to want—to wildly crave—things that are simply out of reach. This works on both the emotional and physical level, as the Willow child—and the Willow teen especially—will demand possessions that are way out of their family's financial range and become embittered by the simple reality of family finances. They therefore must be guided in establishing realistic goals and desires and learn to appreciate what they actually have. In the same way, they will demand attention and emotional obedience from all around them. If positive efforts don't bring them the results they crave, they are quite willing to demand them through negative emotional displays.

This may be a sulking child, the one who withdraws to pout in silence. They are usually unable to tell others that they are sorry for their behavior, even after they have alienated all their friends with their sour behavior. Instead, they blame parents, teachers, and friends for making their own life so miserable. The remedy will help such a child to come out of their huff and learn the give and take of relationships.

It can be very hard for parents, especially a single parent, to rein in Willow children and bring them into emotional balance. These can quite literally be out of control children, who are quite willing to say or do whatever makes them feel better in the moment, no matter how they may silently regret it later. As Hillary Clinton once famously told us, it takes a village to raise a child. In the case of Willow children, this is certainly true. The parent may need the assistance of teachers and school administrators, to say nothing of the police department and juvenile court system, to guide a Willow child safely into adulthood.

### The Willow Adult

The most important aspect of the aging process when considering the Willow type is that the Willow lacks all flexibility. And that, while the Willow demands that others behave as the Willow dictates, the Willow will never change their own behavior pattern for the sake of others.

It is this very inflexibility that dominates the Willow's emotional and physical symptoms as the Willow ages. The years of emotional rigidity begin to show their toll upon the Willow's body, as the aches and pains of age make themselves known. Willows tend to suffer from chronic pains of all sorts, most commonly from joint pain and arthritis. They may have chronic inflammations and chronic urinary troubles as well. The key here is that the conditions that manifest themselves for the elderly Willow tend to be chronic and cyclical in nature. Look for the Willow to take the pain as a given, as yet another in a long line of betrayals, as this time their own body is betraying them. Doctors' offices are filled with Willows in various states of agony.

Many seniors need the remedy Willow. Nursing homes are filled with Willows, whose children are happy to think that their parents are well cared for, but out of their homes. Look for the emotional rigidity of Willows to increase with age and for their need to control their environment to increase with it. They demand obedience from everyone around them. Their families are at the mercy of their needs and wants. And elderly Willows have a particular intolerance for young people. They refuse to consider the fact that behavior patterns have changed with the change in generations, and that the young must behave as if they were young and cannot be held in check by a reprimanding adult.

### The Willow Animal

This remedy can be of help for animals that have been abused, or when you suspect abuse in an animal that acts out aggressively. Think about Willow for aggressive or sulking animals, for the animal that urinates on the carpet or on your bed as an act of revenge when it is angered. It can also be helpful for elderly animals, especially for older animals that are beset with pains, most commonly arthritic pains.

### Willow and the Homeopathic Pharmacy

Two remedies come to mind when considering parallels to Willow.

The first is Ignatia, which relates to the roller coaster of emotions that occur during the first stages of shock and betrayal. Like Willow, Ignatia sheds many tears, and acts out the rage and shame attached to the sensation of betrayal and/or desertion. Like Willow, Ignatia will overreact to stimuli; will be unable to bear strong smells, colors, or light. And, like Willow, Ignatia will be unable to hear words of sympathy and comfort, and is likely, when others express consolation, to respond that the others have no idea what the Willow's pain and plight are like, as no one else has ever experienced such pain.

The other remedy is Staphysagria, which is often considered to have been Samuel Hahnemann's own constitutional remedy. The Staphysagria knows that they have been harmed in some way, and, indeed they have, as the onset of Staphysagria's symptoms always involve some emotional or physical injury that has undermined the patient's sense of well-being. This sense of injustice brings out the foot stamper in Staphysagrias. They unleash rage whenever the sore spot of their injury is touched, or they swallow their rage and display passive-aggressive behavior. Either way, they share Willow's wound and the pent-up rage it has created.

### Issues that Suggest Willow

Aging; apathy; appendicitis; bleeding; blood pressure troubles; bursitis; cystitis and other urinary troubles; death and dying; denial; divorce and marital issues; influenza; jaw pain; joint pain; leg pain; liver problems; menopause; mononucleosis; sciatica; upper back problems.

### In Conclusion

So many negative words apply to the Willow: self-righteous, smug, controlling, hateful, vengeful, malicious, cruel, cunning, scheming, wicked, negative, haughty, overbearing, bitter, offended, disappointed, angry, petty, and corrupt, just to name a few.

Like Holly, this is a remedy with a wide-range of negative states. The bitterness and sense of loss and betrayal can be expressed in many different ways. But the outcome is always the same. The Willow, who seeks two things—happiness and justice—both for herself and others, experiences a life devoid of both. And, in lashing out in response to her loss, she robs everyone else of them as well.

As with all the other remedies, Willow takes what is in essence a just cause and perverts it into a force of negativity. Willow has experienced an injustice or injury in

life and seeks to set things right. The Willow, who once was happy and trusting, has
been robbed of her happiness and wants it back. But the Willow goes about setting
things right in a negative and vengeful way. In doing so, she sets up a negative emotional state in which each new slight, each new loss is perceived as magnifying the first
and, as a result, deepens the dark emotional state.

While the Willow may well enjoy her acts of vengeance during the moment they
occur, she will tend to brood over them and silently regret them later. However, she
will never express her sorrow or regret to the party she has wronged. This creates the
feeling of deep despair that grows within the Willow. The person who, at heart, is not
only decent, but loving, is aware on some level of her acts of destruction and regrets
what she has become, but cannot change her emotional pattern.

## PINE · THE REMEDY FOR THOSE WITH GUILT

Bach writes of Pine that it is "for those who blame themselves. Even when successful
they think that they could have done better, and are never content with their efforts or
the results. They are hard-working and suffer much from the faults they attach to themselves. Sometimes if there is any mistake it is due to another, but they will claim
responsibility even for that."

• **Pine is both an acute and a constitutional remedy.**

### Botanical Information

Commonly known as the "Scots Pine," this tree (*Pinus Sylvestris*) is native to England,
Scotland, and Ireland, but it naturally grows in the wide range of land from Spain to
Siberia. It is the only pine tree native to the British Isles. It is a tall pine that grows up
to forty feet and lives between 150 and 300 years. This is a tree that has offered many
uses to mankind. Its wood is primarily used for outdoor purposes, from fencing to telephone poles. And its needles are the source of pitch tar, resin, and turpentine. The
Scots Pine is somewhat fussy about the soil in which it grows. It prefers a light and
sandy soil and cannot tolerate strong wind or salty sprays.

### Pine in General

There is no remedy type quite so Old Testament in outlook as Pine. Pines believe that
grace cannot be given as a gift—that it can only be earned by good works. Therefore,
the possibility of grace accounts for nothing in their lives, and they tend to see themselves as the children of an angry God. They are the ants, always rather ruefully looking
at the grasshoppers enjoying life a little too much.

What links Pine to the other remedies in this category of Despair is their ongoing sense of discontentment. As Bach puts it, they "are never content with their efforts or the results." Now this is not meant in a capitalistic sense. Pine does not care about the financial rewards of excellence or even whether others judge their efforts to be successful or not. No, Pine has a higher and sterner judge—himself. Pine is both self-judgmental and self-rejecting. Often Pine will be highly responsive to some form of authority, often either governmental/political or religious in nature. But they are great respecters of words that have been carved in stone. They will compare themselves against these words, whether they are carved in the Lincoln Memorial or Moses' stone tablets. Either way, Pine will find himself—in his thoughts, his words, and his deeds—to be lacking.

This is the remedy for those who are controlled by feelings of guilt. Like the other remedies of this "mood," Pine, when in a chronic negative emotional state, tends to be rather compulsive in his behaviors. The motivation for this compulsion is a moral code that has been shaped around a strongly authoritative message. In his Old Testament thinking, Pine will work hard to earn his freedom from guilt, only to find himself lacking again and again. This will, in the end, enhance his guilt and magnify the flaws he finds within himself.

Obviously, in Pine's emotional patterns, we can find echoes of other remedies grouped with it under Bach's category of Despair. Like Oak, Pine has a rigidity of thought and a strong moral compass. But busy Oak has no time for emotions like guilt and is motivated only by his sense of responsibility and accomplishment. Like Crab Apple, Pine sets his goals of personal perfection beyond the grasp of the human hand. Crab Apple, however, focuses upon physical and mental purity as a means by which he can be happy, while Pine instead focuses upon his shortcomings and uses his deep sense of shame and guilt as his sole motivator.

> The patient who needs Pine has been given the message that he has reason to feel ashamed. Once that message has been taken into the patient's heart, it remains. Worse, it festers, until like a cancer, it spreads throughout his system.

This sense of guilt is so strong in the Pine that it can be used to easily manipulate him by anyone who knows his vulnerability. Anyone who can make the Pine feel even the slightest twinge of guilt will be able to motivate him in any way, as long as they offer some relief of the guilt as a reward.

Indeed, the patient who needs Pine has, at some point in his life, been given the message that he has reason to feel ashamed, that he deserves to feel guilt. Once that message has been taken into the patient's heart, it remains. Worse, it deepens and festers, until like a cancer, it spreads throughout his system.

It is important to note that like the ritualistic behaviors of Willow and Crab Apple, the guilt feelings that echo within the mind and heart of the Pine are empty things. They are quite meaningless. This does not mean that each of us has not done things that we should not have, or do not have reason from time to time to appropriately feel guilt. But, just as Willow has locked himself into a hollow and pointless need for revenge, Pine has locked himself into a meaningless sensation of guilt that limits his life and drains his energy and ability. Pines tend to feel that they have done truly terrible things, but they have not. This is the hollow core of the remedy. A person who has done terrible things—abuse, murder, and the like—and who, after realizing the nature of what he has done and who he has become because of his actions, spirals into a deep sense of guilt and shame, is not a person in a Pine state. No, the murderer, in my opinion, behaves appropriately when he feels shame and remorse. But the Pine type can be likened to a petty thief who feels he deserves the death penalty for his crimes. He has locked himself into a torturous prison in his own mind for no good reason. It is because the Pine is acting compulsively and inappropriately that the remedy can help him see the reality of his situation. When brought into a positive emotional state, he may well see the need to make good on some past actions, but having done so he will feel that the slate is at last wiped clean. He can then move forward without regret and without the weight of guilt coloring his every action.

Pine has an excellent use that should be noted here. It should be considered as the remedy of choice for patients dealing with sexual shame. As has historically been the case in our culture, homosexuals, especially young homosexuals, will feel that they are wrong to feel the sexual urges they do. Some raised in religious homes may have received the message that they are sinners because of their sexuality and that they will be condemned for their sins. Because of this, millions of people carry a deep burden of guilt because of their sexuality. They experience an ongoing sense of shame and guilt that may force them to deny their core sexual impulses or live lives of closeted denial mixed with shameful release. Pine can help them work through that guilt and bring emotional balance into their lives. It can help them work through the issue of their personal sexuality and its impact upon their moral code.

In the same way, Pine is excellent as a remedy for children raised in homes in which their family carries any sort of secret shame. Children who are warned not to talk about specific subjects, that they are private topics, or who have been secretly abused or tormented in their home. Children who, for any reason, dread their home and fear going there instead of finding it to be a refuge very often need Pine as a remedy, no matter how many years have passed since they established a home of their own. These burdens of childhood are often carried throughout life as secret shame. Pine can help release that shame and bring the patient's emotional life into balance.

This same sort of secret shame can carry on as a theme throughout the Pine's whole lifetime. The Pine child who has been taught shame and is motivated by guilt by his or her parents can grow up to be a codependent adult who enters into a marital relationship that involves secrets and abuses. And, since Pines are trying to find a behavior that allows them to feel less guilty, they are often quite willing to stay in relationships that others would quickly leave, especially if their mate, like their parents, understands that the Pine can always be motivated by guilt. They foolishly knuckle under when told, "Look what you made me do."

Pine types, therefore, can be seen as rather weak willed and easily lead. And this, in one sense, is certainly true. They respond to authority with knee-jerk respect and tend to do exactly as they are told by anyone they perceive as being in charge, or anyone who is smart enough to manipulate their sense of guilt.

But in another sense Pines can be very strong willed, even pigheaded. They will simply refuse to do anything that betrays their moral compass, or that sends them into deeper feelings of guilt. For instance, if Pines are told by their government to go off and fight a war that their personal code of morality tells them is wrong, it will set off a struggle that most often ends with the Pines defying the external authority for the sake of their internal code. Like others who Despair, Pines can be remarkably strong and stoic when their core beliefs are challenged.

In the acute context, Pine has as many uses as there are people on Earth. All of us have some reason or other to feel some degree of guilt. All of us need help in forgiving others and forgiving ourselves. All of us benefit, from time to time, from a few doses of Pine.

## Negative Qualities of the Type

When in a negative state, Pine is controlled by guilt, by feelings of weakness and cowardice. And by the sensation that, whatever they try to accomplish, they will do the wrong thing. Sin is the terrible state of life for the constitutional Pine. He feels that God would be displeased with him as a person, and that he can never earn his way into heaven. This sense of weight and despair depletes his life energy. The Pine, therefore, feels chronically tired and weak. For this reason, Pine is often indicated for those who struggle with chronic fatigue and other debilitating diseases.

Because of the deep despair of this remedy type, and the fact that it manifests itself both physically and emotionally, most constitutional Pine types benefit from mixing this remedy with a couple of others. Pine blends especially well with Mustard, which is our remedy for depression. The combination of the two remedies can help bring things into balance when the patient's emotional state is shaped by guilt and leads the patient into a state of clinical depression. In the same way, Pine combines very well with Gorse when there is a state of despair in which all hope has been lost. Pine also combines well with Crab Apple when the guilt leads to perfectionism and compulsive behavior. Finally, consider using Pine with Cerato for the Pine type who is easily controlled; who has lost any sense of self-respect because their feelings of guilt undermine their own strength of character. Cerato and Pine together can be very helpful to the patient who exhibits codependent behavior.

### Positive Qualities of the Type

Pines who are in a positive emotional state offer the world the wonderful gift of forgiveness. They know that, in order to be at peace, not only must they learn to forgive others who have done them harm, but they must also learn to forgive themselves. Positive Pines are able to renew themselves and their relationships by offering forgiveness and willingly accepting it. In doing so, they display the true purpose of religious, political, and moral thought: they create a world in which all may be accepted as they are and live in harmony.

No other remedy type is so able to accept and forgive the faults of all humans or, indeed, to understand human nature itself as Pine. When guilt gives way, it gives way to acceptance: acceptance for the whole of the human condition. Pine then can rejoice in the beauty of humanity's successes and quietly work to correct humanity's failures. This last is the life's work of many Pines, work that they no longer find burdensome because they have learned to accept the good with the bad, and success with failure.

Finally, by learning the power of forgiveness, Pines throw off their Old Testament shackles. They learn the aspect of grace they once denied. Once they accept the notion of grace—forgiveness that is freely and joyfully given and not earned, no one so clearly shows the grace of God as Pine.

### The Pine Child

The child who has taken upon himself the burden of guilt tends to be a rather timid creature. He apologizes too easily and too often, and all but refuses to stand up for himself. He often feels guilt by association and even takes on guilt that rightfully belongs to others. He feels guilty if he asserts himself in any way. This is a quiet child, one that is always worried that he has done something wrong. He may even feel he has to apologize just for living.

The Pine child may try and become invisible in school and public settings. Like the Crab Apple type, the Pine child will often feel he is tainted or in some way worse than the other children. But, unlike the Crab Apple, the Pine will not use these feelings as a motivator to push toward excellence. Instead, he will try not to be noticed, and if he must be noticed, he will try to appease others. This child may do other children's homework to feel tolerated. He will have little ability to carve out a niche in the social structure of his school and will, instead, try to avoid any conflict or situation in which he is the center of attention. Therefore, we have in the Pine child a student who will, even when they know the answer to the teacher's question, sit on his hands and hope that he is not called upon.

### The Pine Adult

I find that the Pine state is particularly strong in children. This does not mean that it cannot continue for a lifetime, but as we age, as we gain wisdom from experience, many of us learn to throw off the messages we have taken in during our youth. Thus, many young Pines rebel actively against the guilt and shame messages they received as children—often for the sake of rebellion alone. The fact that an overbearing parent once used guilt against them as a means of control is frequently reason enough for the guilt to be cast aside in young adulthood. Often the secret or shame that was the source of guilt is announced loudly to the world.

In many cases, however, the chains of shame and guilt continue long into adulthood and again we are left with Thoreau's words about those who lead lives of "quiet desperation." Adults who carry the message of guilt and shame with them into the later states of life remain childlike in their willingness to be controlled by any or all who wield guilt as a weapon. Their feelings of inadequacy and inferiority remain a vulnerable point in their emotional armor for their lifetimes.

### The Pine Animal

Honestly, I don't feel that animals have a sense of guilt. Some people will insist that their dog acts guilty when they come home if the dog has chewed the rug while they were out. I don't agree. I think that when animals act contrite they are more concerned with avoiding punishment than they are wrestling with their personal moral code. I personally find no use whatsoever for this remedy with animals other than humans.

### Pine and the Homeopathic Pharmacy

In terms of homeopathic remedies, Rhus Tox most closely resembles Pine. Both are motivated by guilt. Both suffer from feelings of over-responsibility. And both wear down their natural life energy by overworking, by paying too much attention to the details, by fretting over the work that always still has to be done.

Further, no remedy quite touches Rhus Tox for codependent behavior. Like Rhus, Pine will stay in bad relationships far too long out of guilt and will put up with far too much in the way of abuse.

### Issues that Suggest Pine

Abuse; chronic fatigue syndrome; depression; immune dysfunction; genital troubles; headaches; herpes; impotence; pain; sexual dysfunction; snoring.

### In Conclusion

As is always the case with constitutional types and Bach remedies, Pine has taken a natural virtue—the ability to acknowledge when one has done something wrong—and has warped it into a negative motivation.[7] The guilt that Pine takes upon himself is usually greatly disproportionate to anything that he has actually done, as he blames himself more for being human than for any wrongdoing. Culturally, we seem to encourage guilt. The message of personal guilt echoes down to us from the high halls of justice and from our pulpits. Guilt is used as a controlling mechanism in our homes and in our schools. Guilt, therefore, at least in small quantities, is seen as a good thing. Therefore, many of us make the mistake of thinking that the Pine state, while perhaps a bit whiney and morose, is not a particularly bad thing. In truth, however, the Pine negative emotional state can be a terrible thing.

The Pine state at its most negative is highly destructive to the Pine himself and to all those he loves.

The burden of compulsive guilt is exhausting. It drains those who bear it of joy and of freedom of thought and movement, and it physically drains them as well. And those who live their lives in a limited fashion, controlled by a pointless and never-ending sense of guilt, are not only drains on themselves but also on their families. The weight of their negativity and the rigidity of their behavior control not only their sense of freedom and joy, but their children's, spouses', and friends' as well.

In setting himself free from an inappropriate and negative emotional state, the Pine sets free all those who love him, who, like him, have been controlled by his guilt.

## SWEET CHESTNUT · THE REMEDY FOR THOSE WHO ARE IN DESPAIR

Bach writes that Sweet Chestnut is called for in "those moments which happen to some people when the anguish is so great as to seem to be unbearable. When the mind or body feels as if it had borne to the uttermost limit of its endurance, and that now it must give way. When it seems there is nothing but destruction and annihilation left to face."

• **Sweet Chestnut is almost always an acute remedy.**

### Botanical Information

The plant (*Castanea Sativa*) is commonly known as "Spanish chestnut," "European chestnut" or "sweet chestnut." The sweet chestnut tree can grow to be very large—over 100 feet—and live for a century or more. They are known for having both flowers—

---

7. Because of this wrong-headed sense of the "nobility" of his suffering—a thought that what he is doing is religiously based or based in the notion of purifying or bettering himself—the Pine type can be very hard to treat. Like Willow, he may see absolutely no reason why he should change his emotional or behavioral patterns. Remember, like the other remedies for Despair, Pine is rigid in his thinking and slow to see any need for change.

yellow, sticky catkins—and fruit that is prickly and rough to the touch. They are native to Iran and the Balkans, but were naturalized into Europe, especially into Spain, where some of the finest examples of the tree were cultivated. From Spain, it was imported to England, where it is a prized ornamental tree. The sweet chestnut tree is commonly seen in open woodlands throughout the temperate regions of the world, from Europe to Asia to North America.

### Sweet Chestnut in General

The Sweet Chestnut state can be created by any number of external circumstances and it can be embodied in a number of different ways, but some aspects of the Sweet Chestnut state are constants.

First, the patient in a Sweet Chestnut state is almost always at an acute, even a momentary emotional level. Because of the deep emotion involved in this state, and because of the extreme circumstances that create this emotional state, patients cannot exist within its boundaries for long. Patients in the Sweet Chestnut state move on rather swiftly to other emotional states, positive or negative, or return to their natural emotional patterns. The outcome of the Sweet Chestnut state is largely determined by the circumstances that created it, and by the outcome of those circumstances.

The Sweet Chestnut state always involves a sense of deep despair. This state speaks to those times in our lives when we feel that we are "up against the wall," when we have been pushed to our limit and beyond, when we feel totally depleted in our resources and totally unable to cope with present circumstances. The person in a Sweet Chestnut state may have very unpredictable reactions and behaviors. They may strike out wildly, become hysterical, or collapse inward emotionally.

Another key to understanding the Sweet Chestnut state is that it is never a suicidal depression. It is, in fact, quite the opposite. In circumstances that might be life threatening, such as a sudden illness, automobile accident, or physical threat, the Sweet Chestnut patient seeks above all else to survive. In these moments of great duress, life seems very sweet indeed.

The Sweet Chestnut state is also isolating. The patient who feels Sweet Chestnut's total despair also feels cut off from the support system of those who love him. This may be the result of terrible pain that blocks the patient's ability to feel the support of others, or it might be a real physical isolation, with the patient trapped in a circumstance while far from home. Further, the Sweet Chestnut panic and despair often comes on in the middle of the night, when the patient is isolated in the darkness and struggles to make it until dawn. The Sweet Chestnut patient always feels alone and deserted in his struggle for emotional and/or physical survival.

The Sweet Chestnut state is exhausting, both for the patient and for those who are lovingly supporting him or her through the crisis. The drain of emotional or mental strength may be momentary or may leave all concerned in a state of exhaustion for some time to come. In cases where exhaustion predominates or is long-lasting, the remedy Olive mixes well with Sweet Chestnut.

The Sweet Chestnut state is deeply rooted in the past. It is the moment in time when the patient's life seems to flash in front of his eyes. The Sweet Chestnut longs for the past, for the time before present circumstances brought him to what can only be perceived as destruction. Like Jimmy Stewart's character in that old movie, *It's a Wonderful Life,* the Sweet Chestnut patient has arrived on the bridge on a cold, snowy night, his life crumbled around him, his sense of defeat and despair complete, longing for divine intervention.

As with all the other remedies contained in this category of Despair, Sweet Chestnut is a remedy that possesses great rigidity. It is, in fact, the most rigid of all the remedies listed here. In the same way, it is the most negative emotional state of all.

> Like Jimmy Stewart's character in *It's a Wonderful Life,* the Sweet Chestnut patient has arrived on the bridge on a cold, snowy night, his life crumbled around him, his sense of defeat and despair complete, longing for divine intervention.

Sweet Chestnut is a remedy of response. Some catalyst has created a moment of incredible stress. This catalyst may be a long time in building, such as the collapse of a business or relationship in which the patient has invested all his or her strength and efforts. Or the catalyst may come in the form of a serious illness, one that has, for a long period of time, drained the patient of his or her strength and ability to experience life without fear or pain. The catalyst may be sudden, a plane crash or robbery. It is usually targeted upon the patient himself or herself, but it may sometimes actually happen to someone else. The most common example of this is the death of a loved one, especially a sudden and traumatic death, although a slow death from illness may be the catalyst to a Sweet Chestnut state as well. No matter the catalyst, the outcome is the same.

The patient reaches a point at which they can take no more. At which they feel they may literally collapse, either physically or emotionally. The point at which they have used all their strength, their resources, their ability to adapt to the situation, and can take no more. It is this sensation—that they have moved beyond their ability to adapt—that is key to understanding the Sweet Chestnut state. This is where the rigidity comes in.

The Sweet Chestnut emotional state is the response to the external catalyst that has pushed these patients beyond their ability to cope: they simply go rigid. During these moments, they may literally forget to breathe. The features of their faces may be frozen. They can only hold on to one thought: they must resist the catalyst, fight against the circumstances as best they can with what little strength they have left. Like the child that does not want to be kissed by the great, huge adult looming over them, the Sweet Chestnut can only resist by going rigid and turning away.

The remedy Sweet Chestnut cannot undo the current circumstances. It cannot stop the dying from passing on or fix broken bones. What it can do is restore emotional balance. It can help us—both the patient and those who love and support the patient—during the moment of crisis and in dealing with the outcome of crisis. It can, if you will, allow us to put ourselves into the hands of God, and to prayerfully accept what lies ahead.

If the crisis has a positive outcome, then everyone involved tends to return to normal on their own. They begin breathing again and making plans. If the crisis has a negative outcome, however, if, for instance, the illness or accident takes the life of the patient or the loved one, then Sweet Chestnut can be used for a longer duration to help everyone involved cope with the event. In cases that involve death and grief, consider mixing Sweet Chestnut with Chicory to help move the survivors through their broken-heartedness and to help them cope with their loss. In all cases of trauma or sudden crisis, blend Sweet Chestnut with Rescue Remedy, Bach's cure-all for emergencies. In cases that seem particularly hopeless, especially those that involve long illness that drains not only the patient but also those who love and support him, blend Sweet Chestnut with Gorse and/or Olive, to help strengthen and stabilize all concerned.

## Negative Qualities of the Type

As there is no such thing as a Sweet Chestnut "type," it is hard to discuss the remedy in its negative context. In fact, for Sweet Chestnut, there is nothing but negative context. The moment a patient moves into a Sweet Chestnut state they experience what has been called "a dark night of the soul." Circumstances have created a situation in which the patient quite literally feels that things can get no worse. Destruction is all that can be seen. There is nothing about the Sweet Chestnut state that is not negative or threatening.

## Positive Qualities of the Type

Again, as there is no such thing as a Sweet Chestnut "type," it is hard to examine aspects of moving into a positive Sweet Chestnut state. The positive Sweet Chestnut state does not exist. Those who move through the negative acute Sweet Chestnut state throw off the deep despair and move into other emotional states and types. Those who survive the dark moments of life rise like a phoenix from the ashes. They have undergone a transformation and are new people. Their character and power of belief are strengthened, not weakened, by their trauma.

### The Sweet Chestnut Child

Usually the acute Sweet Chestnut state will affect a child in a time of grief, such as at the death of a grandparent. For states of overwhelming grief in children or adults, blend Sweet Chestnut with Chicory to help these patients release their grief and adapt to life without their loved one. The combination of Sweet Chestnut and Star of Bethlehem can also be especially powerful for children, and can help support them emotionally and open them up to the possibility of a better tomorrow at times of crisis or loss.

### The Sweet Chestnut Adult

Age does not dull our ability to feel despair, nor does it improve our ability to deal with life's crises and traumas. Indeed, older patients may have more need for this remedy, as their ability to adapt to and respond to emergencies may be inhibited by age or infirmity.

### The Sweet Chestnut Animal

Sweet Chestnut can be helpful to animals as well as humans. While it can be very difficult to tell when an animal needs this remedy or to differentiate the need for it from other remedies like Mustard or Vervain, there are some solid circumstances that can suggest Sweet Chestnut.

Consider this remedy for the animal that has had issues with food and starvation. First, always think of Sweet Chestnut for a rescued animal that has been underfed or nearly starved. And think of this remedy for animals that will refuse to eat if their owners are not near, or that, because of deep illness, will not eat at all.

This can be a very helpful remedy for animals that are very ill or near death. It can, if the animal's vital force is still strong enough, help revive an animal that has been greatly weakened by long illness and is no longer expected to survive. In these cases, Sweet Chestnut should be given to all concerned—owner and animal alike. And consider mixing the remedy with Gorse when the situation is believed hopeless.

Finally, Sweet Chestnut can be very helpful for animals that fly out of control because of fear or upset. This, again, is especially true for rescued animals that may have spells of panic or manic behavior. If panic is involved—such as wild despair during a thunderstorm—mix Sweet Chestnut with Rock Rose. If the animal acts out aggressively during these spells, or has moments of being out of control, mix Sweet Chestnut with Vervain. In general, Sweet Chestnut mixes best with Olive in cases of deep illness and can help the animal build his strength and fight his way back to health.

### Sweet Chestnut and the Homeopathic Pharmacy

The first homeopathic remedy that comes to mind when thinking about Sweet Chestnut is Aurum, a remedy made from gold. However, the Aurum type is a likely candidate for suicide, and Sweet Chestnut is not. Further, Aurum is most often a constitutional remedy, used for those who are in deep, clinical depressions, while Sweet Chestnut is more commonly needed in acute situations, when a crisis pushes the patient beyond his or her ability to cope.

Therefore, a more apt remedy is Belladonna. Like Belladonna, Sweet Chestnut is an acute state. The illness in Belladonna comes on like lightning and can be life threatening. In both cases time stops—the past doesn't matter and there may be no future at all—so all energy must go into this moment and into survival.

### Issues that Suggest Sweet Chestnut

Abuse; accident; broken-heartedness; death and dying; emergency; failure; heart attack; midlife crisis; sudden illness.

### In Conclusion

The need for Sweet Chestnut is dictated by circumstances and not by status, gender, or stage of life. Therefore, the need for Sweet Chestnut is universal—any life-threatening circumstance that targets either ourselves or those we love is almost guaranteed to generate deep despair. Sudden trauma or sudden illness, moments of great misfortune or physical threat, national emergencies such as terrorist attacks, weather emergencies such as hurricanes or tornados: all these catalysts may create the response of deep despair and fear for survival in one individual or a massive population. But no matter the number of people involved in the emotional state, each feels totally separate, totally alone as they face what seems to be almost certain destruction.

This is important to our understanding of the remedy. The Sweet Chestnut state cuts our emotional connection to others as well as to our experience of our environment. The patient in a Sweet Chestnut state loses his bond to the world as totally as he would lose his sense of vision in total darkness. The total darkness of his despair cuts him off, and he must face perceived attacks from all sides alone.

## STAR OF BETHLEHEM · THE REMEDY FOR THOSE WHO ARE IN SHOCK

Bach writes that this remedy is "for those in great distress under conditions which for a time produce great unhappiness. The shock of serious news, the loss of some one dear, the fright following an accident, and such like. For those who for at time refuse to be consoled this remedy brings comfort."

• **Star of Bethlehem is both an acute and a constitutional remedy, although it is most commonly used in acute crisis situations.**

• Star of Bethlehem is a component of Rescue Remedy.

*Botanical Information*

When developing his system of thirty-eight herbal remedies, Bach was careful that none of his remedies fell into either of two categories. First he was careful that none of his remedies were toxic. This ruled out his use of plants like Belladonna that had long been used medically, both allopathically and homeopathically, because he did not want to risk injury or aggravation of symptoms. Second, he did not want to use any plant that was normally consumed as food, as they would already be a likely part of the patient's system and would therefore be less likely to act medicinally. Bach comes as close as he gets to breaking one of these rules in the remedy Star of Bethlehem (*Ornithagalum Umbellatum*). Star of Bethlehem is related both to the onion and to garlic. It is commonly thought of as a weed and referred to as "wild onion" or "wild garlic." Like the onion or garlic plant, it grows from a perennial bulb with a slender stalk. It has slim leaves with white stripes down the center. It is known for its flowers that are green on the outside and pure white in the inside. The flowers have six petals that, together, resemble a star, giving the plant its name.

Star of Bethlehem is native to Northern Europe but grows in temperate climates worldwide. It is very common in the pastures and on the lawns of North American homes. It flowers in the spring, in April or May, depending upon the climate. Notably, the flowers of Star of Bethlehem open only during the day when the sun shines.

*Star of Bethlehem in General*

This remedy relates to the need for healing in our lives, the fact that we all carry injury that may have happened only yesterday, or that may date back to our childhoods, on every level—body, mind and spirit. As each day brings some insult, some slight stressor, our need for Star of Bethlehem

> If there is one Bach remedy that is truly universal in its need, that can benefit nearly all the people all the time, it is Star of Bethlehem.

grows. Each new layer of hurt, such as having a near miss on the freeway or problems on the job, only increases our need for Star of Bethlehem as we move on with our lives.

If there is one Bach remedy that is truly universal in its need, that can benefit nearly all the people all the time, it is Star of Bethlehem. I think of this remedy as having the ability to allow each of us to feel as if we were wrapped in the warm arms of those we love and those we have loved who have left us. This is the remedy that suggests to us that healing is possible, that life can be gentle, and that our future holds great promise. It gives a positive slant to our daily lives and upholds us in time of true crisis.

Think of Prince Charming's kiss, which awakens the sleeping Snow White and removes the curse placed upon her. In the same way, Star of Bethlehem awakens each of us and opens us to the possibilities around us. This is the remedy of awakening and the remedy that will spark the potential for healing that is innate in each of us.

I have been taught that when you are opening a patient to the power of the Bach remedies for the first time, the best places to start are Holly, for the anger and aggression that most of us carry with us, or Walnut, which helps to find our path in life and the work that will sustain us. But I strongly disagree. The best first remedy I can think of for almost everyone is Star of Bethlehem. As the remedy of awakening, of healing, it is the place to start. It does not demand, but only sustains, soothes, and centers.

It was because Bach understood the universal need for the remedy and the almost limitless amount of good it can do for us as we struggle through the petty stress of our day-to-day lives and the sudden crises we face that he included Star of Bethlehem in his Rescue Remedy. Indeed, before there was a mixture called "Rescue," Bach considered Star of Bethlehem to be *the* Rescue remedy. He called it his "comforter and soother of pains and sorrows."

Star of Bethlehem can cause no harm. And you will seldom fail to hit your target in using it. Each of us carries emotional burdens large and small, so each of us can benefit from one or many doses of Star of Bethlehem.

Remember—and this is key to understanding the full use of this remedy—that it doesn't matter a damn when the circumstances that created the stress or hurt took place. They could have happened moments ago, or they could date back to the birth trauma the patient experienced. Either way, they can be released once and for all through the use of this remedy.

It's not that Star of Bethlehem is my favorite remedy, or even that I think it is possible to have a favorite out of the thirty-eight, but I admit that I find I tend to use Star of Bethlehem more than I do any other remedy, and I find it always has a positive result. I tend to include it in any mixture or "personal rescue remedy" I create. It mixes very well with any of the other remedies, most especially with Aspen, in cases where hurt and stress have led to anxiety, and with Mustard, when the patient feels an ongoing depression based in a stressful situation at work or at home.

Because Star of Bethlehem can speak to and heal nearly infinite old and new hurts and slights when you thought you were giving it just for one specific cause, it can be nearly impossible to judge how long or how often a particular patient will need this remedy. In fact, I feel that the idea of "acute" versus "constitutional" and "mood" versus "type" becomes nearly meaningless when it comes to Star of Bethlehem. Give it without hesitation for as long as it is effective. However many weeks or months it is given, however, be careful not to repeat the remedy at too-frequent intervals. Be sure that the given dose has acted fully before repeating it. The length of time that a specific dose of Star of Bethlehem is effective is largely indicated by the emotional slight or wound it is bringing into balance. A dose of Star of Bethlehem given in an extreme emergency will need to be repeated much sooner than a dose given to help a patient cope with some old injury. This is not to say that you should worry about giving the remedy, but remember, like every other Bach remedy, Star of Bethlehem owes much to Hahnemann and homeopathy. And more cases of homeopathic treatment are spoiled by repeating a dose too often or too soon than by any other mistake. So be prudent with this and all Bach remedies. Trust that they may have impact for quite some time after the dosing. Watch the patient and wait. Let the patient provide input as well. They will often know when it is time for the next dose.

### Negative Qualities of the Type

The negative Star of Bethlehem patient is in a state of paralysis. The patient has received some shock—bad news, disappointment, trauma—at some point in his or her life, and has been wounded by it. No matter when the trauma occurred, the patient remains injured by it, to some degree paralyzed by it, and in need of comfort. And they need to find a way to move forward out of their paralysis.[8]

And yet, the typical Star of Bethlehem patient will not accept comfort.

Like those who are treated with the homeopathic remedy Arnica, the Star of Beth-lehem patient has been traumatized, injured, and yet will want to send the doctor away. They will not want to be fussed over or touched or comforted. They hold their pain within, and form patterns of rigid behaviors around those hurts and pains. As these pains are often small or petty emotional injuries, these rigid or ritual behaviors are also likewise petty. The Star of Bethlehem type may avoid certain places that hold bad memories, or avoid certain colors or foods for which they have unpleasant associations.

But no matter how petty the injury and the resulting behaviors, the Star of Bethle-hem patient's life is, to some degree or other, controlled by pain, by trauma, or by past circumstances. Because of this, they live lives that are smaller and less free than they might be. The remedy can help bring the patient back, awaken him to his fully func-tioning self again, and open the doors within him that he has slammed shut.

Those who have used drugs for a long period of time are often in a Star of Bethle-hem state. They are in a numbness and need great comfort, but are unable to recognize comfort or caring. For this reason, Star of Bethlehem, along with other forms of therapy and treatment can be useful for those addicted to drugs or alcohol.

### Positive Qualities of the Type

In the positive state, the Star person is filled with energy and has great clarity of mind. They heal quickly and adapt quickly to changes in their environment. This new adap-

---

8. Each remedy in this group of those who experience Despair display some form of rigidity. It is in this feeling of emotional paralysis that Star of Bethlehem shows their inner paralysis. As I said above, they need to be reawakened. They need to be refreshed. They need to move forward from their hurts, old and new, if they are to live their lives fully.

tive behavior is the key. When the Star of Bethlehem patient moves from their paralyzed negative emotional state to a more balanced and positive outlook, they take on the wonderful ability to deal with all that life brings them, good or bad.

Perhaps even more important, they display the gift of soothing others, of leading others toward healing.

### The Star of Bethlehem Child

Any child may need Star of Bethlehem for any number of circumstances. It can be very useful for small things: for nightmares, for fear of the dark (mix with either Mimulus or Aspen, depending upon the exact nature of the fear), or for small physical traumas, such as accidents on the playground or skinned knees.

Star of Bethlehem children may have more profound needs as well. The child who feels unsure of his or her place in the home or of his or her parent's love will benefit greatly from the remedy. Mixed with Walnut, it is very helpful for the milestones of childhood, especially for changes in circumstance, such as moving, starting a new school, or experiencing divorce and the breakup of the household.

Remember, just as Star of Bethlehem can be used many years later to help the child (now an adult) work through the traumas of his youth, it can be used during that child's youth to keep the traumas from piling up in the first place. Star of Bethlehem is the remedy of first choice to help your child steer through the traps and traumas of life, especially during those stages when the child is dependent upon the ability and goodwill of his parents for his emotional as well as his physical survival. And think of this remedy as a helper during those times when the child's parents fall short of being the parents they should be, due to their own flawed human nature. In these moments, both parents and child should take Star of Bethlehem. The parents should mix in a little Pine to help them with their feelings of guilt, while the child may need some Aspen added to help with feelings of anxiety.

### The Star of Bethlehem Adult

I believe that just as Star of Bethlehem is of special help to dependent children it is also very helpful for seniors who find themselves without full freedom of movement or the ability to dictate the full circumstances of their life situations.

In fact, anyone who finds that they are dependent—physically, financially, or emotionally—upon others for their survival are sure to need Star of Bethlehem to help them cope with what is always a difficult circumstance. Anyone coping with physical conditions that inhibit their freedom of movement and ability to determine their daily schedule, who are in any way physically dependent upon others for their meals or any other aspect of life, are sure to need Star of Bethlehem as well.

Although Star of Bethlehem, above all the other Bach remedies, is useful for people at virtually any stage of life, I also find that it is of great use to the elderly who are in the last stages of life. Again, it helps heal the old hurts, and helps the patient let go, both of their old guilt (mix Pine with Star of Bethlehem in cases where the patient clings to old guilt) and their old blame. In many cases, Star of Bethlehem will help the patient make things right with family and friends and will help the patient find peace in the last stage of life.

Also, Star of Bethlehem is of great help for all concerned in times when we grapple with death and dying. While other remedies, like Sweet Chestnut in combination with Chicory, help with the wild emotions and deep despair surrounding the death of a loved one, Star of Bethlehem is needed by everyone—the patient moving toward death as well as his or her loved ones—to help soothe as death approaches and help the survivors let go of their loved one while still keeping him or her in their hearts. In the long season of grief, a time when it seems that nothing at all can help, Star of Bethlehem offers some small comfort and opens our eyes and hearts to the unfolding future at a time when we are paralyzed by our grief.

### The Star of Bethlehem Animal

If you have an animal that was rescued, or whose background you do not know, just give it Star of Bethlehem. It's that simple. Just as you cannot know the hurts or traumas the animal experienced in the past, you can be absolutely sure that Star of Bethlehem will help resolve whatever issues there may be and help it move forward. Star of Bethlehem can be helpful any time the animal moves to a new home or is in a new situation. In these circumstances, mix it with Walnut to help the animal adapt.

If the animal displays specific fears, mix Star of Bethlehem with Mimulus. If the animal is jumpy or anxious, mix Star of Bethlehem with Aspen.

Star of Bethlehem can be very helpful for animals in recovery, especially for those recovering from a medical procedure. Think of Star of Bethlehem for any animal after any medical treatment, especially after visits to the vet for animals that are upset by the experience.

### Star of Bethlehem and the Homeopathic Pharmacy

The logical homeopathic remedy to mention in association with the Star of Bethlehem type is Arnica Montana, the homeopathic most often used in beginning the healing process. Like Star of Bethlehem, Arnica is effective whether the trauma occurred yesterday or twenty years ago. And while the remedy Arnica is often associated with physical pain, it can be very useful for emotional pain as well. Classical homeopaths know to give Arnica to the patient suffering from the ill effects of a nightmare or bad news, just as they would give it to the patient physically bruised by trauma.

Along with Arnica, I mention another remedy, Hypericum. Hypericum is another homeopathic remedy associated with pain—specifically pain that travels along the nerves, such as when you slam your finger in a car door, or the pain associated with toothache. Hypericum pain most often comes on suddenly, as a result of trauma. It can be quite intense and long lasting, and in this way, it also mirrors the Star of Bethlehem state.

### Issues that Suggest Star of Bethlehem

Abuse; accidents; animal care; death and dying; emergencies; grief; shock; stress.

### In Conclusion

Bach insists that he found treatments for each of the basic personality types in his pharmacy of thirty-eight remedies, as well as remedies to help each of us deal with specific transitory moods and crisis situations. But if there is one remedy that truly seems to fit all the people all the time, it is Star of Bethlehem. As both a homeopath and a Jungian therapist Edward C. Whitmont[9] tells us, "that which cannot be absorbed on an emotional level leads to physical illness." Thus the use of Star of Bethlehem to help us absorb hurts and injuries within our minds, spirits, and emotions can help us avoid the physical ailments for which they are the root cause. And, further, the use of this remedy, and Bach's other thirty-seven remedies, can and will, as they let us heal on a spiritual level, help each of us let go of the ailments that plague us physically and limit our lives. This was the core of Bach's philosophy of treatment. It was the motivating thought that moved his medical practice from allopathy to homeopathy and on to his own simplified system of healing, which lets us unlock and remove the mental, spiritual, and emotional blocks that lead to chronic ailments of the body. In no other of Bach's remedies is this principle as dramatically demonstrated as it is here, with Star of Bethlehem.

---

9. Whitmont is the author of two books on the philosophy and practice of homeopathy, *Psyche and Substance* and *The Alchemy of Healing*. I strongly recommend these books to anyone who wants to learn more about homeopathy and how it can best be practiced.

# 6

# Considering the Third Mood: The Constraint of Doubt

The idea of discussing the concept of doubt in terms of constraint seems particularly apt to me, in that, in my experience, those of us who chronically feel the emotion of doubt and are motivated by it find our emotions tightened and our lives constricted as a result. This can be true whether the doubt is a small and nagging sensation or the chief feature in a given patient's emotional landscape.

But what are we really experiencing when we say that we are "doubtful?" Like fear, doubt can be considered in two ways. Some of our most common human doubts are based in negative experiences. The woman who once was fooled into trusting a man who then deceived her will not be as willing to believe the next man. She will doubt his every word. And the patient who has already gone from doctor's office to doctor's office without good results will surely doubt the next doctor's ability to bring about a cure, no matter how much that doctor insists that he and he alone has the skill necessary to put things right.

These patients can enter into a chronic negative emotional state that can be very difficult to put back into balance. Their emotional and sometimes irrational self fuses with logic to create what must be considered "rational doubt." Like the Mimulus patient, whose fears are based in past experience, those suffering from rational doubt have based this emotion on actual firsthand experience. Something has really happened to them that created their ongoing sense of doubt. Past experience has informed the patient's expectations of what is to come. And, based on a logical consideration of these past experiences, the patient can only conclude that all similar future situations will have similar negative outcomes.

But doubt can also be irrational in nature. It does not need to be based on any actual firsthand past experience, but can—again, like fear—be more freeform. Doubt can be created by the experiences of others—especially by the experiences of those we love. We can see the hurt a sibling or friend has experienced and decide that experience will never happen to us.

It can even be a cultural thing. Certainly, after Watergate, many American voters began to doubt the veracity of any politician, and even the foundation of American government.

Like fear, doubt is a communicable emotion. It can spread from person to person, group to group, until it undermines the ability of individual or the whole group to accomplish anything. Perhaps more efficiently than any other emotion, doubt stops forward motion and blocks accomplishment. And all the while it speaks to us and convinces us that we are doing the right thing—the only logical thing—in shutting down, in giving up.

Doubt can be turned inward or directed outward. Again, often based on past experience, we can come to doubt ourselves and our abilities. Perceived failures and inadequacies undermine the ability of many of even the most talented and driven patients as they are increasingly controlled by a festering doubt. In the same way, a community or culture can shift its thinking and lessen its goals because of a growing sense of failure and doubt.

And while this idea of combining failure with doubt often seems sensible, it should be noted that success is by no means an antidote to doubt. The person or culture that has become ensnared in doubt's net is quite capable of perceiving something the rest of the world sees as a great success as a terrible failure or a qualified success at best. Like beauty, success is largely found in the eye of the beholder. And the patient controlled by doubt has a very critical eye—an eye that sees the flaws others miss, that will not see how good their present relationship is until it is over. That will fail to see the achievements of an existing government until it has passed into history.

> Doubt keeps us from experiencing the depth and range of our emotional selves. It blocks other feelings and spontaneous actions.

Even an undeniable success can be twisted by the person poisoned by doubt. Even while standing on the stage receiving his or her Academy Award, the doubter can be sure that, any moment now, everyone else will finally see the phony, the loser that he or she truly is, and demand the statue back.

The New Testament gives us two excellent examples of doubt.

The first and perhaps most iconic is, of course, "Doubting Thomas." Here was a man who knew Jesus personally and traveled with him for a period of years. Who witnessed miracle after miracle, who heard the Sermon on the Mount firsthand, and helped hand out the loaves and fishes. And yet, when he experienced the greatest miracle of all, the resurrection of the Christ, his first response and emotional reaction was to doubt. When all the others were falling to their knees (if not passing out altogether) Thomas reacted with what I am sure he considered to be cool logic. While everyone else was reduced to babbling, Thomas kept his wits about him and asked to examine the corpse. Only when his doubts were satisfied could he bring himself to worship. Only when he could confirm to the best of his ability that he was in no way being made a fool of could he release the rest of the emotions his doubt kept in check.

This is the best example possible for one of the negative outcomes of doubt. Doubt keeps us from experiencing the depth and range of our emotional selves. It blocks other feelings and spontaneous actions. It warns us that we must act with caution at all times and in all ways—even when the greatest miracle of all is looking us in the eye. Or we may be tricked, we may be injured, we may be humiliated.

Doubt, then, keeps us from experiencing life. True, it may, from time to time, be a handy tool that keeps us from experiencing embarrassment, but it also keeps us from experiencing joy, hope, and freedom of action.

The second example shows another way that doubt can cripple us. It has to do with the incident when Jesus walked on water. As I remember the story, when the disciples saw Jesus literally walking on water as a demonstration of what was possible through the power of belief, the disciple Peter was so moved and inspired that he jumped out of the boat and began to walk on the water himself. Jesus saw him and beckoned him to come. With this action, Jesus encouraged Peter, assured him that all would work out well. And Peter, like Jesus, actually walked on the water. That is, until doubt began to undermine him and control the results of his actions. No doubt Peter began his walk in a state of great excitement. And his excitement grew as he found his footing and discovered to his delight that he too could actually walk on water. And he walked toward the man he acknowledged as his spiritual Master. Then, something inside Peter awakened. He no doubt thought, "What the hell am I doing?" And, in that instant, he lost his footing and fell into the sea.

Just as doubt can come to control our reactions and our experience of life, it can color and control our accomplishments as well.

Peter was actually accomplishing the impossible, for however long he managed it—a second or a minute. He was walking on the water. And it was not the nature of the water or his physical body that caused him to fall, it was his doubt. It was the nagging voice that asked him, as it asks us all when we are doing the impossible, "What the hell do you think you are doing?" And, with that thought, we are back in the natural world, the world in which the impossible is impossible, and we fall.

What are we doing when we doubt?

Like each of the other six of Bach's emotional states, doubt represents a wound to our sense of self. In this case, our sense of belief has been wounded. The patient in need of any of the remedies in this broad category of emotional states has been robbed of their full ability to believe that their life is moving ahead as it should, that things will turn out for the best, through some experience, some trauma.

Those who doubt face life with a lack of belief, always feeling the need to test—test their world, test others, test themselves. Like Doubting Thomas, they are people who need to see the wounds, touch the wounds, before they can believe that anyone has truly been wounded.

Those in this pattern may lack self-confidence, or may be unsure as to their path in life. Or they may be unsure of others and their intentions. They may be prisoners of hopelessness, or may simply be unable to decide where they should go next in life or what to have for dinner. But what is at the core of this mood pattern is a lack of belief, a lack of trust.

To get back into a state of emotional balance and begin to move forward in life once more, those who doubt must give up their past hurts and, even more difficult, be willing to give up their logical assessments of past circumstances. They must learn that, as the linguists tell us, dog one is not dog two is not dog three. In other words, the doubter must learn once more to risk as they did before doubting became the sensible thing to do.

## Doubt and the Homeopathic Pharmacy

Because the emotion doubt so often wears a nice business suit—because it comes dressed up as logic—it can be a difficult thing to uncover and treat homeopathically. Where some remedies clearly speak to other emotional states like fear or anger or indifference, it can be more difficult to find a remedy based upon a patient's doubt alone without coupling it with physical symptoms.[1]

The Repertory, however, does contain some information on homeopathic remedies that may be helpful for those who doubt.

The first remedy that is listed for doubt is one that has already come up in these pages more than once. That remedy is Lycopodium, and it is not surprising that it would be the chief remedy for those who doubt. The Lycopodium is riddled with issues of self-confidence, which he uses as a jet pack to propel him toward accomplishment. Poor Lycopodium often mixes self-doubt with despair, but would rather die than have anyone else find that out. His life's axiom is "Never let them see you sweat." Instead, Lycopodium works hard so others will see him as intelligent and on top of things. The stress level this creates leads to chronic indigestion and a number of other functional diseases.

Lycopodium can also be among the most cynical of people (cynicism being the vocal expression of the doubtful personality), as can Lachesis, which is a homeopathic

---

1. In reality, this is always the case. Remember, homeopathic medicine is based upon the consideration of the patient as a whole being: body, mind, and emotions. The homeopath, therefore, will need to consider mental, emotional, and physical symptoms before treating any patient homeopathically. For the sake of understanding the parallels between homeopathy and Bach treatments, I include the discussion here based solely upon emotional symptoms.

remedy made from snake venom. The Lachesis tends to be highly verbal and very vocal. They project a highly intelligent persona and use their intelligence to intimidate others. Like snakes, they lash out with their mouths.

Another remedy that tends toward doubt is Sulphur. Sulphur also tends to be intelligent and highly verbal. But where Lycopodium and Lachesis use their verbosity in a highly focused manner, Sulphur tends to have a less trained intellect and to be more naturally curious about everything. Sulphur tends to use words to confound more often than intimidate. But Sulphur shares the tendency toward doubt. He tends to have less focus and less drive than the others, and, as a result, is often stopped in his tracks by an overwhelming sense of doubt that blocks his every accomplishment.

Like the Bach remedies that related to Despair, those listed here tend to be constitutional remedies. They speak to a deeply ingrained emotional state that, over time, has come to control the actions and accomplishments of the patient needing them.

## REMEDIES FOR THOSE WHO DOUBT

- **Gentian**—for those who are discouraged

- **Hornbeam**—for those who are lethargic

- **Gorse**—for those who are without hope

- **Scleranthus**—for those who are indecisive

- **Cerato**—for those with self-doubt

- **Wild Oat**—for those who are unfulfilled

## GENTIAN · THE REMEDY FOR THOSE WHO ARE DISCOURAGED

Gentian types, writes Bach are "those who are easily discouraged. They may be progressing well in illness or in the affairs of their daily life, but any small delay or hindrance to progress causes doubt and soon disheartens them."

- **Gentian is both an acute and a constitutional remedy.**

- **Gentian is one of Bach's original remedies, the Twelve Healers.**

### Botanical Information

Gentian (*Gentiana Amarella*) is unique among Bach's remedies in that the flower used in creating the remedy blooms in late summer and autumn, from August until October. Because Bach used sunshine in potentizing his remedies, he most often selected remedies that bloom during late spring and summer, at a time when the sun is high in the sky and sunlight is strong. It is also known as the "autumn felwort."

Gentian is a small annual about six inches tall. It is a narrow stalk of a plant that takes up only about one square inch of space. It has beautiful tubular flowers that are white at the tip and purple at the base.

### Gentian in General

The patient needing the remedy Gentian either acutely or constitutionally is working from a feeling of rational doubt. Often, the remedy is needed for those who find themselves in a truly bad situation. It can be helpful to those whose usual positive and hopeful natures have been overwhelmed by circumstances like the death of a loved one or a period of unemployment in which their sense of self-confidence has been overwhelmed by the apparent indifference to their accomplishments in the workplace. Divorce can often lead to a period of life in which Gentian is required, either by the husband and wife, if he or she feels that the loss of the relationship is due to his or her own failure, or by the children, especially if they are required to move between their divorced parents' houses or if they decide that they are responsible for the divorce. These can be very difficult emotional states to bring into balance, especially if the patients feel that their negative assessments are the result of an honest and sensible account for the situation at hand. When feelings of doubt lock together with rational thought, the idea of returning from a negative emotional state to a more hopeful outlook for the future can seem silly at best. Indeed, in some cases that require Gentian, the patient's emotional state will not even seem to be the issue. Instead, it will be the patient's *mental* state that is in need of encouragement and rebalancing.

Often those needing Gentian will be innately intelligent people, whether they are highly schooled or not. The sensation of doubt that all but cripples the Gentian type seems to be particularly common in those who are highly sensitive and intelligent. It is very common among artists of all sorts—actors, singers, writers, and painters among them—whose work involves not only the completion of the artistic process, but also the intense scrutiny of producers, publishers, and other business partners who judge the merit of the artist's work in terms of potential sales income. Finally, the artist's work and the artist himself or herself must withstand the scrutiny of journalists and amateur critics, all of whom claim an equal right to voice an opinion as to the merit of the artist's work. Given the likely experience that most artists must undergo, it is not surprising that, over time, many have a need for Gentian that far exceeds the need exhibited by plumbers, groundskeepers and the like. Indeed, anyone who takes on the sort of work that places him in the public eye, including anyone who seeks and holds public office, will have a greater tendency to need Gentian than will anyone whose work allows him the grace of anonymity.

In the acute context, Gentian can be needed by any person who has come up against any sort of life's roadblocks and, because of them, is tempted to just give up. And this is the key to understanding the emotional state that is central to Gentians: they want to give up. Sometimes, they may have what most other people would consider a minor setback, and yet Gentian types will just fold under the pressure. This does not mean that the patient needing Gentian may not have experienced a disaster like the death of a mate that would stop any of us in his or her tracks, but the typical and usual need for the remedy is in the patient for whom each small roadblock seems an insurmountable thing. It is the chronic tendency to be easily discouraged that is central to the type.

Other patients may reveal the other colors of the remedy. Some will seem to be very skeptical people, even cynical people. In my opinion, cynicism is a sign of a deep and constitutional need for the remedy. It reveals a negative emotional state in which the patient has yielded his inner sense of belief and has taken on such a deep state of doubt that discouragement now seems to be a "normal" emotional state. Patients who display cynicism often need the embittered remedy Willow in combination with Gentian to restore their sense of possibility, of belief.

> Gentian types will actually welcome worry, because they know and understand worry. They are uncomfortable when things just seem to be falling into place in their lives.

Another sign of the constitutional need for the remedy is when the patient takes on the role of the pessimist. The deep emotion of doubt here is not targeted toward the self in this case, nor toward others, but toward the nature of the universe itself. The pessimist has moved so far into doubt as to be quite sure that God himself arranged the universe to be a realm in which we are each cursed to try and to hope and to ultimately be disappointed in all we attempt. This Gentian type lacks faith, and has trouble believing in things unseen. This type is like folks from Missouri, the "Show Me" state.

These Gentian types will actually welcome worry, because they know and understand worry. They are uncomfortable when things just seem to be falling into place in their lives, when any "invisible" force seems to be acting in their favor. Ironically, they have no problem when invisible forces seem to be working against them, as this fits into their map of the universe.

Certainly, many of those who need Gentian acutely or constitutionally turn their sense of doubt upon themselves. They start out strong with high hopes, but each of life's setbacks causes them to question themselves and doubt their ability to succeed. Because of these festering doubts, the Gentians' tendency is to be too willing to allow their original vision to lose its focus. They compromise too easily, and too often let the opinions of others be absorbed as facts and not as opinions. This can often lead Gentian types to realize that their original vision has been lost and, as a result, once again want to give up on the whole process.

The patient who needs Gentian as a constitutional remedy may repeat this process over and over again. Sometimes they may repeat it exactly, in the same line of work, or they may move from career to career only to repeat the same process of beginning the new job with excitement and expectation and then have the positive emotions slip through their fingers as disappointments begin to mount up. In cases like these, a combination of Gentian and Chestnut Bud, the remedy that speaks to obsessive behavior patterns, may be needed to restore emotional balance.

Gentian is quite often needed by those who have endured a long illness and now, even though they are in recovery, cannot help but be undermined by any small setback or recurrence of symptoms. Gentians will believe that any ache or pain is a sign that they are about to undergo another bout of illness, even if their recovery is in sight. Mimulus, the remedy for those with specific fears, may blend well with Gentian in cases when the patient is terrified of any sign of his or her illness. If a setback in recovery triggers a sense of hopelessness, combine Gorse and Gentian to restore emotional balance and to encourage recovery.

## Negative Qualities of the Type

Patients trapped in a negative Gentian state tend to be pulled in two directions—by the future and by the past. Gentians are locked into behaviors and opinions that are based upon past experiences, especially upon past hurts that are unresolved for the negative Gentians and therefore still loom large. If they took a chance on love or on success and were thwarted, they lock in on that failure and assume that it will be repeated if they attempt success again in the future.

But they are pulled by the future, and that future often can be summed up by two words: "What if?" And the Gentians' every "What if?" is answered by a negative outcome. They have worry and panic inside, which they push off onto others. They not only affect their own life negatively, but also shape the lives of those around them for the worse.

Because Gentians are pulled by both the echoes of the past and the dread of the future, they tend to not experience the present except as a minefield that combines past injuries with future hurts. They are weighed down by a nagging sense of doubt in the present moment, and it causes them to question every one of their actions and/or opinions.

## Positive Qualities of the Type

Positive Gentians are filled with faith, and can look beyond what exists into the realm of what is possible. They are, therefore, among the finest healers, as they themselves have usually risen from a chronically sick state. They also make fine teachers. The movement from the negative Gentian state to the positive Gentian state involves a true transformation of character. The Gentian transformation is that they learn to trust the universe and let go of worry. When they have attained a positive state they are too involved in every aspect of shaping their world and have become too trusting that things are working to the good to easily yield their success for the sake of doubt. Therefore, they become quite powerful in their resolve and sure of their vision and their success.

## The Gentian Child

Gentian children tend to want constant reassurance. "Yes, the sun will rise again tomorrow." "Yes, the dog is fine, so go to sleep."

Gentian children can go along just fine in life for long periods of time. They are intelligent children, so their grades are good. Their health is fine. But when something negative happens, their whole world collapses. Gentian children seem to lack resources or strength when they are tested. Their faith is only strong when it is not put to the test.

In fact, Gentian can be helpful for children who are afraid of being tested in school and may develop sudden symptoms of illness when a quiz is scheduled, or who, when they do take a test, do poorly even though they know the answers to the questions. These are children who, if they feel that they have done poorly in school, will not want to return to the same school ever again.

They are mild-mannered children who may be placed in the victim role in school, because they will have trouble standing up for themselves. When their opinion is questioned, especially by adults, they will immediately yield their opinion and agree with the majority. They will compromise their goals, not only for the sake of the majority, but also to appease any stronger person, adult or child.

## The Gentian Adult

It can sometimes seem as if adult Gentian patients have never looked for a moment at the whole flow of their lives, but only have seen the individual moments—the good moments and the bad—and have focused only upon the bad. Gentians, as a negative personality type, only sail through the good moments. Their skin is thin and bones brittle; they do not stand up well to any form of pressure.

For this reason, Gentian is often required by elderly patients who have come to feel that they have been beaten up by life. Often they have been widowed and have retired into a state of life in which they have become deeply pessimistic. They are quite assured that their experiences have proven that they are right to hold a negative opinion about life in general and their own life specifically. For this reason, adult Gentians can be very hard to treat, as they will not feel that there is any reason for treatment. Further, Gentians are commonly very hard to treat because they will not take their remedies. There are two reasons why they will not take them (even if they tell you that they are): First, they will tend to have doubts about the Bach remedies themselves, and about Bach's ideas about healing. Even if you can get them to admit that they need help in the first place, and even if they have seen them work for others, they will tend to believe that the remedies cannot offer them any real help. Second, expect Gentians to stop taking the remedy the moment it begins to work. Like Willow types, Gentian types, especially elderly Gentian types, tend to be very comfortable with their negative emotional state and do not want to give it up easily. If they begin to feel changes in their mood because of the remedy, they will immediately put it aside. So if the remedy does not seem to be working even though you are sure it is called for, make sure it is being taken before giving up on Gentian.

### The Gentian Animal

While Gentian is one of those remedies that is almost impossible to see in an animal's behavior, it does have one use that I have found valuable. If you adopt an animal into your home and are aware that the animal was caged while in the shelter, make sure to include Gentian among those remedies you give the animal when first bringing it into your home. Gentian may be combined with Walnut—a remedy commonly needed for newly adopted animals—or with Aspen or any other remedy that the animal's emotional state suggests.

### Gentian and the Homeopathic Pharmacy

Hahnemann's homeopathic remedy Gelsemium seems to parallel Bach's Gentian nicely. In both cases the patient tends to be mild mannered, worried, and literally gasping for air. Gelsemium in particular seems to have a mild buzz of anxiety around their head at all times. They are filled with fears and wracked with mild ache and pains.

Both remedies will help in cases that involve long-term events that are a source of discouragement: chronic illness, long-term unemployment, and similar situations. Both are remedies for discouragement when things drag on and on.

Gentian's lack of strength also can suggest the remedy Silicea, which also can lack strength of character and be deeply distressed by any minor setback, and have an ongoing willingness to give up when faced with difficult circumstances.

### Issues that Suggest Gentian

Accidents; acute illness; chronic backache or neck pain; gout; immune dysfunction; jaw pain; mononucleosis; multiple sclerosis; pain; relapse of any illness; rheumatoid arthritis; weakness—especially weakness of the bones.

## In Conclusion

Just as with Hahnemann's homeopathic remedies, some Bach remedies have a rather narrow focus, like Rock Rose, while others have a wider range of applications. Holly, certainly, is one of the latter, as it can be used for virtually every aspect of negative emotion that is expressed through aggression. In the same way, Gentian speaks to many different behaviors and emotional variations that cluster around the concept of doubt. Gentian is therefore appropriate for the cynic, the pessimist, and the unwilling victim of fate equally, and it offers emotional balance to all who feel crippled by doubt and are all too willing to give up on a goal at the first sign of adversity as a result.

Gentian can therefore be said to offer a sense of belief to those who have put it aside in the face of adversity, and to reinforce the faith that is inborn in us all.

In cases of constitutional need, Gentian represents one of our most negative emotional states, rivaling Willow for its depth of negativity. And, again like Willow, Gentians feel that their emotional outlook is "earned" and are all too willing, when asked to give precise reasons why they feel as negatively as they do. At the very least, they will respond with the back of their hand and a quick "I have my reasons," as their response.

It may be said that Gentian is the polar opposite to Oak in emotional state, given the Gentians' tendency to give up their work and their goals at the first sign of trouble. Both take the idea of attaining goals or embodying a personal vision and create a chronic emotional state from the issues and troubles caused by the struggle to attain those goals. The Oak uses the struggle itself to display his willingness to continue to struggle, even after it has become apparent to everyone else that the cause is lost. The Gentian uses the struggle itself as a reason to yield and give up, even if everyone else involved feels that the setbacks are few and small and that the cause is worth struggling for. Both have taken an issue common to us all—the struggle involved in achieving our goals—and have created an emotional pattern that creates upheaval for themselves and all others involved. Both lack the ability that the more balanced individual uses virtually every day—the ability to judge whether or not the relationship, career, or cause is worthy of the time, effort, and struggle involved to see it through to the end. Whenever our balanced outlook about our daily struggle flies out of balance, whenever we question our talents, our abilities, and our personal strengths and weaknesses, one or the other of these two remedies, which speak to the same issue from opposite directions, is likely to be the remedy that can help set things right for us emotionally.

## HORNBEAM · THE REMEDY FOR THOSE WHO ARE LETHARGIC

Bach notes that Hornbeam is needed by "those who feel that they have not sufficient strength, mentally or physically, to carry the burden of life placed upon them; the affairs of every day seem too much for them to accomplish, though they generally succeeded in fulfilling their task. For those who believe that some part, of mind or body, needs to be strengthened before they can easily fulfill their work."

• **Hornbeam is both an acute and a constitutional remedy.**

### Botanical Information

The Hornbeam (*Carpinus Betulus*) tree, also known as the "European Hornbeam," the "Ironwood," and the "Musclewood," is slow to grow to its full height of sixty feet. It tolerates both sun and shade and has a natural pyramidal shape. The hornbeam is native to Northern Europe and now grows in temperate regions throughout the world. Hornbeam has two types of flowers. The male flower hangs down from the tree, the female flowers are upright and blossom green-brown in mid spring.

### Hornbeam in General

I believe that the remedy Hornbeam, more than any other of Bach's remedies, relates to life in the postindustrial age. I believe that it relates to an emotional state that I call "modern malaise." We live in a time in human history when most of us are not using every moment of the day to gather enough food to eat or fuel for heat and light, so we have to a great extent set aside the struggles that occupied our thoughts and our physical actions for the majority of human history. Instead, we face endless days in windowless office cubicles, unchallenged by anything more life and death than a deadline or a trip to the grocery store. Our media reveals a cultural knowledge of our plight. Stories like Thurber's *The Secret Life of Walter Mitty* and movies like Preston Sturges' classic *Sullivan's Travels* show the sense of creeping despair and discouragement many of us feel as we are faced with a life of endless responsibilities and few real challenges that elicit a creative or joyous result.

> What every lethargic Hornbeam wants is that he or she will, at some near moment in time, experience some sort of excitement. These are people who live in a rut and are never challenged, other than by the voices of bosses and mates, all of whom are expressing dissatisfaction with the Hornbeam's present output.

What every lethargic Hornbeam wants is that he or she will, at some near moment in time, experience some sort of excitement. These are people who live in a rut—who likely eat too much, exercise too little, and are never challenged, other than by the voices of bosses and mates, all of whom are expressing dissatisfaction with the Hornbeam's present output. These are housewives who have to face the fact that Monday—every Monday—is laundry day, Tuesday is for ironing, Wednesday is for dusting, and every day at four o'clock they have to start cooking dinner.

Hornbeam lives in a state of lethargy, a state that combines depression with exhaustion. But this is an exhaustion of an emotional sort. A simple test will often reveal the need for Hornbeam. The patient who appears negative, who seems exhausted and disinterested, but who changes completely when he or she is intellectually challenged, or, simply, made to laugh—whose entire demeanor changes and whose face glows brightly with sudden interest—is the patient who needs the remedy Hornbeam.

We have all experienced the acute need for Hornbeam. We have all felt the dragging sensation when we are called upon to repeat the same tedious process over and over again. And, certainly, modern life is filled with repetition. We have to make the same commute to and from work every day, and deal with the same traffic jams and the same race for good parking spaces. We also tend to have jobs that require the same paper work, the same meetings, and the same phone calls over and over again. We have the same holidays every year and the same meals on our tables night after night. Finally, we see the same faces around us daily, at home and at work. And it is this sameness that is the source of the Hornbeam's lethargy. Where most of us absorb the cycles and repetitions of our lives, Hornbeam has reached the point at which the sameness exhausts him. His emotional and physical strength are increasingly drained by the tedium of his life. In acute situations, the need for Hornbeam can easily be put right. The father who arrives home from a bad day and a worse commute can easily be cheered out of his plight by a room full of loved ones. The worker who feels underappreciated and unchallenged by his work can be cheered by a simple word of appreciation from his or her boss. But as the negative emotional state of lethargy grows over time, it can become a powerful thing.

Where the concept of Doubt comes into play for the Hornbeam type is that he is in a constant state of doubting his own abilities. Because of the weighted sense of lethargy that hangs over his daily grind, the Hornbeam feels that he cannot fulfill the expectations that others have placed upon him, although he is, in reality, perfectly capable of achieving success in all things. The Hornbeam doubts this reality, however, and may feel a good deal of anxiety about his ability to please others, especially others who are in a position of authority. Therefore, the Hornbeam not only feels somewhat bored and trapped in whatever situation has drained him of his natural excitement and joy in life, but he also feels that he is incapable of accomplishing the very tasks that so bore him. He can over time become quite trapped in his fear of failure, even if he has a strong support system at work or at home that reminds him again and again of his inborn abilities.

And so the Hornbeam feels a great deal of stress. First because his life situation has a stranglehold on him. And, second, because even if his situation offers him no creative stimulus or mental challenge, he ironically feels he is not capable of performing on an acceptable level. The Hornbeam who finds himself in this cycle often fails to achieve due to his fear and stress levels. This failure seems quite mysterious to those who know what the Hornbeam is capable of and cannot understand why he appears to be working below the threshold of his capabilities. The bosses of Hornbeams will call them into their offices and issue warnings. Their teachers will send home notes, wondering why they are not working up to their abilities. And the Hornbeams' family wonders why they struggle, year after year, at a job that is in all reality beneath them.

This is the cycle that is repeated again and again by those who need the remedy Hornbeam constitutionally. Those trapped in this cycle may need the remedy Chestnut Bud—the remedy for those who make the same mistakes again and again—in combination with Hornbeam. Other remedies that combine particularly well with Hornbeam, especially on the constitutional level, include Elm and Larch.[2] Elm is especially helpful for those who suffer from deep stress from overwork and who feel overwhelmed by the tasks set before them and incapable of moving to clear away those tasks. Larch is very helpful for those who combine the issue of low self-esteem with the emotional and mental exhaustion common to the Hornbeam.

In my experience, Hornbeam is one of the most all-pervasive of all the Bach remedies in terms of need. And, in my opinion, it is not a natural emotional state. Rather, it is one that has been forced upon us, as we have, in modern society, abandoned many of the natural tasks of life for the sake of a world that has become increasingly abstract, a world in which our only likely contact with the animal world are dogs—an animal that

---

2. I feel that the combination of Hornbeam and Elm is one of the great tonics that can be made using the Bach remedies. The two remedies combine so well that, at times, I tend to think of them as one. I think that this combination speaks to the needs of millions of people who, in this modern age, find themselves almost completely removed from nature and from life as it was lived by humans for hundreds of thousands of years. I remember a science fiction novel I read many years ago, called *Easy Travel to Other Planets*. That book created the concept of "information sickness," a malady that beset many characters in that novel. Overwhelmed by the amount of information that entered their thoughts every day from all sorts of media and the amount of detail required of them in their dreary jobs, these people simply sat down on park benches and started bleeding from their ears. Those characters would have been helped by the combination of Hornbeam and Elm, which lets its users find their passion when it comes to their life's work and focus in on achieving their goals. For those who find themselves flummoxed when it comes to just what that work is, what their goals are, and who are laboring away miserably at something else while they "find themselves," mix Wild Oat with the Hornbeam and Elm.

becomes increasingly anthropomorphized by humans with each passing generation, until they have nearly as many possessions, clothes, beds, toys, and special foods and drinks, as we do. It is also a world in which more and more people are never touched by another, and instead communicate with each other by electronic means. A world in which we can go for days without connecting with anything other than a keyboard and a computer screen. A world in which the food we eat comes wrapped in plastic and the water we drink comes in bottles. In short, the remedy Hornbeam speaks to the fact that we are still animals, living in an increasingly abstract and unnatural world. The malaise of lethargy that is the core emotional state of Hornbeam is the cost, and I think this remedy belongs in every household because of it.

## Negative Qualities of the Type

The "sin" central to the negative emotional state of Hornbeam is the deadly sin of sloth. The Hornbeam finds no challenges in life, and has fallen into the rut of just completing the tasks that he has already mastered, day after day. He complains about the rut, but does nothing to change it. He is a couch potato who comes home exhausted every night only to eat too much, watch TV, go to bed exhausted, and then get up exhausted the next morning.

If the Hornbeam is made to laugh, however, or if he becomes excited about a subject or thought, he is suddenly filled with energy once more, and feels the possibility for change. This usually dissipates rather quickly, however, as the Hornbeam sees what's on HBO.

The Hornbeam, therefore, is another of our pessimistic types. His view of his life is a rather flat vista that stretches out before him, with each day like the one before, identical to the one that comes after.

The behavior pattern common to the Hornbeam that is most likely to drive everyone around him—his bosses, coworkers, and families alike—crazy is the Hornbeam tendency toward procrastination. Because he finds no challenge in the tasks set before him, he tends to put off performing them. Or worse, he performs part of each task but finishes none of them. Thus, the typical Hornbeam makes piles. His desk is covered in piles, as is the floor and every blank tabletop and counter. These tasks allow the Hornbeam to sort through his unfinished tasks and pretend that he is actually performing them. Instead, the piles call out to the Hornbeam and haunt his dreams, but he does nothing to finish them off and file them away.

## Positive Qualities of the Type

The positive Hornbeam is the person who is constantly interested in all that is going on in life. He feels that each day brings new challenges, new possibilities. He is filled with excitement about each new day.

This is not because he has become totally brain-dead and has decided that folding laundry is indeed exciting. It is because he has achieved a clear focus on what he wants to achieve in life. The positive Hornbeam has learned to give the little energy it takes to fulfill the "obligatory" tasks each of us must perform on a regular basis—cleaning the house, filing forms, paying the bills—and to give these tasks no more time or worry than they are worth.

These done, the Hornbeam can then focus in on the tasks that will actually get him to his goal. He will finish school at night if he must, or actually write the book he has always intended to write. And he will begin to find the creative challenge that has been missing in his life.

Hornbeam is one of our most refreshing remedies. Like White Chestnut, it clears the mind of those needing it. Suddenly, they will feel minty fresh, calm, and centered. Once they begin to take the remedy—and it can work amazingly swiftly—they begin to sleep better and find that their sense of humor, which they had misplaced somewhere, suddenly returns.

It is always an agreeable circumstance for all concerned when a patient begins to take the Bach remedy or remedies he needs. But few remedies bring as much joy to the home or workplace as Hornbeam. Suddenly, everyone is happy.

### The Hornbeam Child

If there is one thing that the Hornbeam child needs, it is for his computer or iPod to be taken out of his hands. He needs to be forced to get up and go outside and play. Hornbeams are quiet children, usually overweight, who do not want to move, although they want to eat, they want to read, and they like listening to music.

They also are procrastinators, who will day after day put off doing that term paper and then have to exhaust themselves working day and night to finish it. When faced with any challenge, they just feel exhausted thinking about it.

### The Hornbeam Adult

Adults who need Hornbeam are virtually identical to the Hornbeam child described above. In fact, they are in many ways just large children, who do not want to go to bed on time, who do not want to do their homework, and who want an extra piece of cake. Hornbeam adults may even tend to dress like large children, with shorts, tee shirts and baseball caps turned backward.

Hornbeam is commonly needed by adults of a certain age group: younger adults, from late teens to early thirties. It is the remedy for those who, even if they have been forced from the nest of their parents' home, have moved into apartments with friends—apartments that in many ways resemble dorm rooms—and work jobs that are just that, jobs and not careers. The remedy is of special help to those who seem to be getting older but no wiser, those young adults who seem unwilling to change as they age.

It is also very helpful for couples in their thirties who have bought their home, are raising young children, and feel that they have taken on responsibilities that they are still too young for and that they are unprepared for. They struggle with the reality of their lives, that they have little money and few hopes of getting ahead. That now, as parents, they must put the needs of their children first, ahead of their own needs or wants. They feel overwhelmed and choked by their situation. In this sort of situation, a sense of heavy lethargy falls not only on the husband and wife, but also on the whole family. Each member may need Hornbeam to get things back on track.

### The Hornbeam Animal

I feel that the lethargy associated with the remedy Hornbeam is primarily a human emotion and has little expression in the animal world. However, as we continue to make the lives of our domestic pets more and more similar to our own and our dogs and cats have no more experience of the natural world than we do, some animals may need Hornbeam as well. Think of this remedy especially for dogs and cats that are alone in an apartment or house for the entire day, while their master goes to work. Or for animals raised in city settings; animals that must walk and urinate on concrete and have lost the feeling of grass under their paws. When these animals seem sluggish, especially if they do not have enough mental challenges in their lives and lack the stimulation of contact with anyone other than their masters, give Hornbeam to help them deal with their unnatural life and their boredom.

### Hornbeam and the Homeopathic Pharmacy

Patients needing the homeopathic remedy Carbo Vegetabilis, made from charcoal, also eat too much and exercise too little. They have reached the point in their lives when they feel they are suffocating. They can't digest anything else that is happening to them. Both of these types are living too much in their minds, to the detriment of their physical bodies.

### Issues that Suggest Hornbeam

Allergy; chronic fatigue syndrome; depression; exhaustion; eye pain; hay fever; insomnia and nightmares; overweight; swelling, especially in the feet; thyroid troubles; varicose veins.

### In Conclusion

The need for Hornbeam can manifest itself in several ways. The patient may want to achieve some sort of success or perform tasks of great value to his community. But the patient may be unsure—not of the sort of thing that he would like to do, but of his own ability to do it. Hornbeams can be powerfully caught up in self-criticism. The emotional state that he may believe is based in modesty or realism is, instead, based upon uncertainty about his own value as a human being and a questioning of his own self-worth.

Or Hornbeam might reveal itself in the person who seems lacking in drive or ambition, while still yearning to "make something of himself." He labors on in a job or in a relationship that makes him feel as if he were sleepwalking through his life. He feels numb, bored with the days of his life.

Or Hornbeam may be even more lethargic, and may seem disinterested in work, in accomplishment, and in taking on the trappings of mature life—marriage, house ownership, and parenthood. This Hornbeam may spend most of his time on the couch in front of the television or at his computer, enjoying some aspect of electronic media.

Or Hornbeam can be in a state of being overwhelmed, and can look a bit like Elm. But where the Elm is overwhelmed by challenges and the demands of his work, the Hornbeam is overwhelmed with the tedium of his work. He is quite often overwhelmed not by the actual work but by the effort he exerts to avoid doing his work or accomplishing his daily tasks.

However the negative emotional state of Hornbeam is expressed in the individual, the Hornbeam state is always one of emotional exhaustion and the weight of lethargy. The emotional exhaustion may be mirrored in the physical body, but it can be thrown off quickly when the Hornbeam's intellectual interest or sense of humor is stimulated. The negative Hornbeam state is therefore something of a morass. Like the caged hamster who runs on the wheel in his cage, the Hornbeam feels that he is on the run, but getting nowhere.

## GORSE · THE REMEDY FOR THOSE WHO ARE WITHOUT HOPE

Bach writes, "Gorse is for the person afflicted with very great hopelessness, they have given up belief that more can be done for them. Under persuasion or to please others they may try different treatments, at the same time assuring those around them that there is so little hope of relief."

• **Gorse is both an acute and a constitutional remedy.**

### Botanical Information

The fact that Gorse (*Ulex Europaeus*), native to Europe, grows well in stony ground seems particularly apt to the remedy taken from its flowers, which bloom in the early spring. The flowers are fragrant and brightly colored, often bright yellow. Today it is grown as a hedge or shrub, but it is often considered a weed, especially in the United States.

## Gorse in General

Gorse is an important remedy and speaks to a very common negative emotional state. Gorse is effective for those who have lost a sense of hope. This hopeless state can be turned toward the self—and Gorse is often called for in cases involving long-term or debilitating diseases—or outward toward others, even toward the world.

The Gorse state can be created in many ways, but each of these involves a loss or a number of losses that have, cumulatively, robbed the patient of his or her sense of well-being and trust in the world or in God. Certainly, the events the last few years in human history have robbed many of us of some aspect of hope for the world and for the future. We have seen and experienced much that informs us that there is little reason to hope. And yet, we must remind ourselves daily that there are few greater losses we could experience than the loss of hope itself.

As the Gorse state of hopelessness is an aspect of Bach's mood Doubt, we have a particular difficulty when we wrestle with the Gorse mindset. The Gorse type can always easily give very valid reasons, based on specific personal circumstances or world events, why they have little reason to hope. In fact, many in the Gorse state will be able to build a solid case why it would be foolish for them to hope. They feel, while in the Gorse state, that they are being logical, level-headed, and sensible. They tend to feel that their setting aside of hope is a triumph of the logical mind and not an emotional state at all. As with Gentian and other remedies in this group, patients needing Gorse tend to feel that they are not in an emotional state at all, positive or negative, but that they are in a clear-headed mental state. Hopelessness is not a negative state to the patient who needs Gorse, and for this reason the Gorse type can be very hard to treat.

This is particularly true for the Gorse whose negativity is based in chronic illness, especially chronic pain. These patients carry the daily burden of real suffering, and have been told by the best doctors money can buy that they will have this burden for as long as they live. An argument could be made in these cases that the Gorse state itself was placed upon the poor patient by an idiot of a doctor, who has substituted his small amount of education and knowledge of the human body's ability to heal for something much more powerful—the force of hope. The doctor who thinks he must give his patient the truth as he sees it and, as a result, takes away his patient's natural ability to hope does a terrible thing. And the burden of negativity that he places upon his patient reverberates throughout that patient's home and family and community. In my opinion, that doctor has much to answer for.

But even in extremely negative situations, Gorse does a wonderful thing—it actu-

ally can take a patient who has lost hope, who has given up on ever feeling better or
ever returning to the freedom that he once felt from limitation and pain, and give him
back the will to live. It can take the patient who has given up the struggle with his disease and resigned himself to the most negative outcome possible and allow him to
rally and wish to be well once more. In doing this, Gorse can also stimulate the
patient's ability to heal and help turn around a situation that seemed quite hopeless to
everyone.

In any situation, Gorse can help bring hope back into the equation. Considering
that the New Testament lists hope, along with faith and love, as the three greatest and
most powerful virtues of the human heart, this is a powerful remedy, because these are
the three most powerful tools we have for building and maintaining a full and happy life.
In abandoning hope[3] the patient has abandoned a powerful tool for renewal and transformation. He is forced to approach his illness with one less means of eliminating it.

It is possible to confuse the need for Gentian and Gorse because of their joint tendency toward Doubt, and because of the unique combination of mind and emotion that
each negative emotional state involves. Both seem to be pessimistic people on the surface. Both are negative and can be difficult to be around. Both may seem self-pitying
and complaining.

But stop and think about these two negative emotional states and you will see the
difference. Remember, the Gentian is not completely without hope. In fact, he tends to
enter into each new prospect with a small sense that it will be very successful. This is
true whether the prospect at hand relates to the patient's personal health—perhaps he
has found a new doctor or treatment that inspires some sense of hope—or to a new relationship or job. It is not until some small difficulty arises that the Gentian wants to give
up. His problem is not a lack of hope, but a willingness to throw it away too quickly in
times of trouble. The Gentian lacks the ability to put troubles in proportion and judge
honestly whether or not the struggle at hand is worth the effort. He always feels that
any struggle is not worth the effort or that any confrontation is to be avoided.

The Gorse, on the other hand, lacks hope in dealing with all things. He struggles
on, trying to use reason in place of hope, and finds, to his increasing distress, that his
sense of reason cannot sustain him as hope would.

As Mimulus and Aspen deal with two closely intertwined aspects of fear, the
known fear and the fear of the unknown, Gentian and Gorse are closely related and
intertwined in their ability to work with the powerful negative state of doubt. Just as
both Mimulus and Aspen are often needed to complete a case, either one at a time or

3. I think that the commonly used phrase "abandon hope" is another case in which language, the
way we subconsciously phrase things as a culture, reveals our truths and beliefs. Hope is an aspect of
life, and a link to our faith, that is always with us. It never leaves us; to lose hope, we must abandon it.

combined, Gentian and Gorse are often used together for the patient wrestling with the negative power of Doubt as it embodies itself in the aspect of hopelessness.

Because of the nature of the Gorse state, I believe it is most commonly called for and best used as a chronic or constitutional remedy. Those who need Gorse are likely to need it for an extended period of time. While it may be of value as an acute remedy at times—for a momentary period of hopelessness brought on by very bad news, or a change in situation that seems impossible to overcome—it is most often needed as a constitutional remedy. People do not enter the Gorse state of negativity overnight. They are most often worn down into it by a long struggle with their health, their career, or their personal life. Most of us do not willingly abandon our innate sense of hope. It has to be taken from us, bit by bit, over a period of time.

> People do not enter the Gorse state of negativity overnight. Most of us do not willingly abandon our innate sense of hope. It has to be taken from us, bit by bit, over a period of time.

Therefore, I usually find that Gentian is the most helpful remedy for the small periods of our lives when we wrestle with a loss of hope because of the loss of a job or a relationship and save Gorse as a follow up, if needed. Gorse comes into its full value in deeper, more established cases. It has proven itself a powerful tool for bringing hope to those who are hopeless.

Two other remedies combine particularly well with Gorse.

The first is Sweet Chestnut. Use this remedy for the patient who not only has lost his sense of hope over a period of time, but who now is in a state of desperation due to some new crisis of health or finances or world events. Who quite literally does not know how he will get through the next day. In this very serious situation, the combination of Gorse and Sweet Chestnut will work much more powerfully than either remedy alone.

Another powerful combination is Gorse and Wild Rose. While the patient needing Gorse is in a state of hopelessness, the patient needing Wild Rose is apathetic. He has given up and no longer shows interest in any challenge, great or small. These two very negative remedies combine to form a compound remedy that will help the patient who has just given up, because of their perceived hopeless case. Their interest in any aspect of life is now gone. They have turned their face to the wall.

## Negative Qualities of the Type

Perhaps the most negative thing I have found to be true about Gorse is that those needing the remedy usually have begun to define themselves in terms of their illness (or their otherwise hopeless situation). They seem endlessly fascinated with the disease process and have researched it thoroughly. Disease has taken the place that a calling of some sort should have in their life. They weigh themselves and those they love down with the weight of their disease, giving it name, face, and body. Their hopelessness has almost made a demon of the disease, allowing it to possess them in body and soul.

Even for those whose Gorse state does not relate to a particular disease, the utter negativity of the state itself is toxic to everyone in their environment. Like many other deeply negative emotional states, the Gorse state actually seems communicable. It spreads from person to person as the patient lays out his well-researched and reasoned case showing that events are now in control, not the people involved in those events, and that everyone would do well to accept this.

The negativity of the Gorse state can bring darkness into the sunniest mind and bring all potential and forward motion to a screeching halt. It is a powerful and negative mindset that can have terrible results. When dealing with it, it is important to remember that, terrible and negative as the Gorse state is, even it is not hopeless.

### Positive Qualities of the Type

The Gorse patient who has moved through the negative to the more positive state of being becomes somewhat of an evangelist. These patients become motivators, natural healers. They believe in miracles of all sizes, shapes, and colors. They use hope as a force that can power profound changes in our lives. They are charismatic in the true sense of the word, spirit-filled individuals who can persuade the most negative person that good will triumph and that everything will come out right in the end.

### The Gorse Child

The Gorse child is a fairly rare type. But it does occur, most often in seriously ill children. They tend to be children with dark circles under their eyes. They live in an environment defined by the limitations imposed by their disease and enhanced by their parents' and doctors' fears, as well as by medical equipment and medication. They see their disease as their function in life, and must be taught that, no matter how hard the struggle, they need not allow their souls to become ill even if their body faces serious illness.

Other very stressful situations can create a Gorse state in childhood. Children who have experienced war or who have been caught up in tragic world events, such as the Great Depression, can become trapped in the Gorse mindset.

Generally children who need Gorse seem older than their years and have concerns—about finances, about the world around them—that are somewhat uncommon in other children of their age.

### The Gorse Adult

Like Oak and Willow and other long-term negative emotional states, Gorse is most common in middle-aged and elderly patients. Most of us are able to take our health for granted when we are younger. It is not until we reach our middle years that we realize that our health must be cherished just as those who are loyal to us must be cherished, and that those things given to us by life must be appreciated. Often it is not until it is too late that this lesson is learned.

Many of us feel that we have been betrayed by our own bodies when they suddenly begin to succumb to chronic and painful conditions. We fail to see that the decline in our health was not a sudden thing at all, but the outcome of years of neglect and ignorance. Our lives take on a new chapter with the onset of chronic illness. We play by a new set of rules, and anyone who has entered the frightening world of doctor's offices and medical labs knows firsthand that the rules we play by are not our own. Illness often includes more than just limitation or pain. It includes a loss of self and of our natural ability to determine our future. We must, to one extent or another, turn over our personal power to others and hope for the best.

When the best does not happen, when we are told to expect the worst instead, a wound is created in our ability to hope, and that wound may never heal.[4]

Often in these cases, especially in older patients, the Gorse state will link with the negative Willow state, making for bitter patients who find themselves highly dissatisfied with the outcome of their treatment and lacking hope for any future positive outcome. Our medical industry has created millions of Willow/Gorse types, both by the failure of their largely allopathic treatments and by the way medical personnel—doctors, nurses, and technicians all included—speak with and treat their patients.

## The Gorse Animal

This is another remedy I find to be almost useless for the treatment of animals. Not because I think animals cannot give up hope in times of deep distress, but because I lack the ability to "read" animals well enough to know when it can be of help. You might consider using Gorse for an animal you suspect has had terrible abuse in the past, that seems disconnected from its present situation, as if it had given up hope.

## Gorse and the Homeopathic Pharmacy

The homeopathic Phosphoric Acid has much in common with Gorse patients. Like Gorse, they are chronically ill and beaten down by the process of illness. They are needy for both treatment and attention from medical practitioners, family members, and friends alike.

---

4. While I use chronic illness as my example, you may substitute anything here that might cause a person to lose hope. They may be terribly betrayed by their life's mate, or they may put their whole heart and soul into a particular work and find failure instead of success. The important point is that their sense of hope has been wounded—once or a thousand times—and that the wound festers and does not heal.

## Issues that Suggest Gorse

Aging; AIDS; apathy; cancer; chronic fatigue; chronic illness of all sorts; death and dying; depression; lymph troubles; lupus; multiple sclerosis; pregnancy.

## In Conclusion

One important aspect of the remedy state remains to be answered, and that is: What can we expect Gorse to do when it is used correctly?

Too often, I think, we want Gorse to do more than help the patient cope with his situation, see it honestly with both his mind and heart, and move through it in the best way possible. We also want the remedy to fix the situation, whatever it is.

Again, the problem when working with Doubt remedies is that the patient experiencing doubt is trying to balance a sense of hope—a force that informs him that he need not always yield to his present situation, however terrible it is, but that he may see some external force improve his life—with a sense of logic built on the circumstances he witnesses daily with his eyes, his ears, and his mind. When we are in a state of proper balance, we can use the information we receive through our senses to inform our minds without draining our hearts of a sense of hope. We are able to move forward doing our best, battling when we can, and yielding when we must. Hope and reason work together to build a better world.

The patient in a Gorse state has lost the message of the heart and has only the message sent by his mind. He is, therefore, out of balance. In his present negative state he receives only a negative message that reinforces itself over and over again. And, as the negativity reinforces itself, the possibility of a negative outcome intensifies.

Remember, Bach wrote again and again that his patients' emotional states moved from negative to positive and their physical maladies faded away as he treated them with his remedies. When we use Bach remedies today, we tend to think that they don't really affect the body, that they only calm the mind. But perhaps we are limiting their capabilities because we have lowered our expectations of what these remedies can do.

What I am saying is this: When you give Gorse to a person who lacks hope, you are helping him hear the message of his heart once more. That he is in the right place. That all is right with the world. That things will turn out for the best. Those messages, at the very least, will help the patient look at his present situation—which may in all reality be hopeless—so he can face squarely what is ahead and live the life he has in the best means possible. All that he has lost emotionally can be restored. Humor can return. Belief can return. Hope can return. I cannot say for sure what that will mean in terms of physical health or financial success. I only know that it might, it just might, be enough to make the difference.

## SCLERANTHUS · THE REMEDY FOR THOSE WHO ARE INDECISIVE

Bach writes, "Scleranthus is for those who suffer much from being unable to decide between two things, first one seeming right then the other. They are usually quiet people, and bear their difficulty alone, as they are not inclined to discuss it with others."

- **Scleranthus is both an acute and a constitutional remedy.**
- **Scleranthus is one of Bach's original remedies, the Twelve Healers.**

### Botanical Information

Given the emotional state of the remedy, it should come as no surprise that the plant called Scleranthus (*Scleranthus Annuus*) features both multiple stalks and a weak root system. It is a very small annual plant that is often considered a weed.

Scleranthus is native to Northern Europe, where it is commonly found in railway yards, fields, and roadways. It now grows in temperate regions worldwide.

The plant also shows its duality in its flowering. It often flowers in March and again in October.

### Scleranthus in General

The negative emotional state suggested by the need for Scleranthus is fairly simple and easy to understand. The Scleranthus type has difficulty making choices in both the acute and the constitutional state. Even if the Scleranthus manages to make a choice between two alternatives, he or she will have even more difficulty sticking with their decision and not changing their mind. Scleranthus begins the decision-making process by narrowing the field of choices (think of these choices as being like the entrees listed on a restaurant menu) down to two. This is, for the Scleranthus, a simple process. The Scleranthus then has a great deal of difficulty selecting between these last two choices. Each will seem appropriate or desirable in its way, and each time the Scleranthus decides that choice A is definitely better than choice B, choice B will again begin to look pretty good. Scleranthus is trapped in a loop, constantly vacillating between two possibilities.

On first glance, Scleranthus seems to be a narrow remedy of less importance than the other Bach remedies, especially when compared to the others grouped here as aspects of Doubt. The fact that the poor Scleranthus is having trouble deciding between two jobs, two loves, or, indeed, two entrees, seems a rather minor thing and perhaps not even worthy of treatment. You have to look beneath the surface dither common to the Scleranthus type to get a better picture of the remedy and its implications.

First, this is a remedy that deals with self-confidence and self-worth. The Scleranthus patient on a fundamental level simply cannot or will not trust himself. He feels he is incapable of making strong decisions for his own benefit. He has turned his sense of Doubt, which links all the remedies grouped here, inward upon himself. Because of this, the Scleranthus type is often easily led, not only when it comes to the decision at hand, but in all things. Those who need the remedy in a constitutional manner are often shy and quiet people, people who welcome abdicating their decisions to other, stronger personalities.

At the same time, the Scleranthus type will be eager to mask his inner sense of doubt. He does not want others to know how much stress—even torment—he feels when he is asked to make the same decisions that others make so easily. And so the Scleranthus often just does nothing. He waits, hoping that someone else will make his decisions for him. If he is told that the chicken is much better than the fish, he will smile agreeably and order the chicken, much relieved that the onus of the decision has been borne by another.

> Scleranthus types are able to narrow a decision from infinite possibilities to just two: two entrees, two lovers, two gift ideas. But then they are unable to make the final commitment to just one choice. And that is the great fear inside Scleranthus— making a commitment.

Scleranthus is also a remedy of duality. There is something of fissure that has formed within the emotional being of patients chronically struggling with Scleranthus' self-doubt. In their love life, they will quite honestly find themselves loving two very different people at the same time. Each speaks to a different aspect of their duality. One may strengthen their desire to settle down and buy a house; the other may make them want to move to Greenwich Village and live in a loft. Each life path speaks to an aspect of the Scleranthus' dual desires and brings joy to an aspect of their dual natures. Scleranthus types are forced, however, to make a choice—either of which is virtually guaranteed to bring them at least some aspect of joy—and cannot.[5]

Scleranthus types often are perceived as being erratic, even foolish, but they are more intelligent than they appear. The Scleranthus lacks internal balance and a defined sense of self.

---

5. Many constitutional Scleranthus types will find themselves locked into this pattern—it is perhaps the most common for them. In most cases, the situation resolves itself in time without the Scleranthus actually making a decision. As usual, he waits, juggling the two loves until they either tire of his lack of commitment or find out about each other. In the end, both usually leave him, making his decision for him. In some cases, one will walk away and the other can claim the Scleranthus, who rather passively remains in the relationship, until another love enters the picture at some point in the future. Either way, the cycle is bound to repeat itself once more with Scleranthus again dithering between two loves.

They are able to narrow a decision from infinite possibilities to just two: two entrees, two lovers, two gift ideas. But then they are unable to make the final commitment to just one choice. And that is the great fear inside Scleranthus—making a commitment.

They will not even want to commit to one topic of conversation or stand up for one side of an argument, but will discuss opposing viewpoints with equal fervor.

These are patients who are victims of their own failure to commit. This may even be embodied physically and they may move in a jerky manner, as if unable to commit to the next forward step. They may also tend to be somewhat clumsy, and their energy level will vary as greatly as their mood vacillates. For this reason, Scleranthus is often a remedy that can offer help to patients with physical ailments that involve muscle wasting, such as multiple sclerosis.

In the same way, Scleranthus is also often needed to help patients with either acute or chronic inner-ear problems that rob them of their sense of balance.

Scleranthus patients can be very difficult for their physicians to treat, because their symptoms can seem as vacillating as their moods or choices. Scleranthus patients' aches and pains tend to constantly change and evolve, leaving the poor doctor to wrestle with a physical condition that seems to defy logic and medicine as he understands them.

The patient who chronically needs Scleranthus can become something of an extremist over time. He will swing like a pendulum from one extreme state to another, passing over all the more moderate states in between. He will drink to excess for a period of time, only to abstain completely when he becomes convinced that it is bad for him to drink. In the same way, he can move from being thrifty to spending wildly, seemingly overnight and without reason. And that can be key to the experience of those who know the Scleranthus and, especially, of those who love him. The Scleranthus seems an erratic, unstable person, who appears to flit from one stand, one idea, one relationship, one undertaking to another, apparently without reason.

The Scleranthus trapped within this pattern can seem a very weak person. He can resemble the patient needing Cerato, another remedy for Doubt. Both of these types are shy and rather weak people and both are easily led. There is one difference, though—and this difference explains why these two remedies are very seldom mixed together. When choosing a remedy for a patient with a weak sense of self and self-trust, you will often choose between them.

The Cerato will ask the help of everyone he knows. He is society's natural polltaker, going from person to person soliciting opinions, often with no real interest in that specific person's ideas. The Scleranthus, on the other hand, is rather stoic, even though he is equally plagued by Doubt. He chooses not to ask for help even when it could easily be supplied. Instead, he waits and wrestles with himself over the decision at hand. And since life is made up of a good many decisions, the wrestling match can be a long one.

Thus, life can be very stressful for the patient who needs Scleranthus, either acutely or chronically. No other type wants to "have their cake and to eat it too" so much. Think of all they are quietly balancing: their fear of commitment, their lack of self-worth, their constant belief that they will be making the wrong decision whatever they choose to do, and, on top of it all, their strong desire that no one else suspects they are having difficulty with the issues that torment them. Like Mimulus (a remedy that often is used in combination with Scleranthus), the Scleranthus will expend a great deal of energy to make sure no one suspects that they are as indecisive as they are.

We all need the remedy Scleranthus from time to time. Not only for those moments when we must choose between the chicken and the fish, but also for the moments of distraction. Scleranthus can be very helpful when we are having trouble concentrating, not because of boredom, but because our minds seem inundated with new ideas and tremendous possibilities. When we are in a dither, when we lack focus,[6] when we don't know how best to move forward, either in the moment or with our lives, Scleranthus is the remedy that can help.

Most of us only need Scleranthus in passing, and a dose or two will help us get underway again. But those who suffer chronically from a lack of commitment and coherence in life may need to stay with the remedy for a time, or combine it with other remedies.

Scleranthus is commonly combined with either Aspen or Mimulus, or with Wild Oat or Clematis. Most often, if fear mingles with the Scleranthus emotional state, you will have to choose between Aspen and Mimulus. I find that Mimulus is especially helpful to the fearful Scleranthus, who expends so much energy trying to deny his negative emotions. But the vagueness of Aspen's anxious fear can show itself in Scleranthus' chronic vagueness.

Scleranthus often combines with Wild Oat for patients in the midst of a real life crisis who have no idea as to who they are, what they want, and how to move forward

---

6. The word "focus" reminds me of another use of this remedy that relates to the physical body. Scleranthus is of tremendous help for patients who have amblyopia, or what is commonly called "lazy eye." For most of us, our eyes form with a natural bond between them. They are "yoked," as doctors call it, taking in information as a team, and wired to supply the brain with a three dimensional image from which it can extract information about its environment. The person born with a lazy eye tends to see with one eye at a time, which results in a flat, two-dimensional environment. Because of this lack of yoking, patients with lazy eye will often move into a Scleranthus mode, and sometimes even develop two strong dual natures, each responding depending upon which eye is dominant. When Scleranthus amblyopes move from a left eye to a right eye stance, seemingly overnight, they tend to undo decisions they made before and swing from one extreme lifestyle to another. For this reason, those with amblyopia have been considered to suffer from a form of schizophrenia in the past.

in life. This can be the case with the patient who has lost a loved one or a career—anything that makes the patient feel as if the rug has been pulled out from under him, and leaves him in a state of frozen confusion.

Use Clematis with Scleranthus for the patient who is the vaguest of the vague. Since the Clematis state is one of indifference and Scleranthus speaks to Doubt, this combination is needed when the patient has reached a state in which he is in an almost constant state of daydreaming and withdrawal from dealing with life and its commitments.

### Negative Qualities of the Type

Those who are trapped in the negative emotional state of Scleranthus are pile-makers. They litter their thoughts and their desks alike with ideas, projects, and possibilities. Constitutional Scleranthus types often start several projects at once, knowing that they are incapable of finishing all of them. In the same way, they start several potential relationships at once, knowing that they cannot dedicate themselves to all of them. They do this with the hope that all will resolve on their own, that the need to commit or decide will be taken from their own shoulders and placed upon someone else's.

Some of the signs that you are dealing with a Scleranthus include chronic lateness, chronic confusion, and an irritating inability to finish anything or commit to anything, including a simple lunch date. Those needing Scleranthus may be very pleasant and, on the surface at least, quite willing to work with you and give you their full attention and best efforts. Underneath, however, they are unsure as to whether or not they ever want to work with you or see you again.

Thus, in its chronic phase, Scleranthus patients display perfect passive-aggressive qualities. They will tell you exactly what they think you want to hear, often will promise anything to get you to hang up the phone or leave, and then will do exactly the opposite of what they have told you.

Like Ceratos and other "weak" personality types, Scleranthus hates confrontation and cannot understand why he seems to elicit so many of them. He does not realize that others are unaware of his inner vacillation. They cannot understand why he does not say what he is going to do and do what he promised he would. The more the Scleranthus feels pinned down, the more he will struggle to get away. And yet, he will continue to be unable to take real action. When he wants to end a job he will seek to be fired, rather than have to take responsibility for his decision. When he wants to leave a relationship he will seek to get dumped, so someone else has the responsibility for ending it.

### Positive Qualities of the Type

Scleranthus can be brought into balance if they can move from a negative to a positive emotional state. While they will still possess the duality that lives within us all, they will be able, by balancing the opposites, to see all the potential positions that lie in between.

This balanced position opens the Scleranthus up to all the potential thoughts and ideas that lie before him, and allows him to have a refreshed and creative viewpoint brimming over with innovative ideas. These ideas, which once so easily overwhelmed the Scleranthus, are now a wellspring of possibilities from which he is able to select. And once he has decided on his choices he is able to take full responsibility for both his successes and failures.

Also, Scleranthus types develop—while remaining a person capable of seeing all sides of an issue—a great gift of concentration and mental focus. They will not be dissuaded from their path once they have chosen it, because they have learned to trust their own mind as the best guide in all situations. Gone is the self-punishment linked to Scleranthus' inability to make a commitment. Gone is the self-doubt that once controlled their lives. These are replaced by the joy they feel from knowing they have moved ahead in life having made the choice that was right for them.

### The Scleranthus Child

The Scleranthus child will often physicalize his emotional duress. Look for this child to have travel sickness, vertigo, and mood swings. This is a hesitant child, who will look to his parents with the hope that they will tell him what to do instead of making up his mind for himself. The Scleranthus child needs to be taught that life is filled with decisions. That we all make, in the course of our lifetime, some very good decisions and some very bad ones. And that, either way, we must accept the responsibility for our decisions and act accordingly. The Scleranthus child must learn that they will gain nothing and often risk everything by avoiding decisions and the commitments that decisions bring.

Further, parents must be careful not to instill or enhance a Scleranthus state in their child by robbing him of the opportunity to make decisions, or by allowing him to avoid the responsibilities of his decisions. An overbearing parent often raises a Scleranthus child, who has learned to give over his own rightful decision making power into the hands of a dominant figure.

### The Scleranthus Adult

This is one of the Bach types in which the childhood state and the adult state are much the same. This does not come as a surprise, since there is something rather infantile about the Scleranthus type's inability to trust himself and make his own decisions in life. Scleranthus types often present themselves as childlike. They may be quite youthful in their language, dress, and behavior.

In the most extreme form of the negative emotional type, the Scleranthus patient can display a strong duality, as if two minds were living in the same body. Scleranthus types are usually strongly introverted people who do not share their troubles with others, but sit silently wrestling with themselves. To others they seem flighty, disconnected, and emotionally out of balance. Often the Scleranthus type will have any number of health problems, and will drive their doctor crazy with their bizarre number of troubles.

### The Scleranthus Animal

I have never found an acute use for this remedy for an animal. However, it can be very helpful for animals that have a strong pattern of erratic behavior or a dual nature. For the animal that is docile and quite friendly at times and very aggressive at others, think about Scleranthus.

### Scleranthus and the Homeopathic Pharmacy

Many would put Pulsatilla in the category of Scleranthus, and I can see why: they have much in common in their erratic moods and lack of self-confidence.

But I also see a strong parallel with the homeopathic remedy Mercurius. Both have a specific duality of nature, an inability to hold a consistent level of energy in their body or mind, and an inability to cope with changes in their personal environment—changes as simple as minor fluctuations in temperature. Mercury, as a substance, is unable to hold its own shape and adapts endlessly to environmental changes. Perhaps because of this, as a remedy type it suggests a patient who is easily overwhelmed—who loses emotional shape—and who is wildly sensitive to a change of any sort, particularly to changes in weather and temperature.

### Issues that Suggest Scleranthus

Amblyopia; asthma and other breathing problems; constipation; diarrhea; eating disorders; exhaustion; fevers of unknown origin; inner ear problems; insomnia; vertigo; irritable bowel syndrome; morning sickness in pregnancy; muscle-wasting diseases; psychosomatic illnesses; travel sickness.

### In Conclusion

One more thought about Scleranthus: the Scleranthus type will most often avoid decisions because of a very specific fear—the fear that anything, once decided, cannot be changed. The fear is a fear of being locked in, closed in. For this reason, you will often find that the patient needing Scleranthus, especially in a constitutional manner, will have severe claustrophobia. He may also fear the dark, in that it also represents a trap. Or he may manifest his fear in a fear of deep water, even of crossing water in a boat or on a bridge.

The Scleranthus does not want to be trapped, but his avoidance of decision making tends to attract stronger personalities who make his decisions for him. He thus becomes quite literally trapped, in a situation he feels he cannot survive. So the Scleranthus uses his innate indecision as a way out—finding some other equally strong type who offers the promise of a new life and a new way of doing things. And the Scleranthus sets up his pattern of "double-whammy," escaping to a new life only to have the past repeat itself in new surroundings.

Like most of the constitutional Bach types, Scleranthus, in working as energetically as he can to block a particularly dreaded situation, will, in the end, only succeed in creating the very thing he dreaded. Because he fears both the decision and the commitment that it brings, he yields his power of decision-making to another and, as a result, ends up having a commitment forced upon him—a commitment to a decision made by another.

Scleranthus types locked into this passive-aggressive mode of living usually respond well to the combination of Scleranthus and Chestnut Bud, as the Chestnut Bud helps open their eyes to the patterning of their lives and helps them find new strategies for success and survival.

## CERATO · THE REMEDY FOR THOSE WITH SELF-DOUBT

Bach comments, "Cerato is for those who have not sufficient confidence in themselves to make their own decisions. They constantly seek advice from others, and are often misguided."

- **Cerato is both an acute and a constitutional remedy.**
- **Cerato is one of Bach's original remedies, the Twelve Healers.**

### Botanical Information

Also known as "Palmgold," the Cerato (*Ceratostigma Willmottiana*) plant is a small shrub that grows to two feet tall. It is native to the Himalayas but has been cultivated in the Western world. It has cobalt blue tubular-shaped flowers that bloom in fall, usually in September. It is known for the golden color of its leaves, which in combination with the red stems of the flowers and the blue flowers themselves, makes for a striking addition to any garden.

### Cerato in General

Of the six remedies grouped under the "mood" of Doubt, two are rather similar and can be confused for each other. The first of these is Scleranthus, the remedy that precedes this one in this text. The other is Cerato.

Both Scleranthus and Cerato turn their Doubt inward. Both lack a sense of self-trust that would allow them to act decisively in life and give them the freedom to reach for their goals. A third remedy, Wild Oat, is another Doubt remedy that follows Cerato in this text. This remedy also turns Doubt inward but, in doing so, undermines the patient's ability to actually form goals. Both Cerato and Scleranthus can set goals and have solid wants and desires, but neither can direct themselves to achieve those goals. Both types tend to be rather shy and can be perceived by others as being passive and weak.

The difference between these two types—both sharing a fear of simply telling other people what they want and of working hard to get it—is that the Scleranthus hides his indecision and tries to protect his weak will, while the Cerato all but advertises the fact that he is unsure of himself and his abilities.

> Cerato is the remedy for insecurity, either as an acute emotional state, or as a chronic condition that undermines a patient's ability to live their life fully and creatively.

Ceratos lack confidence in themselves and do not try to overcompensate because of it. Instead they take on a victim role, walking through life looking for help, testing out every decision and idea on anyone willing to play along. Ceratos seek to push off their personal responsibility onto those others. They are, in essence, always seeking a way they can honestly say that their failures are not their own fault. They are looking for others they can turn and say, "Look what you made me do."

Cerato, therefore, is the remedy for insecurity, either as an acute emotional state, or as a chronic condition that undermines a patient's ability to live their life fully and creatively. The riddle that the Cerato negative emotional state presents is that the Cerato[7] wants to please, wants to get the job done right, but just doesn't know how. This mindset allows a great many mistakes, multiple high jinks, all without any actual personal responsibility for the Cerato, who is trying his or her very best to get things right. At their most maddening, Ceratos come across like Lucille Ball on *I Love Lucy*, especially when she worked behind the conveyor belt at the candy factory. Ceratos tend toward that same expression of dumb surprise when their attempts fail, and tend to require overpowering Cuban bandleader husbands to keep them on budget and in line.

The Cerato sticks out like a sore thumb in the dynamic of every family or every

---

7. I had to resist the urge to type "poor Cerato," instead of just "Cerato" in that sentence. I refused to write it because that idea of "poor" is part and parcel with Cerato's negative state. Ceratos tend to see themselves a victims, as people who are attempting to do everything right but just don't know how. In this way, they tend to project their insecurity onto others. Others, as a result, tend to refer to the Cerato as the neighbors on *Knott's Landing* did when they kept calling one sweet, dumb character "Poor Val."

office. He or she is the one tires are changed for and dishes are washed because, in the end, it is easier just to do it yourself rather than have to redo it after the Cerato is done.

We tend to both enjoy and encourage the Cerato state in women, especially in love relationships. The "man's man" may enjoy the almost infantile state the woman retreats into when she leaves all responsibility for finances, lifestyle, and personal decision making up to her husband. In men, we culturally tend to find the Cerato state rather disgusting and inappropriate, since men in our society are supposed to be strong and uncomplaining.

And Ceratos do complain. They love to tell their troubles to anyone who will listen. They can be very clingy when they are ill or in distress. For this reason, the remedy Cerato blends well with Heather when Ceratos are at their most insecure and needy—especially for situations that I think of as being on the "dawn patrol," when the Cerato needs to be sat with and counseled throughout the long, dark night.

Cerato is often combined with either or both Mimulus or Aspen—two of our most-used fear remedies. Ceratos can have severe phobias—being alone and being in the dark are two of the most common—and therefore often benefit from combining Cerato with Mimulus. They can also need Aspen in cases where their fear is more free-form and more of a dread of what will happen next. Ceratos often lock onto a pattern of overconcern for others, especially for those upon whom they are dependent, and will tend to worry constantly. In these cases, combine Cerato with Red Chestnut.

In the constitutional Cerato type, the patient will lack an inner voice, a sense of self-direction. In some cases, this sense of inner strength and guidance is totally lacking. In other cases it exists, but the patient has entered into a mental and emotional pattern in which that voice is drowned out by the chatter of the patient's own inner dialogue, leaving the patient unsure of himself and unable to direct himself as he should.

This leaves the Cerato type vulnerable to stronger and more directed types. The Cerato who comes under the influence of a Vervain, a Vine, or a Rock Water may soon find himself living in the California desert in some sort of commune and eating a strict vegetarian diet. He may also find that he has divested all his worldly goods to the commune after having been led out of a personal crisis by the Vine, after having been moved emotionally by the charismatic words of the Vervain, or after having had his diet turned upside down by the Rock Water. In any of these cases, and in others like them, the Cerato is likely to yield much of his personal power to a more dominant personality for one simple reason: that person seems to be surer of himself than is the Cerato.

Now, to be sure, the above examples are extreme, but in truth Ceratos will seek others to whom they can yield their personal power and responsibility. For this reason, they will marry much stronger personalities, they will take jobs with critical and overpowering bosses, they will join the military—anything that will give them their path in life and lay out for them, step by step, what they are to do and when and how they are to do it.

Even more common are less extreme examples of Cerato behavior. Any time we do not trust our own judgment, any time we consider ordering some product from television just because a supposed expert tells us that it is the latest thing for weight loss, we should consider a dose of Cerato. Any time we are directed externally, listening to a loud voice in our ear instead of that "still, small" inner voice, we need Cerato.

We all lack a sense of ourselves from time to time. Sometimes we are insecure about ourselves, our abilities, and especially our appearance—that's the hook by which many of us are caught. Some people can be incredibly secure in their minds, their abilities, but fall apart when it comes to their weight or their jowls. These people need Cerato just as much as the overly-chipper girl who moves from desk to desk at the office, trying to get someone to advise her about her new boyfriend.

This brings up another strong factor in Cerato's behavior—false cheerfulness. As I have said, Ceratos do not mask their insecurity as Scleranthus will. Instead, they mask the sadness, even the despair they feel as a result of the mistakes they have made due to their insecurity. Ceratos have decided, somewhere along the way, that if they laugh at themselves first, others will laugh with them and not at them. And they take on a rather heartbreaking tendency to use a syrupy sweetness and mock joy as their emotional mask. Ceratos certainly want to be liked. They want to be everyone's friend. This is a very important need for Ceratos—they must exist in a place of goodwill to function at all well.

Another tendency of Cerato types is that they talk too much. They ask too many questions, sometimes out of a real desire for knowledge (Ceratos tend to crave knowledge and information, but lack the ability to put it to use), sometimes just to talk. Lacking an inner voice, they can come to love the sound of their physical voice.

It may be necessary to look below the surface to get it right when selecting the appropriate remedy for an overly cheerful type. False cheerfulness and a tendency to talk too much can cause Cerato to be confused with Agrimony, a remedy for oversensitivity that masks emotional aches and pains with a cheerful mask and an oft-repeated set of "humorous" monologues. But Agrimony lacks honesty with himself and others. He often has some specific terrible memory he is trying to escape (often with the help of alcohol or drugs), but he does not lack a sense of self.

## Negative Qualities of the Type

Simply put, the negative Cerato emotional state is a drain upon the patient's own energy and the energy of all those around him. The Cerato wants advice, he wants approval, and he wants self-definition. And he will ask for all of it every day, all the time. As a result, something inside you may turn to stone when you hear his voice on the telephone, because you know this will be a long, draining phone call.

Cerato also has the irritating need to play stupid, to act as if he has no inkling of what to do, when you both know that Cerato knows very well what to do, but refuses to act upon what he knows to get the job done alone and get it done right.

The pattern of behavior common to Cerato types is one of the most alienating of all the behaviors associated with the Bach remedies. After a while the fact that they are pleasant and (apparently) mean well does little to offset their constant talking, constant questions, chirpy attitude, and emotional neediness. As a result, they tend to alienate the very people they wish to draw close to. Like many other Bach types, they end up creating the very situation they wished to avoid and are left alone and grappling with their inner sense of chaos.

### Positive Qualities of the Type

The Cerato gains the independence he once lacked when he moves from a negative to a positive emotional state. He no longer has to seek guidance externally, but can depend upon his own good judgment instead. He can trust his own ability to learn from life's lessons and use those lessons to refine his approach to life.

No one is more impressive than the positive Cerato in his approach to work. No other worker is as diligent. Where the Cerato once colored his constant failures with a rather giggly expressed desire to do well, he now can take great pride in his ability to master tasks and be counted upon to attempt them with a cheerful attitude and a positive result.

The amorphous nature of the negative Cerato becomes, in the positive aspect, a valuable ability to fit in to almost every group dynamic. The positive Cerato is the worker who can work for virtually any boss and any coworker with great success.

Finally, look for the positive Cerato to cast off his old need to keep up with the latest looks and cutting edge fads. An assured and independent Cerato will seek out the fashions and possessions that are right for him and that fit his sense of taste and lifestyle, instead of adapting his life and budget to attain the latest gadgets.

### The Cerato Child

These are the children who are always asking the teacher if they are doing the project right. They just want to keep checking in—with parents, with teachers, with anyone they perceive to be in authority—because they are sure they aren't capable of getting anything right. These children are natural born mimics who will copy the attitude, clothing, and style of others. Parents need to instill a strong sense of self in the Cerato child.

Often the Cerato state begins as the child grows older. It can be the result of the child becoming overwhelmed by his or her schoolwork. A child who falls behind in school can take on the Cerato role as he or she flounders when trying to catch up.

In the same way, many children move into a Cerato state as they become teenagers. These are the children who are "pleasers." They are often impressed by the attitude of the "in group" and will try anything to fit in with that group. They will follow every new fad and quickly adopt the latest style. The child who tells his parents that he must have a new cell phone because others he wants to impress have it is a child speaking from a Cerato lack of security. Even in later life, once this pattern has been established, the Cerato will want to join the right country club and own the latest clothes, cars, and other possessions.

### The Cerato Adult

Age certainly may bring experience and some sort of wisdom, but it seldom changes an ingrained lack of self-direction and a Cerato behavior pattern. We therefore find Ceratos of all ages, all genders, and in all economic groups. It is more common in females than in males. The same insecurities tend to be directed into Scleranthus patterns in males, since a lack of independence of spirit is looked upon as a terrible thing in men.

It may, in fact, be a bit more common in richer people, who have not been forced by a simple lack of money into taking charge of their lives and directing themselves toward success. Those who have not been sufficiently challenged by life or those who have failed to meet those challenges may fall into a Cerato pattern.

Ceratos seem to be something of a Zelig,[8] a chameleon that changes in accordance to the situation. Since they have no strong sense of self, the self that they do have is fluid and mutable.

Ceratos lack the inner truth that guides most of us and must be very careful where they turn for guidance. They are the prey of the latest "gurus" who hold all the secrets of the universe. They will style their hair, clothes, gestures, and language after these people, and will buy their tapes as they go through the lobby after listening to them lecture.

### The Cerato Animal

This is an excellent remedy for animals—dogs, mostly—that have had their spirit broken by an overbearing, over-training master. These dogs lack the ability to initiate activities without a command.

### Cerato and the Homeopathic Pharmacy

This state reminds me of the homeopathic Cannabis state. These are the walking confused, who are looking to others for guidance.

But the most troubling thing about both Cerato and Cannabis is that they will ask for advice again and again, but neither will follow the advice given. It is as if the asking itself were some sort of ritual and not a real search for information.

8. You remember Woody Allen's movie by the same name, don't you?

*Issues that Suggest Cerato*

Allergies; anxiety attacks; breathing problems; colds; cysts; diarrhea; fainting; glandular troubles; hives; hyperventilation; leg pain; nose bleeds; overweight; post-nasal drip.

*In Conclusion*

Some books refer to the Cerato type as the "Cerato Fool." This seems to be a harsh judgment of what is, after all, no more a perversion of a natural sense of being than we see in the overly-responsible Oak state or the bitter Willow. But Cerato, like the perfectionist Crab Apple, is one of the negative emotional states that seem to fascinate us as a culture.

Our culture even seems to encourage the Cerato state in some cases. Women especially may be burdened by it, and even have it thrust on them when they are told to not "bother their pretty little heads" with the important issues in life. Luckily, there has been some advancement in this area in recent years. Women in our society are moving beyond the infantilization associated with Cerato's behavior pattern, however grudgingly or hesitantly that change has been allowed.

And I do believe that the core issue of Cerato—like Scleranthus (which I consider to be the male equivalent of Cerato, although either remedy may be needed either acutely or constitutionally by either sex)—is that the patient has not achieved a true understanding of himself and his personal power, and therefore lives in an infantile state. Both types can, like a child, be quite literally dependent upon others although they are well beyond the age of maturity. And both can function as adults in many ways but still function as children emotionally. Either way, these are our remedies for the stunted personality, the person who lacks self-knowledge and trust, who must turn to others for information that should be innate. Both the Cerato and the Scleranthus can be as completely crippled by their negative emotional state as the Mimulus is by his quiet fear or the Agrimony by his hidden torment.

The "Cerato fool," therefore, is nothing to laugh at.

## WILD OAT · THE REMEDY FOR THOSE WHO ARE UNFULFILLED

Bach writes, "Wild Oat is needed by those who have ambitions to do something of prominence in life, who wish to have much experience, and to enjoy all that which is possible for them, to take life to the full. Their difficulty is to determine what occupation to follow; as although their ambitions are strong, they have no calling which appeals to them above all others. This may cause delay; and dissatisfaction."

• **Wild Oat is both an acute and a constitutional remedy.**

- **Wild Oat is, along with Holly, one of Bach's "Primary Remedies."**

### Botanical Information

The flowers of the Wild Oat (*Bromus Ramosus*) are hermaphroditic, containing both male and female aspects, and are contained within the scales of the plant's spikes.

The Wild Oat is most often considered to be a weed. It grows by roadsides, in fields, and in woods. It invades yards and gardens.

The Wild Oat prefers damp soil and partial shade or full sun.

### Wild Oat in General

The core issue of the remedy Wild Oat is ingrained in our culture. We assume that each of us will go through a process of self-discovery at some point, usually in early adulthood. This process will help the individual define his concept of self and explore his options in terms of career and adult relationships. This is the time when we exert an extraordinary freedom of thought and movement, when the young adult may literally explore geographically by driving across the country or studying in Europe.[9] We even talk of sowing one's "wild oats" when we talk about the process by which young people experiment with various aspects of life—religious, work related, sexual, and social—during the transition from childhood to adulthood. So we should not be surprised when we learn that the Wild Oat type is a person who seems ever-youthful, ever unconventional, and ever ready to do anything—except settle down.

Life is an adventure to Wild Oats. They will go into the new situation, the new relationship, the new career, truly believing that this time it's forever. But soon they are bored. Soon they manage to get caught cheating, or make a major mistake at work, so that they can be on their way again to something new.

For, while Wild Oats may see life as filled with excitement, they also see it as lacking meaning. When they take on a new topic of study, a new work project, a new relationship, or a new cause, they do so with the fervent hope that this new one will be truly and deeply meaningful, unlike their other explorations, which tended to come to dead ends. When it fails to resonate as it should, it too is abandoned.

Like the other remedies for Doubt, Wild Oat takes what should be an internalized

---

9. As with Hornbeam and other remedies related to Doubt (Scleranthus and Cerato come to mind), the Wild Oat negative emotional state is, in my opinion, largely a creation of the modern age. Before the onset of the Industrial Age, young adults had much fewer options and tended to simply stay where they were raised, take on the same work as their parents, and marry as their families desired. Only in the modern age, which literally offers the whole globe as a potential home and a wide range of sophisticated choices for career and lifestyle, does an adult have such a vast selection of options. This can be literally paralyzing, which creates the Wild Oat state of Doubt where doubt is turned inward, undermining the concept of meaning in life.

aspect of life and externalizes it. Wild Oat lacks an inner sense of meaning in life and is not in touch with that aspect of self that would supply a sense of meaning to the tasks of life. Therefore, the Wild Oat searches in the external world—geographically, politically, emotionally—for what is lacking in himself.

> The Wild Oat searches in the external world—geographically, politically, emotionally—for what is lacking in himself.

Because of this lack of meaning in life and the rootlessness it creates, commitment frightens Wild Oat types, whether it is a commitment to another person or to a team of people at a job, or to anything else, for that matter. After all, in the Wild Oats' mind, commitment equals locking yourself into a task, a job, or a relationship that is ultimately meaningless and dull. Committing to anything other than that one undiscovered, meaningful thing means trapping yourself in a situation in which you can never find peace, creative excitement (after the initial wildly exciting phase), or satisfaction.

While Wild Oats fear commitment they do seek satisfaction. They can think of nothing better than that future moment when they will be able to lie back knowing they have at last accomplished something of real importance, of real meaning—not only to them, but to others as well. They are driven by the deep desire for accomplishment and for recognition of their accomplishment. They often feel, especially in youth, that they are destined for great things, but they cannot find the path that will lead them to these things. And they lack the ability to continue on any path once it has been drained of its initial excitement and has "revealed" itself to be just as dull and detail oriented as the others.

Because of this dynamic, Wild Oats tend to drift, if not physically—and many of them do move restlessly from place to place—then emotionally and intellectually. They will try many things and are open to many explorations, especially sexually and philosophically, as they attempt to fill the void within. Wild Oats are very vulnerable to drugs and alcohol and may turn to them, either as part of their general exploration of life or as yet another means of filling their inner void. They often become dependent upon them.

Wild Oat types must be very careful about the crutches they use to help them along their way. They may, as I have said, use drugs or alcohol as a crutch, using them to avoid their inner doubt. They may use relationships as a crutch in the same way. They will move quickly from one love partner to another, as they drain each partner emotionally and, often, financially. They also may use religion as a crutch. You will find many religious retreats packed with those in a Wild Oat negative state, searching, searching, searching for meaning, excited by the potential of a new idea, a new group, and ultimately always being disappointed.

No matter how many times as they have watched it on TV, Wild Oats have failed to understand the message of *The Wizard of Oz:* that courage, heart, intelligence, and, above all, a sense of home, are things that we each have inside of us. They cannot be found on any journey. But instead of looking inward, Wild Oats just move onward and outward.

Time is also a great issue with Wild Oats. Because of their inner restlessness, they tend to feel that time is passing more slowly than it really is. This is an aspect of their tendency toward boredom. Because they honestly feel that hours have passed when, in fact, only minutes have gone by, they can get bored very easily and feel trapped by anything that requires them to sit still for very long. Therefore, many Wild Oat types are labeled as hyperactive. Their innate interest in all things new, new toys, new electronic devices[10] (especially these), new feelings and experiences, and their over-responsiveness to their environment—to color, sound and motion—tends to make them seem out of control, especially when they are young. They can be very difficult for a teacher or parent to manage, and for this reason, many young Wild Oat types are on toxic allopathic medications today, to rein in their exuberance.

For this reason, Wild Oat is often mistaken for and blends exceptionally well with Impatiens. Both types bore easily and are always interested in anything that takes their attention away from the thing that bores them, even for a moment. Both tend, for different reasons, to flit from thing to thing, person to person, concept to concept. Together, these remedies are a powerful tool for the patient who is hyperactive, intelligent, and hard to control.

Because time is so important to the Wild Oat—and how could it not be, since he feels he is meant for a great and important work, and yet cannot even begin that work until he finds it—he often "gives" his time as a present. The Wild Oat will dole out his time and attention to his supposed love ones—especially the loved one he is about to abandon in his search for a better, more meaningful relationship—as if minutes were diamonds. Songs have been written about this idea—"All I can give you is my time." Because the Wild Oat literally perceives time as the ticking of his life clock, it is of great value to him. You will find him, again and again, to be totally unwilling to give his time to anything he has concluded lacks meaning for him. He is on a clock, after all, and has to move on to better things.

Passion is also very important to the Wild Oat. He is attracted by passionate people and takes them very quickly as lovers, mentors, or gurus. He will meet this person with equal passion, at least for a time—he will remain totally engaged as long as the passion

---

10. You will find that Wild Oat types love the most cutting edge things and have a special affinity for new discoveries, especially for electronics. Many love science and science fiction. Many love math. But all want the latest computer, the newest electronic toy. This is particularly true in youth, but you will find a parallel for this in middle age, when the older Wild Oat type, who perhaps entered into the state with the onset of his midlife crisis of meaning and life's path, craves cutting edge toys once more, often bright shiny sports cars.

lasts and the voyage the two share is one of discovery. When the initial passionate stage begins to dissipate, however, the Wild Oat may reach a point of crisis, when he must decide whether or not this new idea, this new cause, or this new relationship has enough meaning for him to work to instill it with fresh passion.

More often than not, it is at this point or soon after that the Wild Oat will move on once more.

The patient who needs Wild Oat constitutionally leads a "binge and purge" life. He latches on to some new thing, idea, or person and literally binges on the object of his attention for as long as time allows and passion lasts. Once the meaning promised by the encounter has been exhausted, the Wild Oat purges himself and moves on.

The amount of time that passes between purges can differ greatly from patient to patient and situation to situation. And the intensity of the Wild Oat's purge will be determined by the amount of time and passion that he invested in the situation. A Wild Oat may stay in a marriage of five years or more, only to conclude one day that the marriage is boring and meaningless. And because he has invested a good deal of time and effort in the relationship, he will tend to feel very angry and betrayed when he "discovers" the meaninglessness of his situation. He will likely feel that he had been tricked or manipulated into staying. He may even feel that he has betrayed himself by doing the one thing he never meant to do in committing himself to marriage.

The same dynamic can take place in the workplace or in the Wild Oat's church. And once the Wild Oat has decided that the object of his time and passion is unworthy or lacking in meaning, nothing that is said or done will change his mind.

Some constitutional Wild Oats will drift often and will change the direction of their lives and the objects of their time and passion very frequently. Others will tend to stay in one place for much longer times and will truly dedicate themselves to a selected path, only to abandon it quite surprisingly one day when they decide it is the wrong path for them. However often the cycle of binge and purge repeats itself, it is quite capable of crippling the life of the Wild Oat and will keep him from ever achieving the important tasks that are the target of his search. The chronic Wild Oat negative emotional state can also be highly toxic for those involved with the Wild Oat in any way. To place your trust in this type—to make him a business or love partner—is to court disaster. The likely outcome for those who do is that one day they will find themselves abandoned and with a real mess on their hands. When the constitutional Wild Oat leaves, he often takes the contents of the joint bank account with him.

In most cases, the constitutional Wild Oat state occurs when the patient is a young adult. It often resolves itself as the patient explores, makes his conclusions, and moves to a set path in life. In other cases, it suddenly appears in midlife, or at a time of great change, such as when a person who has been dedicated to a particular career suddenly finds himself out of work. Sudden, shocking change can force a patient to revaluate his life and find it lacking in real meaning. He suddenly feels that his work is unimportant, even meaningless, that his relationship is nothing but rote. Suddenly he feels hollow inside. In midlife and beyond, this feeling may be enhanced by a strong notion that their life is finite, that time is fleeting, and that he will likely not manage to do the great work in this lifetime that he had set out to do. This hollowness is coupled with a deep feeling of dissatisfaction, even betrayal, and the patient begins to rebel against all that he had done before. After all, he feels, playing by the rules got him nowhere, so perhaps he should begin to break some rules to get ahead. And suddenly the thrifty patient spends money that he cannot afford. The sedate man or woman tries to look more youthful, more filled with energy and potential. Less limited by time.

Any life change that pulls the rug out from under us can trigger a period when we question all meaning in life. A divorce or the death of a loved one. The loss of a job. Sudden illness or physical injury that makes us realize we are mortal after all. All or any of these can trigger a crisis of Wild Oat meaninglessness.

In daily life the remedy can be used for those moments of listlessness or boredom when we feel that all this work we are doing, all the tasks at hand, are just meaningless, that our lives are small and unimportant. When we feel frustrated, we would do well to reach for Wild Oat.

In times of simple frustration or boredom, mix Wild Oat with Hornbeam to bring a new vigor into life.

Wild Oat also combines especially well with Walnut. Walnut is the remedy of choice for the moments of true crisis, when we feel as if we lack the strength of will to move forward. Any crossroad in life can be helped by Walnut. The two remedies, therefore, share a certain rootlessness and sense of dissatisfaction. Those who are trapped in bad marriages or who work in unsatisfactory jobs would be helped by this combination. Those needing this particular combination often need to continue taking it for many months before they can build the strength to move forward in life.[11]

Wild Oat also combines well with Wild Rose. Wild Rose is the remedy for resignation, so the patient who needs this particular combination feels the deep sense of meaningless, but has abandoned the search for meaning. He has become overwhelmed by the lack of purpose in his life. In abandoning his search, he often replaces it with dependence on drugs or alcohol and disappears into a constant state of haze.

---

11. Walnut and Wild Oat can be easily confused. Remember, Wild Oat is self-directed, even though they lack an inner sense of direction and meaning. Walnut, on the other hand, lacks self-direction. They are easily influenced by any external stimulus. Perhaps this is most easily understood by describing Walnut as a "yin" type, who pulls energy in and is passive in nature, while Wild Oat is "yang" who sends life energy outward. Wild Oat is very active by nature and can be quite an exhibitionist, quite domineering.

## Negative Qualities of the Type

Sadly, Wild Oat patients lack the ability to channel their innate great talents into accomplishments. Often, they undermine themselves simply because they lack the ability to deal with the day-to-day drudgery of attaining their goals. They become bored midway through the activity, and let themselves and others down when they choose to turn and walk away from any given project or relationship. When they move on, they leave others—those who trusted them—to pick up the pieces and clean up the mess they left behind.

Because of this, Wild Oat types can be quite toxic to others. They create havoc in the workplace and real suffering for those who trust and care for them. Because they lack a sense of meaning in life, they lack an understanding of those who do not share their meaninglessness. Often, they interpret other people's ability to work slowly and steadily toward a goal as a lack of passion, as a negative state.

Few other types can create such suffering for those they supposedly care about as the Wild Oat who is in a deeply negative emotional state. He will ignore the feelings and needs—financial, emotional, or otherwise—of all but himself when he is flailing against a perceived commitment trap or toward some new source of excitement and passion. He will say anything, do anything, and take anything that will help him be on his way.

The Wild Oat feels alienated by life itself. He feels he does not fit in. Over time, this belief that he is "different" ceases to be an interesting trait of a young person and becomes a pathetic trait of a middle-aged person. The Wild Oat watches friends marry and settle down as time passes. He watches the same friends buy houses and cars, while he is still living out of boxes and driving an old wreck.

This is the person about whom others scratch their heads and wonder why such a talented guy never made it in the world. Or how such a great guy could be such a jerk.

## Positive Qualities of the Type

When constitutional negative Wild Oats move into a more positive state they begin to turn inward for the sense of meaning they once sought externally. And, in doing so, they realize that they have expended far more time and energy in searching for the perfect and meaningful situation than it would have taken them to create it from within themselves. They realize that they can focus their energies into day-to-day detailed work with the same joy they used to jump from place to place.

In the same way, they show others that life has infinite possibilities. And they will excite others that it is possible to do more than one thing at a time or have more than one dream at a time.

## The Wild Oat Child

The Wild Oat state is, in a way, natural for the older child and young adult. In our culture, which offers myriad possibilities for lifestyle and life's path, young people are encouraged, especially by their college experience, to explore life and accept and reject specific aspects for their own future life.

For most of us, this Wild Oat phase is a positive thing. We may flirt with our moral boundaries, but we do not cross them often or abandon them if we step over the line. For most of us, this phase of "sowing our wild oats" yields in time as we select our life's mate and our life's work.

For some, however, the Wild Oat state becomes the norm, and the restlessness and lack of achievement common to the state become their life. Those who enter into the chronic Wild Oat state become large children instead of growing into adulthood. Their interests remain those of youths and their dedication to their life's path remains as frail as a teenager's dedication to his job at the local Burger King.

### The Wild Oat Adult

If young adulthood is the first natural age for the onset of the Wild Oat mood, then midlife is the second. The milestones of midlife—menopause, milestone birthdays, the moment of confronting personal mortality—all can create a Wild Oat negative emotional state. As we reexamine our lives at the halfway point or beyond we tend to find them lacking, more often than not. We see our mate as the lump he or she has become and not the passionate, intelligent being we married. We find our work dull and meaningless. In the word of Peggy Lee, we ask ourselves, "Is that all there is?"

We all play out this phase with varying degrees of restlessness and disappointment. And as in youth, most of us in midlife tend to absorb our crisis on an emotional level with some simple form of acting out. Some people go out and repurchase the baseball cards or comic books they had in their youth. Others buy a car. Still others have affairs. Many—the wise ones—go back and enhance their education or take on new interests that reinvigorate their lives. But most of us get through it and move on.

But as in youth, some do not move on. Some freeze in the Wild Oat state and, in doing so, become rather pathetic. They struggle with their age and not only try to look young once more, but actually be young. They need to be found exciting, sexy. And, in doing so, they can make great fools of themselves.

Worse, those who suffer from a deep midlife crises can undermine all that they have actually accomplished in life. Their dissatisfaction can derail a good marriage or a solid career, and bring great suffering to those who trust them.

Of course, we can enter into a Wild Oat state at any time or stage in life as our inner sense of meaning and our external environment dictates. That state can be a simple acute phase or a chronic state, depending upon the particular patient's persona and innate sense of personal meaning.

## The Wild Oat Animal

I have never found a use for this remedy with any animal I have known. They do not seem to share our feelings of dissatisfaction and don't seem to waste time and energy on the issues related to Wild Oat.

## Wild Oat and the Homeopathic Pharmacy

So many homeopathic remedies come to mind when you think about Wild Oat: Phosphorus, Ignatia, and most of the other Tubercular remedies, as well as the deeply Psoric and self-defeating remedies, like Sulphur. But one remedy, Onosmodium, actually has the riddle of Wild Oat to work out—they want to accomplish great things in life, but have no idea what those great things are. Therefore, they go through life miserable, on an ongoing search for their life's work.

The ultimate remedy for Wild Oat, however, is Thuja, which shares the ultimate diffused state with Wild Oat. Thuja, like Wild Oat, does not fit in. Thuja seems "other" than the rest of us, seems unable to focus in on living his life like the rest of us.

Wild Oat, like these homeopathic remedies, does not realize the truth in the old maxim that genius is 1 percent inspiration and 99 percent perspiration. They are still waiting for the muses to strike them with total visionary inspiration and easily become bored with the perspiration part.

## Issues that Suggest Wild Oat

Adolescence; alcoholism; digestive disorders; drug abuse; foot pain; gas pains; glandular disorders; hay fever; menopause; midlife crisis, premenstrual syndrome; pregnancy; sexual dysfunction; sciatica; sexually transmitted diseases; toe pain; unemployment.

## In Conclusion

Little is left to be said about the Wild Oat type. Except this: be very patient when treating a Wild Oat. Even the Wild Oat type who is given the remedy he needs will likely have to take that remedy repeatedly for months or longer before it brings him back into emotional balance.

Some Bach remedies work more quickly than others. You will see immediate results with some, especially those that deal with sudden events and their immediate consequences, like Rock Rose. You will see slower results with a remedy that deals with a slower building and more chronic state, like Elm or Oak. You will see the slowest results of all with those needing Wild Oat (and with those needing Chestnut Bud), where the patient must wrestle with a deeply instilled emotional state before he can move past it. Often it seems that nothing is changing at first, and no balance is being achieved. But be patient. With time, balance will come.

# 7

# Considering the Fourth Mood: Self Versus Others: Oversensitivity to the World

Life is a process. It is a process of learning. It is a process of stimulus and response. Throughout our entire lives, from birth onward, we take in impressions, and those impressions shape our experiences on an emotional, mental, and physical level. These experiences—which are born from our individual and unique responses to the stimuli that constantly assault us—teach us the realities of the world around us. Further, they suggest to us the way we should live and instruct us about the rules of conduct and behavior by which life is governed.

Whether we live in a big city and are constantly assaulted by traffic, noise, bright lights, and the crush of the crowd or in a rural environment, our minds and bodies are confronted each day with new sensory stimuli. Each day we have new thoughts and new moods, and undergo a wide range of fleeting emotional states. Our responses are broadly based upon our experiences as well as on our environment and the stresses and challenges that it offers. No matter how beneficial or stressful our environment, we are in a constant state of action and reaction.

We are taught this as a principle of physics, as one of the fundamental tenants of the universe, in elementary science class: *for every action there is an equal and opposite reaction*. And so it is with most of us—we tend to govern our responses to stimuli by the nature of the stimulation itself. We naturally balance our responses to make them equal to the stimulation we have received. Thus, those that do us a great good receive great thanks, and those who slightly injure our feelings usually receive a slightly negative response before we move on with our day.

Our lives, therefore, may be said to be a balancing act. We try our best to shrug off the stimuli that affect us only slightly, either for good or bad, and pay closer attention to those of greater import. Our emotions and minds, therefore, may be said to function as our bodies and their immune systems do. Just as a healthy immune system will know which stimuli to ignore (or be overwhelmed by the sheer number of those stimuli) and which to react to, a healthy emotional or mental self will be able to make similar decisions and, having made them, move on to judge the next impression or stimulation.

But just as our physical immune system can fall out of balance and, as in the case of allergies, begin to respond to things that pose no threat, our mental and/or emotional "immune systems" can fall into an unnecessary state of extreme sensitivity as well. In this state it becomes all but impossible for us to understand which stimuli present a potential serious impact and which do not. And because we do not know or understand the impulses we are receiving it becomes impossible to know how we should respond to them.

> Just as our physical immune system can fall out of balance and, as in the case of allergies, begin to respond to things that pose no threat, our mental and/or emotional "immune systems" can fall into an unnecessary state of extreme sensitivity as well.

Such is the case for those who fall into the emotional states central to the four remedies listed in this chapter. And, the four remedies in this group are somewhat unique within the realm of Bach flower treatments, because they represent a state of oversensitivity to their environment rather than an easily classified emotional state.

The other thirty-four Bach remedies are more easily defined than these remedies. The rest of our Bach pharmacy speaks to emotional states like anger, fear, and bitterness. The remedies in this group share a state of rawness, a state of confusion, but each acts out differently in its response to this oversensitivity.

This oversensitivity can be experienced in myriad ways. Some are overly sensitive to sensory impressions. The typical Holly, for example, may be very sensitive to noise and unable to adapt to very noisy situations. The Holly, who has trouble enough getting to sleep in the best of times, will end up enraged and pounding on the door of his upstairs neighbor who is playing his stereo too loudly at night.

Others may be too sensitive to the influence and opinions of others. Agrimony is deeply sensitive to other people's opinions of him and may be all too willing to shape his behavior around his need for approval. Centaury, in the same way, is very sensitive to suggestions from others and to the way others think he should live his life. The Centaury has a particular difficulty saying the word "No" to anyone.

But of these four remedies, Walnut most clearly displays a general state of over-sensitivity. Walnut is to this "oversensitivity mood" what Mimulus is to the "fear mood." Walnut types are overly sensitive to life itself. They are easily moved and swayed, easily manipulated. The chatter in their minds, the chatter of the world, and the chatter of the past all conspire to bind the Walnut in place and keep him from moving forward in life.

Our remedies for oversensitivity show us the various behavioral traps we can fall into when we lose our emotional balance and when we are crippled in our innate ability to respond rationally to the stimuli, stresses, and crises that life brings us.

## Oversensitivity and the Homeopathic Pharmacy

The homeopathic repertory seems to get far more specific on the subject of oversensitivity than Bach did.[1] There is a giant rubric labeled "Sensitivity, General," but most of the useful information concerning mental and emotional oversensitivity is contained in specific subrubrics with labels like "sensitive to light," "sensitive during a chill," and "sensitive children." Therefore, you are likely going to need some specific physical symptoms to join with the mental and emotional symptoms, even if you follow the path of classic homeopathy and are repertorizing the emotional/mental effects of oversensitivity.

Still, some remedies are particularly linked with the idea of sensitivity. Nux Vomica looms large when it comes to sensitivity, and will be discussed in more detail in the section of this book dedicated to the Bach remedy Holly. Pulsatilla, a remedy known for mood swings and a certain vagueness of character, is another remedy associated with states of oversensitivity. Often the kind-hearted Pulsatilla will have what is known as "air hunger," and will be overly sensitive to warm rooms or enclosed spaces. The Pulsatilla will need to be taken outside into cooler open air to be able to breathe or to recover from fainting.

Other remedies are overly sensitive to weather changes. Phosphorus and Rhus Tox are both extremely sensitive to storms and will feel the onset of thunderstorms, either in their bones and joints (Rhus) or in their sinuses or ears (Phosphorus). Mercurius, on the other hand, is very sensitive to temperature change.

Some remedies are also very sensitive to seasonal changes. Rumex, for example, has a deep vulnerability to spring and fall, and will often become very ill during those times of year when days are warm but nights are cold.

When it comes to sheer emotional sensitivity, however, two remedies stand out. The first is Ignatia Amara, a remedy common to those who feel they have been emotionally betrayed. The Ignatia has wild mood swings and will be seen as both unpredictable and frightening by those around her. It is a remedy commonly needed by those who have been recently widowed and who have become trapped in their erratic state of grief.

The other is a remedy commonly needed by those who have been abused, especially by those who have been sexually abused. Staphysagria is a valuable remedy in cases of both emotional and physical vulnerability. The Staphysagria will often experience physical pain that feels like a knife blow, sudden, deep, and sharp. In the same way, the Staphysagria will experience abuse and betrayal as an emotional stabbing.

---

1. To be honest, I sometimes find this category of remedies to be something of a catchall, a place where Bach put the remedies that he couldn't quite fit in anywhere else. I picture him sitting by his desk, rubbing his chin and wondering, "What do these four have in common?"

The homeopath is perhaps at a distinct disadvantage in having to physicalize a patient's state of oversensitivity. After all, the ability within each of us to balance external stimuli with our internal monologue is central to our ability to survive, live our lives, and achieve our goals. The remedies in this category do just that. They bring our internal selves into balance with our external environment, and allow for the rational and successful interplay of action/reaction and stimulus/response.

## REMEDIES FOR THOSE WHO ARE OVERLY SENSITIVE

- **Agrimony**—for those with false cheer
- **Centaury**—for those who are weak willed
- **Walnut**—for those who are in upheaval
- **Holly**—for those with anger, hatred and/or jealousy

## AGRIMONY · THE REMEDY FOR THOSE WITH FALSE CHEER

Bach writes of the Agrimony type as, "the jovial, cheerful, humorous people who love peace and are distressed by argument or quarrel, to avoid which they will agree to give up much. Though generally they have trouble and are tormented and restless and worried in mind or in body, they hide their cares behind their humor and jesting and are considered very good friends to know. They often take alcohol or drugs in excess, to stimulate themselves and help themselves bear their trials with cheerfulness."

- **Agrimony can be an acute remedy, but more often is taken constitutionally.**
- **Agrimony is one of Bach's original remedies, the Twelve Healers.**

### Botanical Information

Also known as the "Sticklewort," or "Church Steeple," the agrimony plant (*Agrimonia Eupatoria*) is native and grows widely throughout the British Isles, except in Scotland, whose harsh climate limits its growth.

Agrimony is a perennial plant related to the rose, although its yellow flowers, which grow in spikes, neither look nor smell like a rose. In fact, the flowers are said to smell like apricots. The flowers bloom in mid to late summer.

Agrimony is considered to be a medicinal herb as a tonic and diuretic, which makes it somewhat unusual among Bach's flowers, as he tended to avoid any plant that had a history of medicinal use.

## Agrimony in General

Like the friends and family of Elwood P. Dowd, the protagonist of the play *Harvey* (who is a drunkard with a six foot tall invisible rabbit as a best friend), many close to an Agrimony type might find that they would choose to leave him as he is if they were offered a drug that could completely cure him of his emotional negative state and return him to a normal, rational mind.

The typical Agrimony is a very supportive, funny, and extremely docile type who would do anything, offer anything to avoid a confrontation.

Agrimony types offer jokes in place of anger, smiles instead of sorrow. They are the stuff of Hollywood comedies—often played by the likes of Rosie O'Donnell—the funny best friend with a heart of gold, whose needs and wants are as completely ignored by the movie plot as she is by her celluloid best friend.

The problem with the humor an Agrimony displays to the world is that it is not real. It is a mask. Those who need the remedy Agrimony, especially on a constitutional level, are those who have learned the lesson—often in youth—that their best survival tool is humor, and that humor is often most effective when it is turned against one's self. You will, therefore, often find Agrimony types who assume that if they make fun of themselves, if they target their own weight, features, or hairline, then no one else will.

Agrimony is the remedy needed by patients in a very fragile state. Something in their life has left them with an emotional wound that will not heal, and the mask they have developed to protect that wound is one of pleasantry. Agrimony types are always pleasant, always giving. On first glance, they seem to possess a huge reserve of energy to share with others—they will happily give of their time, their emotions, even their possessions, often without even being asked. They will support their friends with what appears to be true concern and true interest. They will make the tea and put the cookies on the plate while listening to their friend pour out her heart about her most recent breakup. They come when they are needed, bring chicken soup to the sick. Why would anyone want to cure them?[2]

Because this remedy's negative emotional state is embodied in a patient who cannot be true to self, who cannot look at the negative aspects of his life and covers his denial in a blanket of assumed happiness. Unfortunately, because the Agrimony type uses denial as a tool, rather than truly facing and working through his life's troubles, he ultimately creates more troubles through his constant denial. Unlike other remedy

---

2. I know this all sounds really good, but let me note right here—and this is important—that as pleasant as he is, the Agrimony type is not motivated by a real sense of compassion for others or a real interest in giving help or support, no matter how freely he might offer it. His apparent desire to support and please others is a false behavior. Agrimony is, in truth, motivated by denial of inner hurt and by a strong desire to avoid any conflict or stress in life.

types in this category, Agrimony is not particularly sensitive to other people's troubles—which is, perhaps, why he is able to listen to them so easily—nor is he so concerned with the judgments of others that he shapes his life around community standards. Agrimony is, however, overly sensitive to anger, to tension, and to any emotional upheaval in his environment. This oversensitivity is due, in great part, to the emotional upheaval Agrimony feels within himself, the same upheaval that he is investing so much energy in denying. This constant stress and energy drain makes Agrimony an easy target for alcohol and/or drugs.

The Agrimony's almost inevitable drifting toward drugs or, especially, alcohol is one of the great weaknesses of the type. If the Agrimony were as happy as he pretends to be, he would not need chemical assistance to maintain his facade. But Agrimony's almost manic need to uphold his pretense of a happy, calm self creates an ongoing state of inner stress. The patient who is, deep within, very unhappy and, at the same time, overly sensitive to any form of tension or stress, has created for himself an increasingly stressful situation in which he is role playing every minute of his life. As the Agrimony state takes hold, the patient is placed, with each passing minute, in a false state of being in which the reality of his emotional life and its presentation are in direct opposition.

One of the best ways to uncover whether or not a friend or family member is in an Agrimony emotional state is to ask yourself just how much you know about him. Even those who consider themselves to be a very good friend of an Agrimony type will often realize that, upon reflection, they really know very little about him. If they think about it, the Agrimony's best friends will realize that the Agrimony is something of a cipher even after years of friendship. In memory, his features fade into a blur, just as his real needs, wants, and motivations remain a total mystery. A friendship with an Agrimony type is a friendship based in falsehoods. An Agrimony is very good at deflecting attention away from himself, and at protecting his hidden emotional self. Because of this, he will usually end up knowing a great deal about his friends without ever revealing very much about himself.[3]

This is not to say that Agrimony types don't talk much. They are, in fact, among

> One of the best ways to uncover whether or not a friend or family member is in an Agrimony emotional state is to ask yourself just how much you know about him. Even those who consider themselves to be a very good friend of an Agrimony type will often realize, upon reflection, that they really know very little about him.

3. This is an important key to understanding Agrimony: while the Agrimony type is very friendly, he is emotionally unavailable. He keeps his hurts deep inside. He can be, at the same time, apparently approachable and completely remote.

the most verbal people. Often they are very well spoken, with very quick wits. And when they drink too much, they tend to be happy drunks, who entertain their guests by telling the same humorous anecdotes they told the last time they were drunk. And the time before that. And the time before that as well.[4]

The core issue for the Agrimony type is one of dishonesty. Because he is motivated by a strong need to avoid conflict—internal or external conflict—he sets increasingly sophisticated mechanisms in place whereby he can appear to be completely different than he is.

Were I to select the group or "mood" into which I would place this remedy type, I would select Despair. I see the Agrimony type as essentially despairing and often clinically depressed. He is so unwilling to face the truth of his life and his behavior and so dedicated to his insincere behavior modifications that his essential self is lost somewhere in the mix. He may be quite successful in avoiding the conflicts of the world and the conflict that rages within, but he does so only at great cost. Often the Agrimony is the patient who has to "hit bottom" before he can gather the courage to face the truth of his life and replace his insincere affectations and alcohol consumption with a life that is lived with candor.

In my experience, Agrimony is one of those remedy types that is needed far more often on a constitutional basis than an acute one. Also, it is a remedy that works extremely well on its own, and it can bring about a remarkable change as it helps the patient trapped in a negative emotional state work through his issues—often with the help of other adjunct therapies and professional counselors.

But in the acute context, Agrimony is a wonderful remedy to consider in times when we feel embarrassed, for situations in which we have been publicly humiliated and just want to disappear into the floor. Agrimony can help set our emotions back in balance and help us match our emotional reaction to the actual seriousness of the situation itself.

Because it can help us when we are being overly sensitive emotionally, you should also consider Agrimony for any situation in which you feel you are not presenting your

4. This brings to mind the idea of Agrimony and inhibitions. Agrimony types who have some shame or perceived hurt to hide are often very inhibited people. Just as alcohol will loosen their tongue, look for it to break through their inhibitions as well. The drunken Agrimony is the one with the lampshade on his head or who is out on the dance floor kicking off her shoes and unbuttoning her blouse. Often the Agrimony will shed his sexual inhibitions as well, or may ignore common sense and/or the law and drive while under the influence. Both instances, and others like them, can bring disastrous results.

While I have said above that, more often than not, a drunken Agrimony is a happy Agrimony, this is not always the case. Because Agrimony tends to shed his inhibitions as he drinks, and because this type, while always happy on the surface, is often quite angry and antagonistic deep inside, alcohol can also unleash an aggressive monster.

authentic self. It can be very helpful for those visits with our parents when we feel that we are acting as if we were children instead of adults.

Agrimony also has an interesting "medical" use. Along with Impatiens, it is very helpful for those suffering physical pain. It will help the patient deal more easily with physical discomfort and heal more quickly from it.

Remedies that are commonly used in conjunction with Agrimony include Beech, Larch, and Centaury. In each case, the Agrimony mask of false cheerfulness adds to and enhances the negative emotional state of the type. For those needing Beech and Agrimony, the mask involves a happy face and good works, and the patient combines a denial of real issues of self and his harsh inner judge to present a double-thick mask to the world: the patient seems supernaturally serene and totally dedicated to reshaping the world into a place of peace and fairness for all, by political or religious means. When the issues of Agrimony and Larch combine, Agrimony's happy mask covers a deep pit of insecurity, and what little independence Agrimony possesses is drained by Larch's lack of self worth. The case that requires a blend of Agrimony and Centaury is one in which the smile is quite frozen on the patient's face. The cheerfulness of this patient will be almost pathological.

### Negative Qualities of the Type

The true issue and most damaging reality of Agrimony's negative emotional state is that it is based upon a lie. And as the pattern of presenting an insincere happy face to the world and feigning an insincere interest in the lives of his friends continues, more and more of the Agrimony's actual life is built upon that same lie and a denial of the true self. Some Agrimony types are more skilled at delivering the lie than others, but, in all cases the very foundation of the Agrimony's projected persona, and, indeed, of his relationships is a falsehood.

And this always leads to disastrous results.

As noted above, the Agrimony must turn to a number of tools to be successful in his sham. Often chief among these is alcohol, but very often the Agrimony who does not turn to drink will turn to food as his coping mechanism. Agrimony types are binge eaters and/or drinkers. We have stereotyped them in our movies and television shows as the "fat best friend" to the more attractive, more interesting slim lead character.

Living a lie also requires the Agrimony to stuff down his own hurts and disconnect, as best he can, from confronting and dealing with the emotional wound that so frightens him. This leads to a tight reining in of his natural personality and an ever-growing number of inhibitions of his natural emotions and behaviors. As a result, these straitjacketed inhibitions tend to break loose dramatically upon occasion, especially when the Agrimony overindulges in food or drink.

The simple fact is that the Agrimony yearns to be the person he pretends he is.

And yet, he knows, deep within, that the face he presents to the world is a false mask, and this knowledge torments him. What the Agrimony refuses to understand is that he must first confront himself and work through his issues to honestly be the person he wants to be and free himself from his constraints and the fear of what lies inside. What lies within is quite often the same warm person he once seemed to be, but now that person is genuine, compassionate, and a true friend.

## Positive Qualities of the Type

There is much to praise in the Agrimony character who has moved from the negative to the positive emotional state. They are social people and genuinely like others. They are naturally optimistic and are natural peacemakers. They would make the best sort of diplomats and lawyers, restoring peace where discord reigns. Once Agrimony types have reached their positive potential, they can look at their own troubles clearly and honestly, while still retaining their hopeful disposition and cheerful outlook.

## The Agrimony Child

The Agrimony negative emotional state often develops while the patient is in childhood, especially when the child has been taken in hand by an adult who has told him to keep a stiff upper lip no matter what. That it is expected that he will never complain and always be polite. Agrimony children have also often heard the message that they should be seen (and seen to be neat and pleasant) and not heard.

The Agrimony child is the child who is always in a good mood, always smiling and happy. Often the Agrimony child will be so good at displaying this good mood that the parent or teacher will not see any sign of inner turmoil. Therefore, this remedy often must be given on the basis of what the child does *not* have—anger, fear, grief, and other negative emotions—rather than on the basis of what the child does have. Agrimony will comfort the child who feels he must always hide his negative emotions. It will allow him to become truly happy, rather than feeling that he must behave as if he *was* happy.

## The Agrimony Adult

Mirroring the child, the Agrimony adult appears to be filled with happiness, enthusiasm, and peace. But the cheerfulness is a denial, a suppression[5] of reality, rather than a tool for healthy living.

5. The homeopathic idea of suppression is important to understanding the Agrimony type. In homeopathic medicine, we teach that medicines, by their actions, either suppress or express a patient's symptoms. Allopathic medicine, what we think of as "Western Medicine," treats by suppressing a patient's aches and pains for a brief period of time while the patient's own immune system does the heavy lifting and brings about the actual healing. Homeopathic medicine, on the other hand, works

The Agrimony state can develop at any time of life and is not more common to one stage than it is to another. In my experience, however, I find it is often more common in one gender than it is in the other.

I have noticed that Agrimony is more often needed by adult men than it is by adult women, perhaps because men are trained in our culture not to show their true feelings. While women may be willing to cry when hurt or angered, men try to put forth a strong face and act as if all is well. A man who has determined that he will be rewarded not only for actiing strong, but also for acting pleasant (and, as a subtext, as if he is rather invulnerable to emotional injury and can face anything you can dish out with a smile) is likely to move into an Agrimony negative emotional state. And, along the way, they begin to see invisible giant rabbits.

## The Agrimony Animal

I have never found an application for this remedy with an animal. I suppose that a case could be made for a rescued animal or one who has been abused that tries overly hard to please. But this is not a remedy I would recommend for regular use or consider necessary to have on hand for the treatment of animals.

## Agrimony and the Homeopathic Pharmacy

While there is no absolute comparison to be made among homeopathic remedies, Agrimony has much in common with Pulsatilla. Both have a weak sense of self, and both will do much to avoid anger and tension. Pulsatilla also will often deny her own pain, both physical and mental, and will greet the world with an unflinching "happy face," no matter her true sorrow.

Another remedy to consider is Arnica, which has also been shocked out of a true sense of self, and also feels wounded. Like Agrimony, Arnica will insist that nothing is wrong and will rejoin the world, if allowed, as one of the walking wounded.

## Issues that Suggest Agrimony

Accidents; addictions; adrenal disorders; amnesia; bleeding gums; cramps; eating disorders; midlife crisis; peptic ulcer; postnasal drip; restless legs; sleep disorders.

---

by helping the patient "express" his symptoms, to quite literally shed them, so that, the patient is permanently cured once they are gone. Homeopaths believe that suppression of any sort is a terrible thing on any level of being, and that it weakens the immune system and the whole being over time. (The other thing that homeopaths have against suppressive treatments is that they cure nothing. Any headache, joint pain, or other ailment that is treated suppressively will recur.) So when I note that, in presenting a happy face to the world, the Agrimony is suppressing his real emotions behind a false mask, I am also saying that he is weakening his emotional well-being, and causing himself a great harm.

## In Conclusion

To this point, I have written nothing about whether or not Agrimony is successful with his ruse; whether he, more often or not, manages to fool the people around him into believing that he is happy, happy, happy when he is not.

The answer is that it depends upon how closely the people in his environment look at the Agrimony. On first glance, his mask is highly effective. The Agrimony looks like the perfect *bonhomie*, a being of good humor, warm regard, and open arms. On second view, however, things begin to be a bit askew.

Even those who may not be able to put it into words (other than the simple thought that "He's such a phony!") will often still feel that something is not right with the Agrimony's behavior. Often they can see the hurt or sorrow in his eyes, even while his face is smiling.

## CENTAURY · THE REMEDY FOR THOSE WHO ARE WEAK WILLED

Bach says that these are "kind, gentle, quiet people who are over-anxious to serve others. They overtax their strength in their endeavors. Their wish so grows upon them that they become more servants than willing helpers. Their good nature leads them to do more than their own share of the work, and in so doing they may neglect their own particular mission in life."

- While Centaury has its acute uses, it is of particular value as a constitutional remedy.

- Centaury is one of Bach's original remedies, the Twelve Healers.

### Botanical Information

The Centaury (*Centaurium Umbellatum*) is an annual plant that is often considered a weed. It grows to a height of one foot and stands long, thin, and tall. It tends to grow in poor soil, along roadways and dusty lanes, and in abandoned lots. It also can tolerate salty soil and, for this reason, it is commonly found along the Atlantic coastline in the United States.

Centaury is native to Northern Europe and grows throughout Great Britain. It flowers in full summer and displays small pink flowers in clusters at the very top of the plant.

### Centaury in General

Those who would benefit from a few doses of the remedy Centaury would also benefit from learning a new word for their working vocabulary. That word is "No."

Ask a Centaury type to do something and they will do it. Whether they have the time or energy or not. Whether they want to or not. They will do it simply because they were asked to do it.

This remedy and Walnut, which follows, have much in common. Both have tenuous links to their life's work. Where the remedy type Wild Oat has no idea as to his most meaningful path in life and flails about trying to find it, both the Walnut type and the Centaury type have found their meaningful work, but both of them are willing to put it aside far too easily. The Walnut type feels that he or she is at a cross-

> The core of the issue is that Centaurys, while they may seem to give too freely and, perhaps, even inappropriately of themselves, they do not give with an open and happy heart. They give because they lack the strength of will to say "No."

roads, that life is changing, and those changes feel threatening. The issue that confounds the Centaury is different. The Centaury is an emotionally open, even a kind and generous type of person by nature (in this, they may seem like the Agrimony, who projects an ever-pleasant façade). But the Centaury takes this virtuous behavior too far. Instead of merely serving others, the Centaury literally becomes a servant to others, swallowing down his or her own needs and wants and putting aside his or her own work so that some other person will have all he needs and can accomplish his goals.

There is a loss of self in the Centaury type's negative emotional state. A loss of what might be called "appropriate" or even "creative" selfishness. While we are called by our religious beliefs to be each others' brothers, and required by our culture to be responsible and compassionate members of our community, we are not and should not be asked to relinquish our life's vision for the sake of another's.

The core of the issue is that Centaurys, while they may seem to give too freely and, perhaps, even inappropriately of themselves, they do not give with an open and happy heart. (In my opinion, such true self-sacrifice would not be the representation of a negative emotional state.) They give because they lack the strength of will to say "No."

This is why the Centaury state, for all its apparent purity, is a negative and damaging thing for the Centaury and those around him. The Centaury cannot find joy in his giving, especially after the initial bounce of "doing good" yields to a long, drawn-out period in which the self-sacrifice unfolds into days of menial tasks and nights of wondering what might have been.

Just as the Agrimony state is a false presentation of boundless joy and an almost uncanny interest in others, the Centaury state is likewise false. The Centaury wears a mask of willingness—he would have us believe that he has nothing better to do than the work that we ourselves don't want to take on. That he has no ambitions in life other than to serve us. And that his almost frighteningly cheerful demeanor hides nothing other than a happy heart.

And, indeed, no one else can be as cheerful as the Centaury. No one else can seem so glassy-eyed and inane. "Chirpy" is perhaps the best word to describe the typical Centaury's behavior pattern. He tends to surround himself with icons that help him maintain his happy face. He will love happy mugs and smiling faces, stickers, shiny things, and places tiny heart-shaped dots over his i's.

But, like Agrimony, the joyful state presented by the Centaury is often in direct opposition to the reality of their feelings. The patient has put aside his inner critic in assuming the Centaury state. He has silenced the inner voice of judgment, which, when it is kept in balance with the rest of our emotional selves, is a valuable tool. In silencing his inner critic, the Centaury loses his ability to judge the value of the cause he has undertaken. Because of this, many Centaury types, sadly, link themselves to relationships and causes that are far beneath their capabilities. They slavishly dedicate themselves to work, but it ultimately yields results that are far less than they could have achieved if they had developed their own vision and talents.

The friends and families of constitutional Centaurys often scratch their heads as these types marry inappropriate partners and then serve them on hand and knee. Centaurys often support the household financially and also make it home on time to clean the house and get dinner ready. In the same way, they may dedicate themselves to jobs and overbearing bosses that bring little in the way of satisfaction or reward.

As the Centaury can be something of a masochist by nature, he will deny himself nearly anything that brings him joy. Watch out for the Centaury who discovers a Vervain or Vine sadist, because together, the two will intertwine in a dance of destruction.

In general, Centaury types wish to give their responsibility for self to another. And, therefore, these types are particularly vulnerable to other more dominant personalities. At the time of life when they should be developing their own calling, they turn their full attention to another person's life calling. They make that calling—or the process of helping that person attain his or her goals—their own pseudo-calling in life. Centaury types can dedicate their whole heart and being to another person, to a political cause, to a religious movement, all with apparent fervor and joy.

Now, our society is based on the hope that we all have some degree of Centaury in us. We hand over some of our right of self-government to have a government that controls the actions of all. If we were all able to achieve our goals in a positive and mature way, there would be no need for government.

But the true Centaury takes things further, and perverts a virtue into a destructive emotional pattern by doing so. He hands over his life energy to another person or to a cause. This is a person who is particularly vulnerable to cults and cult mentality. He searches for gurus who will enlighten him as to how he should live and think, instead of exploring the nature of life on his own and drawing his own conclusions.

But, something eats away at the Centaury beneath all his work and his vibrantly cheerful demeanor. In his core being he knows that the assumptions he has made for how he can best live his life are wrong. Even if he has lost touch with his own sense of selfishness, even if he has convinced himself that the loss of self is the path to bliss, something remains that tells him that he could do better, he could do more. That he could still find a way to be true to himself.

This dynamic—the apparent struggle between selfless and selfish behaviors and the needed balance between the two—creates a great deal of discomfort for the Centaury type. For all his cheer, this is a person who experiences a great deal of stress. In fact, many Bach practitioners feel that the Centaury, along with the Aspen, represents the most sensitive of all emotional states. Where the Aspen type is "on edge" and very sensitive in his anxious state, especially to variations in temperature, light, weather patterns, and other changes in his physical environment, the Centaury is the most emotionally open and empathic of all the Bach types. The Centaury type is incredibly sensitive, especially to the suffering of others—the homeless and the sick are particular targets for their emotional response, as are children and animals. Organizations directed toward helping these groups will be largely staffed by Centaury types, either in positive or negative emotional states. The difference will be that the Centaury types who have evolved into a more positive emotional state do their good works while still finding time and energy to tend to themselves, while the more negative types hand over their lives to their causes.

The patient trapped in the negative emotional Centaury state has lost his ability to bring his life into balance. He hands over his life's work to another so he can hand over the responsibility for his life's work to another. Thus he will not have to be responsible for success or failure, he will not have to make the hard decisions that life requires and then live with the results of those decisions.

I cannot stress enough that, while the Centaury's motivations may seem positive, even pure, the truth of the situation is that they are out of balance Centaury has taken a pure urge to do something good with his life and has handed that life away instead. And how can he—or any of us—say he has achieved something in life if, in reality, he has never lived it? Instead, he has lived someone else's vision and has hidden himself away from the world, its temptations, and its stresses.

In hiding under a bushel, in hiding his secret goals, wants, and needs away from all eyes, and by falsely insisting that he really *has* no needs or wants, the Centaury creates an elaborate falsehood that becomes his life. Is it any wonder then, that he is never truly happy with the results?

There is a certain resignation that haunts the Centaury type. He will, in odd moments, tend toward flashes of what he might have done if he had not done this, but usually the Centaury type will not want to explore these thoughts. He will avoid them and push them away, just as the Agrimony will when faced with the reality of his life.

Because of the weight of this resignation, consider mixing Wild Rose with Centaury to help the patient achieve emotional balance.

Chestnut Bud, with its slavish continuance of habits that even the patient himself admits are no longer working, is another remedy that blends particularly well with Centaury. This combination can help him break old patterns of thought and behavior and move ahead to a new life.

Pine is the other remedy that I think blends best with Centaury. In many cases a deep sense of guilt is at the root of or intertwined with the Centaury's pattern of weak will and slavish behavior. Often a sense of shame and guilt pushed upon a child will produce the weak personality that is common to the Centaury type.

In its acute use, Centaury is helpful for those moments in our lives when we feel we lack the strength to say "No." It can help us stand up for ourselves when more dominant types are being too demanding. Also consider this remedy when you are putting on a happy face but don't feel it, when you are using false cheer to cover a real desire not to be bothered.

Centaury is truly a universal remedy that we all need from time to time. It helps us find our voices and our backbones when we misplace them. And it helps us to be honest to our true selves when we are tempted to yield.

## Negative Qualities of the Type

At their worst, Centaury types become professional victims, never taking responsibility for their actions. They are too passive, too underdeveloped as people. They often live in a constant state of martyrdom. And a constant state of exhaustion.[6]

## Positive Qualities of the Type

When in a positive state, Centaurys are people who are able to say the word "no" when necessary, but often enjoy saying "yes" as an act of encouragement and support. These are the people who make our society function by their willingness to be "team players." By their gift of working with others and allowing all to shine.

Further, the altruism of the positive Centaury type is a shining example to the rest of us, who demonstrates what we might do with our lives and what can be accomplished in this world, if we can lift our eyes from our own needs and wants and elevate our ambitions for the good of all.

---

6. This sense of exhaustion is one of the chronic issues of the Centaury type. Left unchecked, the Centaury inevitably seems to move into chronic illness, often into chronic joint pain. In cases where the Centaury has worn himself down into illness, the remedies Oak and/or Olive can be used to help the Centaury find his strength and his ability for inner healing once more.

### The Centaury Child

These are passive children who are walking targets for the schoolyard bully. They will find it impossible to stand up to this bully; they look for others to assist them instead. They have good imaginations, and are sensitive to the point of being psychic. These are good children, who will play quietly with their toys for hours and always do as they are told. However, be aware that the Centaury child will be an easy target for anyone he believes is stronger than he is. He would, for instance, be an easy target for a molester who simply tells him to get in the car.

Parents of Centaury types need to nurture their child's strengths to help him to find his own talents and voice, and to stand up strong, both on the playground and at home. Parents who fail to help this child trust himself and his own will, and especially those who use guilt as a means to control this child risk creating a dangerous dynamic that can cripple the child for many years to come.

### The Centaury Adult

There is little difference between the Centaury child and the Centaury adult. Centaury adults are still rather shy, rather passive (or passive-aggressive) people. They still lack the ability to say "No." They still retain the psychic nature they had in childhood. These are very sensitive people who lack a strong core self.

The adult Centaury lives in a state of confusion. He does not understand that those who choose a position of service need a strong sense of self and cannot use service to others as an excuse for not developing this core sense. As the Centaury state continues to overwhelm this person, more and more of their energy goes into having to please their guru and less and less energy is available for their own life.

This confusion is often reflected in the Centaury's home. That home may be neat and tidy to the eye, but it, too, will be in a state of confusion. The Centaury, whose vagueness of character is often reflected in a weak memory that is covered over with giggles, will have trouble finding things, paying bills and balancing checkbooks, and running an efficient home.

Centaury is not a remedy that is linked to a particular time of life. While most of us will move beyond this remedy by middle age, there will always be those—who often seem much younger than their years—who continue with their false façade well beyond their youth.

There is a strong gender link for this remedy type, however. This remedy and Agrimony both deal with the same underlying issue of living with authenticity in the world. And because our culture imposes such strong strictures of expectation for the behavior of men and women, I believe that more women than men fall into the Centaury pattern and more men than women fall into the Agrimony pattern of false cheer joined with emotional unavailability.

This is not to say that men and women alike won't need both remedies acutely. I also am not saying that you won't find a man in a Centaury constitutional state, or a woman in need of Agrimony as a constitutional treatment. I am merely sharing a pattern I have noticed.

### The Centaury Animal

This remedy is a real help for the dog that is the "runt of the litter," or any animal that is having trouble standing up for itself. For animals that take on the submissive role.

It is also helpful, especially in combination with Olive, for animals that are exhausted or have endured a long illness and are having trouble in finding their physical strength.

### Centaury and the Homeopathic Pharmacy

The homeopathic remedy most similar to Centaury is Silicea, which is created from pure flint. And as Centaury hands over their life energy to another, so, too, does Silicea lack "grit," and the moral fiber that would allow them to live their life with strength and individuality.

### Issues that Suggest Centaury

Abuse; aging; arthritis; chronic fatigue syndrome; hypoglycemia; lymph ailments; motherhood; myopia; nose bleeds; perfectionism; rheumatoid arthritis and sciatica; toothache and chronic tooth and jaw pain.

### In Conclusion

Nothing much has been said, to this point, about the anger I have found in some Centaury types. They tend to project an almost pathologically cheerful nature, but this does not mean that, on some level, they are not aware of their plight.

The happy and passive natures of many Centaurys mask a strong tendency toward passive-aggressive behavior. The seemingly blissful Centaury finds a way to make his underlying dismay known through these behaviors.

Chief among these behaviors are an almost constant tardiness, in which the Centaury will seem to live by a different clock than anyone else,[7] a verbal skill that often leaves others wondering if the Centaury said "yes" or "no" in response to a simple question, and an awesome skill of obstructionism. By this I mean that the Centaury will tell any dominant type whatever it takes to get the pressure off him in that moment. He

7. Variations on this are procrastination, in which the Centaury will be totally unable to get anything done on time, and a general confusion that pervades his life so that he can never be expected to accomplish anything without being given a great deal of warning and a total lack of pressure.

will agree to anything, but the other person will realize at some future point that he will avoid giving any indication of when he will do what was asked, or how well he will do it, or how completely he will fulfill the task.

When all else fails, the Centaury who is pressed will simply lie—or in his thinking, "make up a story"—to avoid conflict or confrontation, and to avoid having to deal with the reality of any situation. No one can beat a Centaury for making excuses. They can weave a web of excuses that, like their promises, is a wonderful web of confusion, detailing everything while explaining nothing.

With these behavior patterns, the Centaury, while remaining blissfully cheerful and totally subservient, holds on to some control in his life and manages to grab some sort of revenge upon those who tower over him. Many of these behaviors can be associated with the relatively dependent and powerless stage of childhood. But Centaurys, who continue to feel powerless and dependent in adulthood because of their inner turmoil and lack of self, continue these behavior patterns.

## WALNUT · THE REMEDY FOR THOSE WHO ARE IN UPHEAVAL

Walnut, says Bach, is the remedy "for those who have definite ideals and ambitions in life and are fulfilling them, but on rare occasions are tempted to be led away from their own ideas, aims, and work by the enthusiasm, convictions or strong opinions of others. The remedy gives constancy and protection from outside influences."

Bach also wrote that Walnut is the remedy for "those who have decided to take a great step forward in life, to break old conventions, to leave old limits and restrictions and start on a new way."

• **Walnut is both an acute and a constitutional remedy, but more often than not, it is used acutely to help us deal with times of transition in our lives.**

### Botanical Information

The Walnut tree (*Juglans Regia*) has been greatly revered throughout human history, even worshipped, in an odd sense. It grows to over 100 feet high, and thrives in protected areas, especially orchards. It prefers moist soil and cannot grow in the shade.

It is native to Southern Great Britain, and now grows throughout Europe, Asia, and North America.

Walnut trees are androgynous, with male and female flowers growing on the same tree. The flowers bloom in spring, in April or May.

The Walnut tree and its flowers and fruit have long been considered to be highly medicinal. It is perhaps for this reason that it has been considered to be such a valuable plant for so long.

### Walnut in General

I most certainly agree with Bach that all of his remedies will be needed by all of us, to a greater or lesser degree, at one time or another in our lives. I cannot help but notice, however, that some remedies are more universal than others. Some remedies are needed more often than other remedies, and some remedies are needed by more people at any given time than are other remedies. Walnut would have to be one of the remedies that is most often needed by the greatest number of people in both of these categories.

> Think of Walnut for all of life's situations in which we feel that we are in upheaval. In the same manner, think of Walnut for all of life's milestones and for all its many entrances and exits. Walnut is an excellent remedy for puberty, for menopause, for birth, and for death.

Think of Walnut for all of life's situations in which we feel that we are in upheaval. Think of it for physical transformations, from birth itself to teething, when a child is learning to walk and talk, and for the other milestones of infancy and youth. Think of it for the emotional milestones of youth as well, for the first and the last days of school, for changes of home or changes in the home, like the birth of another child, or divorce, or death.

In the same manner, think of Walnut for all of life's milestones and for all its many entrances and exits. Walnut is an excellent remedy for puberty, for menopause, for birth, and for death.

Because this is one of Bach's remedies for oversensitivity, it relates to the times of life in which self-doubt can overwhelm our ability to adapt and change—when we are tempted to cling to the familiar, just because it is familiar. When the devil you know takes precedence over the devil you don't.

Walnut is a great remedy to use during any time of transition, from changing jobs to moving to a new home. And make sure to dose all those in your household with the remedy, including the pets and houseplants, during this time of transition. It will make the transition easier for everyone involved. In fact, I have found over the years that Walnut is almost always best used when it is used for a group and not just for an individual (like many other Bach remedies). Also, because this remedy is rather amorphous in its actions, it combines with other remedies better than most. Chestnut But and Star of Bethlehem are the two other remedies I have found to always "play well with others." These three remedies seem to find harmony and balance with the others, no matter the patient's mood or the situation for which the remedy is used.

Remember, the patient needing Walnut is not in a state of paralysis, nor are they unsure of who they are or their goals or vision in life. The Walnut state is one in which, in spite of a patient's set goals and strong sense of self, he is having a moment in which he is too sensitive to the world around him: to the constant chatter of friends and family, to the opinions of his critics, and to the roadblocks that seem to arise when he sets out to accomplish anything—especially something of value or something innovative. Walnut can help the patient screen out the noise and listen to his inner voice instead. It can help bring strength in times of emotional crisis. It can help the patient find his way when he can perceive no set path in front of him.

Certainly, there are other Bach remedies that seem to echo the issues that Walnut presents. Some are listed in this same group of remedies, for those who are overly sensitive. Both Scleranthus and Centaury types feel many of the same weaknesses and insecurities as the Walnut. Other remedies will reflect the same loss of self-direction as well. Elm, in its state of being emotionally frustrated and overwhelmed by work, can look like Walnut. So can Oak, as the Oak type breaks down from his driving sense of over-responsibility. And certainly Cerato, with his inability to say no, can seem like Walnut.

If you think about or reread the specifics of each of these remedies, however, you will find that each related to a very specific emotional state or life experience. Each represents a pattern of reactive behaviors that, over time, become set lifestyles. Something has happened in each case that has caused the patient to take on a pattern of behavior that is a very successful survival technique at first—it makes the patient feel better or better able to adapt to a bad situation—but over time, continues as a locked-in behavior even after it ceases to be successful. Even if the pattern of Doubt or Despair or Oversensitivity no longer helps the patient feel better about himself or herself, even if it has actually become a destructive pattern to the patient and his or her relationships, the patient continues on with the set pattern of behavior.

That is what makes some of these patients—to say nothing of their patterns of behavior—so very difficult to treat. The behavior gradually becomes all they know.

The same cannot be said about Walnut. Because it is a less specific remedy, because it speaks to the idea of entrances and exits, the times in life when, whether we like it or not, jobs end, relationships finish, and loved ones die, its use does not require any set pattern of thought, speech, or behavior on the part of the patient.[8]

Think of Walnut for the moments of life in which we feel weak—not in will or in vision or even in the physical body, but in personality. It can be a great acute remedy for the moments—and I mean the literal moments—in which our attention is caught, not by our own work or goal, but by the excitement that is happening in the other room. Reach for Walnut when you lack focus and concentration, when you are just

---

8. This does not mean that the other remedies mentioned—and Bach's other thirty-seven remedies, for that matter—cannot be needed acutely and that the mood state of the remedy cannot come and go quite quickly. But some remedies, like those mentioned here, are more often needed on a constitutional level and speak to a very specific range of emotions and behaviors, while Walnut is less specific and often less constitutional in its actions.

too vulnerable to the fudge brownie, the fireworks, or the laughter down the hall to stay on task.

This is the remedy for all the times in life in which we find ourselves at a crossroad. When circumstances, the will of others in authority, or fate itself has dictated that the rules by which we have lived our lives to this point are changing. It doesn't matter a damn whether we like it or not, whether we are comfortable with change or not. Change is shoved upon us. The way in which we react to this change and the amount of time it takes us to roll with it and get on with life can be greatly enhanced by the use of Walnut.

In homeopathic medicine, we have the concept of "miasms." The word miasm literally means "taint." It was coined by Samuel Hahnemann, the father of homeopathic medicine, when Hahnemann reconsidered the cases that he had failed to cure with his medicines. He had had many successes, but the failures plagued him and, ultimately, led him to a great discovery. That was the miasms.

For Hahnemann (and you have to remember that he was working two hundred or more years ago, long before Mendel and long before the idea of gene therapy), miasms were the weights that pulled us down into illness. They are, if you will, the predisposition to illness. Some of his miasms, like Syphilis and Sycosis, are the result of venereal disease and, especially, of the suppressive allopathic treatment of these diseases.

And then there is Psora. Psora is the miasm that Hahnemann felt was at the root of all chronic disease. Psora is the result of generations of suppressive medical treatments that have driven simple ailments ever deeper into our systems, generation after generation. Psora is the root especially of all functional diseases—those that cannot be isolated with any test, that do not, at least in the beginning, have any pathology; those diseases that we are told we shall have to "live with." Psoric or functional ailments are those that limit our lives, and may even shorten them if they get to be severe enough, but do not, on their own, end them. Things like skin conditions, allergies, migraines, joint pains, nerve pain, and chronic fatigue all fall into the category of functional disorders. And all are Psoric conditions as well.

I explain the idea of Psora so that I can make the simple statement that Walnut is, in my opinion, Bach's best Psoric remedy (along with Chestnut Bud, which I think is the most underutilized of all of Bach's pharmacy).

Just as most of us suffer from one or more of the illnesses that would be classified as Psoric, most of us suffer from a lack of will in our lives. Most of us can be fairly easily swayed from our path, by offers of food, money, sex, or fun. Most of us are dying to know what is causing the laughter down the hall.

For this reason, Homer Simpson has become one of our most recognized characters. Recognized not only for his four-fingered, yellow-skinned, bald-headed appearance, but also recognized on an emotional level. We love the Simpsons because we are the Simpsons. We all want donuts and cable television. And we all, some of the time if not most of the time, are willing to sell ourselves short to get it.

The Romans, I think, were the first to take advantage of this human characteristic. The Roman government noticed that its citizens were getting a little restless with their lot in life and with the general incompetence of their leaders. They decided to give the citizens something to keep them happy, and invented "bread and circuses." They gave away some free food and entertainment and found that, to their great joy, it pretty much placated the population.

And societies have offered variations of bread and circuses ever since.

Whatever your point of vulnerability, whatever causes you to divert from your path or sell yourself short, Walnut can help to bring you back into balance.

My experience with Walnut leads me to believe that, while there are some of us who can stay in a Walnut state for long periods of time, most of us need this remedy only acutely. It is often a remedy state that, if it goes ignored and untreated, transitions into one of the others mentioned above—longer-term patterns of aimlessness in which the patient takes on the specific attributes of a type. Walnut is a shallower, more transitory state of being. Think of it as the "gatekeeper" to those other remedies.[9]

Often Walnut is most helpful when the cause of the emotional state is an external one, such as when a patient loses his job for reasons that have nothing to do with his own efforts. Perhaps the company falls on hard times and has to lay off part of the work force. Walnut can be of tremendous help to the patient while he copes with the loss of the job and its income, and through the period of time while he scrambles to survive financially and find a new job. The patient finds he no longer needs Walnut once he is back at work.

And so it goes for this remedy. The length of time it is needed is often determined by circumstances rather than the behavior of the patient. But it can be of tremendous value at any time of transition, during any period of upheaval, or at any moment of confusion or lack of focus.

Walnut combines with all the other remedies. It combines especially well with Wild Oat, for patients who are rudderless, who have lost direction, or have yet to find direction in life.

It also combines very well with Mimulus, for patients who seem shell shocked, who are riddled with fears that have made them very wary and very timid, so that they lead very small, very frightened lives. It is also great with Olive for patients who have crum-

---

9. As I have said before, Walnut combines well with any other remedy, virtually any time. Never hesitate to combine it with Elm or Centaury or Cerato or any other remedy, as long as the patient is feeling the lack of focus and/or will associated with Walnut, or as long as the patient is going through change or upheaval in his or her life.

pled inward due to physical circumstances and have become so physically exhausted that they are very vulnerable to the opinions of others and seem to lack a will of their own.

Think of combining Walnut with our three great weak willed types. It combines very well with Scleranthus, Cerato, and Centaury for any cases in which the patient seems especially weighed down in his emotional pattern or when the pattern has been very long established.

Finally, use Walnut and Star of Bethlehem together in any case that looks like a Star of Bethlehem case at first, but the remedy by itself fails to rally the patient, or for any patient who is left bewildered, confused, or overly sensitive to others because of an emotional or psychic injury.

### Negative Qualities of the Type

The person in the negative Walnut state is not sure of what to do next. His or her normal strong opinions have melted into confusion and hesitation.[10] The patient is at a moment of life when he or she is simply too open to the opinions of others, especially others who loudly issue warnings of the terrible things the future might hold. This is the remedy for those who, finding themselves at a crossroad in life, just want to sit down and wait for someone or something to pick them up and show them the way. Or for those who, while walking down the pathway of their lives, find themselves confused and distracted by some shiny object or another that captures their attention.

### Positive Qualities of the Type

In a positive state, the Walnut type can move through life welcoming change and staying true to himself. The pressures of change and fear of the future never drive the positive Walnut to behave in a manner unlike his true nature. While he is open to others, to the world, and to the future, he is able to choose which opinions he will listen to, and which stimuli will have impact on his life.

### The Walnut Child

Childhood is a stage in life that certainly contains moments in which Walnut is needed. All major stages of growth are appropriate moments for the use of this remedy, as are the times when changes occurring in the household will affect the child's inner strength. Events such as divorce, career change, or job loss are all times when a child will need Walnut to help him deal with changes in his parents' lives.

---

10. This is a great remedy for those moments when we need a good swift kick in the pants. When we know what we should do and what changes we should make, but we can't quite get ourselves to make the move into a new and better life. Walnut helps us gather our wits and our strength and physically make the transition that we have already made emotionally. For the moments when it is "all over but the doing."

Walnut children know what they want to do, know the correct answers to the questions the teacher is asking, but fail to display their knowledge or act upon their abilities. They can be talked into doing things they do not really want to do. Walnut helps these children find the strength within themselves to do what they want and not what they are being talked into doing.

### The Walnut Adult

Usually Walnut comes into play when we find ourselves at a major crossroad in life and are unsure of just which way to walk. That is the general use of the remedy.

But it is perhaps even more useful for those crises in life when we are dealing with times of true change and/or true transformation—crises that are often thrust upon us, against our will, by strong external forces. This is the remedy of choice when we are on the verge of becoming new people, but something binds us to the past. Think of Walnut for the abused wife who is ready to leave and yet does not. For the smoker who wants to quit and yet can't quit. Walnut is a remedy that can be very useful at these times to push us through the doorway and on to a new life.

### The Walnut Animal

Use this remedy when a new animal is brought into the household. Give Walnut not only to the new animal but to all the other animals as well, including yourself and your family. It will help with the transition.

Walnut is also useful for animals, as it is for humans, during all the major milestones in life. But most pets have one milestone that humans do not. Give Walnut after a pet has been spayed or neutered.

In a sad vein, this remedy is a helpful one when we deal with the dying process for a beloved animal. It should be given to any animal during the dying process or before euthanasia, and upon its death it should be given to everyone who loves that animal.

### Walnut and the Homeopathic Pharmacy

Walnut reminds me most of the homeopathic remedy Ignatia as a remedy that allows us to break ties with the past and move on into a new way of living with new energy. Ignatia is known best for being a grief remedy, but it is for anyone who is trapped by past betrayal or grief and who cannot get beyond that grief. Their life is frozen. They can see others who have "moved on" with their lives, but they have been unable to do so. A dose or two of Ignatia, and they can let go of the past and move on to a new life.

Like Ignatia, Walnut tends to be an acute remedy. There are few true Walnut types, just as there are few Ignatia types. Both are people who usually are another type but have become emotionally frozen by overwhelming circumstances.

On a more constitutional level, no other remedy parallels Walnut's confusion or lack of direction better than Sulphur. Sulphur is Hahnemann's great antipsoric remedy, one that is so often used that American homeopathic J. T. Kent once commented, "When I prescribe, I prescribe Sulphur."

Sulphur is the great homeopathic remedy for functional illness, allergies of all sorts, skin conditions, digestive disorders, and aches and pains. For patients who are caught in a cycle of self-destructive behaviors and those whose inherent interest in anything new greatly outweighs their concentration for finishing tasks or mastering their studies. For philosophers who allow their philosophy to overtake their whole lives.

For any great confusion that can, like philosophy, take over our lives, no homeopathic remedy better parallels Bach's remedy Walnut than Sulphur.

### Issues that Suggest Walnut

Abuse; addiction and treatment; adolescence; bad habits; birth; career changes; codependence; death and dying; developmental disorders; digestive disorders; eating disorders; graduation and job search; headaches, especially migraines; hormone imbalances; joint pains; immune disorders; medical treatments—give before and after anesthesia, during and after long hospitalizations; menopause; midlife crisis; milestones; moving; muscle pains; pregnancy; puberty, skin conditions; teething; transitions; unemployment.

### In Conclusion

I have read that some Bach practitioners believe that there are two remedies that can be best used for opening constitutional cases for Bach treatment.

By this I mean that, when you are sitting across from a patient and you know they can benefit from Bach treatment but are unsure just where to begin, these practitioners believe that one of just two remedies will always work. They use Holly for patients who are aggressive and Wild Oat for patients who are passive.[11]

I totally disagree with this concept and think it is a bastardization of Bach treatment. Just as many practitioners have tried to find shortcuts with homeopathic treatments, this cookie-cutter approach to Bach treatments is lazy at best. You are robbing the patient of his or her ability to get well as simply, easily and safely as possible when you offer anything other than appropriate and individualized treatment.

There is no remedy or combination of remedies that can always be used to begin treatment. But, if there *were* . . . it would be Walnut.

---

11. This idea is based, no doubt, in the fact that Bach himself considered Wild Oat and Holly to be his two "primary essences." They are primary because Holly is the remedy that deals with a fundamental disharmony inside oneself, while Wild Oat deals with this same fundamental disharmony when it is placed between self and the world. While this is a very interesting concept, I question whether it is a valid basis for an actual treatment.

I have found over the years that some remedies have rougher beginnings than do others. Holly is one of these. Crab Apple is another. Willow is a third. Because each of these states suggests a rather aggressive behavior pattern and a very negative emotional outlook, I have found that they can create some rather severe aggravations—emotional and physical—when they are first given. They are often best used in combination with other remedies and after other remedies have opened doorways within the patient's emotional blocks.

Walnut, however, is always benign. And, since it is the closest thing we have to a truly universal remedy—by this I mean one that is good for all the people all the time—chances are that it will do a great deal of good no matter who you give it to and no matter when you give it.

So, if I were to say that there was one remedy that was the "best" remedy to open a case—acute or chronic—I would say Walnut. Or Star of Bethlehem. Or Chestnut Bud. Something like that . . .

## HOLLY · THE REMEDY FOR THOSE WITH ANGER, HATRED AND/OR JEALOUSY

Bach tells us that Holly is the remedy "for those who sometimes are attacked by thoughts of such kind as jealousy, envy, revenge, suspicion. For the different forms of vexation. Within themselves they may suffer much, often when there is no real cause for their unhappiness."

Bach stresses the almost universal need for the remedy when he comments, "Holly protects us from everything that is not Universal Love. Holly opens the heart and unites us with Divine Love."

- Holly is both an acute and a constitutional remedy.
- Holly is, along with Wild Oat, one of Bach's two "Primary Remedies."

*Botanical Information*

The English Holly (*Ilex Aquifolium*) is a perennial tree or shrub that can grow up to fifty feet in height. It likes full or partial sun and dry soil. It cannot tolerate poor drainage. It also cannot bear high humidity, bitter cold, or exposure, and often has to be well protected if it is to survive.

Holly flowers in May or June. The flowers are small and white, and only very slightly fragrant. Holly is known for its bright and shiny green leaves and its bright red berries. It is often used as a decoration during the traditional holiday season because of these characteristics.

Perhaps more than any other plant, Holly has a long mythology. It is of particular importance to the Celts and the Druids, for whom it was an icon for a "battle-waging spear." Holly was believed to represent the fierce side of human nature. Further, it was believed to have the power to bring light into dark places, even into the underworld.

Holly, therefore, has traveled through history with the concept that it is a powerful, even brutal creation, but one that offers the possibility of redemption as well.

As Holly is of particular import to the British historically, it is not surprising that Bach would include it among his remedies.

## Holly in General

Holly is Bach's remedy for a panoply of negative emotional states and patterns of behavior. Chief among the emotions common to the Holly type are: defensiveness, irritability, anger, rage, suspicion, mistrust, jealousy, paranoia, envy, revenge, hate, aggression, and destructive behaviors of all sorts. In short, this single remedy is used to balance and subdue a wide-range of explosive behaviors, especially those that occur explosively without premeditation in a single moment. It is both an acute and a constitutional remedy and one of the most commonly called for of Bach's pharmacy. Indeed, as we shall see, Bach considered it to be one of the "primary" remedies.

Because of the intensity of the emotional states it treats, the remedy itself can elicit a powerful response. My experience with the Bach remedies has shown me that three of them, Holly, Willow and Crab Apple—each a remedy for a powerful and intense emotional state—can create initial aggravations, both physically and emotionally.

The term "aggravation," when used in homeopathic medicine, refers to a temporary increase in symptoms that can often be seen in the initial stages of treatment, especially with acute treatments. As the homeopathic remedy begins to act, the patient's symptoms may be stirred up and intensify for a brief period before they greatly improve. It is important to understand the nature of aggravations so patients—especially frail patients—are not forced to undergo a cure that is more uncomfortable than necessary.

In the case of Holly and the other Bach remedies, I have seen that the remedies for the more volatile emotional states can often create an emotional upset that mirrors the patient's own when they are first given. They may also, especially in the case of Holly and Crab Apple, have physical symptoms such as an upset stomach or headache. When this passes, it will not recur. And, with the passing of the aggravation, you can expect to find that the patient's emotional state has greatly improved.

But because of Holly's tendency to aggression, often physical as well as emotional, it is important to avoid any aggravation if at all possible. Therefore, I do not think Holly should be used as the first remedy in cases involving a constitutional type with an ingrained pattern of aggression and hostility. Instead, the case can be opened with a simpler remedy, such as Star of Bethlehem, and Holly can be phased in once the patient is used to Bach treatments and understands how they affect him.

I also find that Holly is best used in combination with other remedies. Some remedies work well by themselves. In fact, some remedies work better alone than they do in combination with others. Holly, however, works best when it is used in combination with other remedies, especially when it is balanced with remedies that speak to other aspects of the patient's character.

I would, for instance, tend to mix Holly with Star of Bethlehem, as mentioned above, or with Mimulus, if the patient has fear underlying his anger (this is a very common combination and a very helpful one).

But I would not mix Holly with Impatiens, Vervain or Vine initially, as each of these types tends to be volatile and the mixture may simply be too much for the patient. In time, of course, each or all of these remedies can be rotated into the mixture of remedies blended especially for that patient.

While I'm on the subject, I have found that one of the best combinations for the Holly type is White Chestnut. (And, again, I am speaking primarily of constitutional types here. When you are using the remedies in a simple acute situation, any or all remedies may be safely mixed or used singly in any order.) I often find that White Chestnut can help the Holly type who is clinging to some slight or reason for revenge let go of (or perhaps forget is a better word) the reason for his anger while the Holly calms the anger itself. This combination can leave even the angriest patient in a state of calm repose in a remarkably short period of time.

One other use of Holly that combines the emotional state of the patient with his physical health has to do with allergies. Consider blending Holly with either Beech or Crab Apple when allergies come on in an explosive manner, and even for cases of allergy-based shock.[12] If the patient is somewhat blocking the reality of the situation, "I don't know what's happening to me," give the Beech with the Holly. If they are announcing that they have been poisoned and their response is quite aggressive, moving about, or thrashing, give the Crab Apple. Beech and Crab Apple are powerful remedies for allergies and poisonings, so both are of great value here. And any situation that elicits an explosive, aggressive response—physical or emotional—suggests Holly.

But what are we talking about in terms of emotions and motivations when we talk about the Holly type? And why, in a pharmacy of just thirty-eight remedies, did Bach dedicate five to different aspects of Fear, six to Doubt, and seven to the concept of Indifference, while he only dedicated one to all the different negative aggressive emotions?

The answer to this is that Bach felt that Holly was, along with Wild Oat, one of his core remedies for the human condition.

---

12. I know I just said that I would not blend these two remedies as an initial treatment, but I was considering constitutional treatments at the time. Here we are talking about an acute crisis.

Now, I know the combination of these remedies seems odd. Holly is a remedy for a vibrant, explosive type, who is most often locked into a deeply destructive emotional pattern, whether he acts upon his impulses or not. Wild Oat, on the other hand, is a benign type, and is a remedy that speaks to situations more than to moods. It is a remedy that can help us rise up when we would prefer to lie down.

But Bach wisely understood that, in the simplest terms, we can only be out of balance in two ways. We either are disorientated with the world or within one's self. Wild Oat is the remedy (again, generally speaking) for the times when we are out of balance with the world and are unsure of who we are in it. Holly is the remedy for when we are out of balance within ourselves, when we lose touch with our essential self, and lose touch with our most essential and creative emotion, love.

Therefore, if one were to remove thirty-six of the thirty-eight Bach remedies and leave only two, one for each of the two most basic states of emotional imbalance, those remedies would have to be Wild Oat and Holly.

It is for this reason that some Bach practitioners rather slavishly believe that these two remedies should, therefore, be used to open any case. If the patient is pale and withdrawn, they give Wild Oat. If the patient is ruddy and aggressive, they give Holly.

While I find Bach's concept of two basic or "primary" remedies, each of which balances the other in a "yin/yang" sort of way—Holly being the most active and emotionally direct of Bach's remedies and Wild Oat being nearly its opposite, passive and emotionally vague—I do not hold with the idea of giving either Wild Oat or Holly in every case, because (if for no other reason) Holly is not always tolerated particularly well at the beginning of treatment, as I have noted above. But, more important, I oppose this method of remedy selection because patients are not so easily defined that their motivations can be reduced to being either Holly or Wild Oat. Bach created his other remedies to fill in the colors of our emotional spectrum that lie between the two.

Given this, what are we treating when we use Holly? When is it appropriate for use? And how can one remedy be used effectively to treat so wide a range of emotional states?

> Holly is the remedy for the most negative of all human emotions: anger, hatred, envy, and jealousy. All of these are states in which the love we should be able to share and enjoy in life has been cut off and we feel neither loved nor loving.

Perhaps the reason is because Holly is not used to treat each of the aggressive, individual states listed above. Instead, it may be more realistic to say that it is used to treat the absence or perversion of the most powerful positive emotion, love.

Holly is, after all, the remedy for the most negative of all human emotions: anger, hatred, envy, and jealousy. All of these are states in which the love we should be able to share and enjoy in life has been cut off and we feel neither loved nor loving. This void is filled with negative emotions that, while destructive to self and others, are perceived by the Holly type as being preferable to indifference or to a lack of any emotion. Therefore, the emotions felt and explosively displayed by Holly types are a warping of their natural desire for love. Perhaps no other type is as loving. Certainly, no other type yearns so much for love or is so willing to be loved. And yet, something—some emotional wound or event—has cut off the Holly type from a sense of loving and being loved.[13] And, as a result, no other type so drains those in the environment around him of peace, hope, or joy.

I have used the word "explosive" again and again in describing Holly types and this speaks to one of their great attributes: they are spontaneous people. Where Willow types, motivated by bitterness, tend to take a longer-term approach to getting what they want (revenge, or what they would term "justice"), the typical Holly tends to be a short-term thinker, if he thinks at all. Hollys are, even when they attain balance and a positive emotional state, very spontaneous people. They live in the moment with little consideration of the consequences of their actions.

They use this natural spontaneity to act without thought of consequences when they are in a chronic emotional state, and as a result will tend to be perceived as walking landmines by others. Often family members, friends, and coworkers will not have a clue as to what will "set them off." From the outside looking in, Hollys are seen as half-crazy. When they suddenly erupt into rage, or fits of jealousy, or even in a simple burst of irritability, they do so without warning and often without apparent cause. Hollys may feel much put upon for a period of time before they fly into what they feel is a justified response. But once they erupt, they tend to give themselves carte blanche in their actions and words. Thus, Holly types are often abusers. They can be physically or emotionally abusive. They can be both. They often tower physically over the victim of their wrath as they spend their pent-up rage in aggression. Once their anger is spent, they feel much better. The others around them, understandably, feel worse. One Holly who gives himself full permission to behave as he feels he must to expend his pent-up rage can undermine the peace of a whole village.

The Holly type will, in moments of calm, often feel a great deal of remorse for what he has done. Some will freely apologize for what they have said or done. Some will swear that it will never happen again (it will). Some will not. Some Holly types instead internalize their regret, sulking to themselves or covering over the reality of their behavior with a simple, "Look what you made me do."

---

13. Again, as with so many other Bach remedy types, this is a matter of perception. The Holly has lost his ability to feel love, either the love he feels for others or the love they have for him. This may be true chronically, or it may be true only in the moments of pure rage in which the Holly blocks all of what he considers to be "weak" emotions, in order to feel the pure surge of his rage. Either way, the Holly who yearns to be loved cannot feel it, even if, in all reality, he is surrounded by loving support.

Given all this, it seems odd that Bach has decided to group the remedy Holly in this section, with the other remedies for oversensitivity, and not with the remedies for Despair, where it could live next to the remedy that is its cold-blooded sister, Willow.[14]

But the Holly type is overly sensitive, to an almost unbelievable degree.

Physically, Hollys will be sensitive to everything, to every change in their environment, to every sensory impression. They tend to be particularly sensitive to sound. Emotionally this will come out as a sensitivity to what is being said, and whether or not others are talking about them, and what they are saying (it will be presumed that it is negative and damaging). Physically, they cannot stand noise. Loud music will send them pounding on the door of the offender. High-pitched voices will irritate them. Dogs barking will send them into a rage.

In the same way, sound can soothe Holly types. Listening to the music they love can calm and center them. Hearing a voice they love will bring them peace as well. They will often learn best by hearing, and will often have a love of the quiet sounds of nature and the outdoors—things like birdsong and running water—that far exceeds others.[15]

The Holly type will also be very sensitive to light, and can become irritable if he has to cope with glare. In the same way, temperature can irritate the Holly, especially cold temperatures. The Holly who becomes uncomfortable because of cold is a Holly who is going to get very agitated as well.

The Holly type will be sensitive to everything in his environment and quite intolerant of anything that offends him. This often gives rise to a wide-range of physical ailments, chief among them digestive disorders and chronic allergies, especially food allergies. Holly types often cannot tolerate alcohol, although they may crave it because they will incorrectly believe it calms them down after a stressful day.

And no one deals with stress worse than a Holly type. Things that would only mildly upset others will paralyze the Holly with anger and a need for revenge. Road rage, therefore, can be described as an example of the Holly negative emotional state, as can any behavior pattern to which the word "rage" has been attached by the media.

Obviously, the Holly state has its physical consequences. The Holly type will often

14. These two remedies can certainly resemble each other from time to time. They both can have acid tongues that can greatly injure those who love or trust them, and both can seem to take pleasure in causing others to suffer. Sometimes the dividing line is as simple as this: Willow takes her time in getting revenge, Holly just explodes and gets it over with. Willow is cold emotionally, Holly is hotheaded.

15. It is not for nothing that the various sound-soother machines used to calm those who are agitated and irritated by noises tend to have nature sounds built in. This helps the wound-up Holly get some sleep.

fall prey to heart disease and hypertension. They are also known for their sudden high fevers, their severe infections, and their chronic pain, especially nerve pain.

Emotionally, the Holly is equally sensitive. Suspicious by nature, Holly will be overly sensitive to everyone's opinion. They often will feel judged by everyone in their environment and are quick to ask, "What did you mean by that?" and even quicker to take offense even when none is meant.

The sensitive Holly will feel as if all eyes are on him and will often become quite agitated in any sort of group situation. He will, therefore, need to feel constantly supported by others, especially those that he counts as friends (the world, for the Holly type, is divided into black and white, friends and enemies—this will hold true on personal, political, and religious levels) and will be totally unable to bear the offense should a friend fail to publicly support him. The Holly that experiences such an offense in a business meeting will hardly be able to contain himself until the meeting's end, at which time he will lash out at the offending friend (and most likely place him on his personal enemies' list).

Many of Holly's outbursts, therefore, can be said to come from his oversensitivity, and his agitated state needs to be fully understood by anyone who lives or works with him. If any remedy type needed to come with an "owner's guide," it is Holly.

We all need Holly from time to time in acute circumstances. Think of Holly when you are in a bad mood, seemingly for no reason. When your family or friends are getting on your nerves. When your neighbor is repairing his car in the driveway next to your house in the early hours of the morning or when the neighbor's dog is barking long into the night. For life's irritations, and for those moments when you are tempted to give way to anger and to give yourself permission to speak your mind or do as you like, try Holly instead.

### Negative Qualities of the Type

Where do you start when it comes to the negative traits of the Holly type? Well, there's his almost constant state of agitation. There is his unpredictability. His distrust of others. His jealous streak. His mean mouth. His tendency toward violence and aggression. His paranoia. His willingness to always believe the worst of others. In short, the Holly type behaves like a dog that has been kicked too often.

The Holly type is in thrall to his emotions, and reacts to nearly all stimuli with one of three highly negative and highly aggressive emotional states: anger, jealousy, or paranoia. These negative emotions poison the Holly and block him from expressing or receiving love. Holly dislikes it when others succeed and loves to see others fail. Holly explodes in a rage spontaneously. Often he chooses to misunderstand the words or deeds of others as an excuse for revenge. He blames others for his anger. Holly chronically feels hurt or injured by others, which again gives rise to anger. He tries to make others feel like failures so he can feel better about himself. He is suspicious. He is vindictive. And he holds grudges.

The negative emotional state of Holly is perhaps the most destructive found among the thirty-eight Flower Remedies (perhaps it's a toss-up with Willow). He certainly is the most difficult to be near.

## Positive Qualities of the Type

In a true positive state, no remedy type is as loving as Holly. In its best incarnation, Hollys embody the universal force of love. And as such, they are among the most creative of all types. Positive Holly types live in harmony with all creation, have the gift of truly loving others, and find joy in the success of others.

Hollys have two other positive aspects as well. First, little has been said to this point about the fact that Holly types tend to be very truthful. Even when they are destructive, they tend to tell the truth. Bluntly, to be sure, but they tell the truth nonetheless. That is why their words are so painful—because negative Hollys have a powerful gift for perceiving the truth and then using it for destructive purposes. They will tell you that you have spinach in your teeth just before you go on camera. They will undermine the abilities of others by using truth as a weapon. So, when Hollys move into a more positive state they are capable of using the truth, and using it creatively, to enlighten and guide others.

And then there is the spontaneous nature of the Holly type. Even when in a positive state, they will tend to live in the moment. This makes them fluid in their thoughts and creative in their actions. This spontaneity, used appropriately, is a source of innovation and achievement.

## The Holly Child

The archetypal Holly child is a classic bully, filled with hatred, jealousy, and a desire for revenge. This Holly child has feelings of his own inadequacy and vents these feelings by trying to make other children feel worse about themselves. The Holly child will be envious of other children's families, of their pets, their grades, and their toys, and will seek to humble or harm the other child.

Holly is an excellent remedy to consider using for any child who is aggressive in his actions or speech. It blends especially well with Aspen and Mimulus for children who mask their fears with aggression. It can also be mixed with Vervain for children who seem hyperactive and who, in their agitated state, tend to break everything they touch.

Holly can be an especially important remedy for use with teenagers and young adults. While the human mind does not mature until age twenty-five or later, the human body reaches adult size around age eighteen. (The brain, scientists believe, actually matures from the back to the front. Since the part of the brain that controls

our actions and impulses and lets us pause and consider our actions and their consequences is located in the front of the brain, it is slow to develop.)

The mix of adult strength and immaturity only makes matters worse. The Holly
child is held in check by parents, by teachers, and by society in general. The Holly
young adult, however, allows himself to fully explode with anger and violence should
the situation, in his mind, suggest it. So Holly is often the remedy of choice in combat-
ing the "hair-trigger" impulses of the young. In these cases, it combines especially well
with Impatiens, which will help the patient slow down, take a breath, and think about
what he is about to do.

### The Holly Adult

Because Holly speaks to one of the great frailties of humanity, the tendency toward
anger and jealousy and revenge, the faces of those who need the remedy are faces that
reflect every age, both genders, every level of society, and every race. If there is a remedy that is needed by everyone at every age, adult or child, it is Holly.

### The Holly Animal

This remedy is a great gift to anyone who has to deal with an aggressive animal. And it
can work wonders for animals that lash out, especially if their behavior is sudden and
without apparent cause.

But aggression in animals may be based in fear. For this reason, the remedy Mimulus may be needed in cases where Holly is given. Consider using Mimulus first if the
animal in question has a history of abuse or a background that is unknown. If it does
not work, either replace it with Holly or combine Holly with the Mimulus.

Also use Holly for cases involving the sudden severe illness of an animal, such as
sudden fevers or infections.

### Holly and the Homeopathic Pharmacy

Holly very clearly parallels the homeopathic remedy Nux Vomica, a remedy made from
the poison nut, or rat poison. This remedy, too, feels a lack of love and great depression
around that issue, and covers it with anger and often violence. Both remedies have too
much push—are too willing to argue, vocally or physically. Both make the world a
worse place for those unfortunate enough to have to deal with them.

Another remedy that comes to mind when thinking about Holly is Lycopodium,
which shares Holly's spiteful ways. Sepia, too, has the resentment and anger of Holly.
Ignatia shares Holly's envy of others and explosive behaviors. These are chief among
our many homeopathic remedies for anger and envy. The total list is long because the
homeopathic pharmacy, unlike Bach's, does not have just one remedy that can speak to
such a wide-range of emotions and behaviors.

## Issues that Suggest Holly

Allergies, especially food allergies; arteriosclerosis; bad breath; boils; burns; conjunctivitis; earaches; fevers, especially sudden high fevers; heart disease; hypertension; infections of all sorts; joint pain; laryngitis; lockjaw; nerve pain, such as sciatica; numbness; polio; rabies; sprains and other injuries; toothache.

## In Conclusion

Holly is an easy target. Holly types are often the villains in our plays, movies, and soap operas. We all feel it is an easy type to understand and, in understanding it, to hate. Often the moral hero of the movie will, at some point near the end, put his arm around the Holly's victim and warn her not to pull the trigger and kill the Holly, who is, at last, at someone else's mercy. "Don't kill him," the hero will say, "Because, if you do, you will be no better than he is."

The implication is that the Holly's victim is, just by nature, "better" than the Holly. In our thinking there is no one worse than the Holly type.

And yet, if we are honest, we would have to admit that each of us has some Holly in us. The victim obviously has some Holly in her just by virtue of the fact that the hero has to stop her from pulling the trigger. We all do.

And yet, if there is a remedy that you will have trouble getting anyone to admit they might need, it is Holly. If you sit with a patient and go over the remedies with them, tell them a little about each, most will say that they need a remedy or remedies that will help boost their confidence. Or they will often want either Hornbeam or Olive, because they feel tired. In other words, they want a tonic. Nobody wants to admit that they have feelings of hatred, jealousy, or paranoia.

And yet, Bach thought that this was a "primary" remedy, along with Wild Oat. One that so speaks to the human condition that it actually speaks to our core, the part of ourselves that motivates us in all we do and all we perceive to be true about ourselves and others.

The primacy of Holly speaks to just how far we have fallen from the Garden of Eden, to how wrong we can be in our perceptions of right and wrong, truth and lies, reality and fiction. And how distorted our reactions to the world around us and the feelings within us can be.

Again and again, as you study the Bach remedy types, you will see that each remedy is acting in error. Something has caused them to come to the wrong conclusion about a specific emotion or about a perceived threat or challenge. And once the error of thought or emotion has been made, it is reinforced repeatedly even after it has been proven to be an error.

Thus, Bach's two primary remedies, Wild Oat and Holly, allow us to see our greatest errors. Wild Oat can open our eyes to the ways in which our perception of the world, the way it works, and our part in it are in error. And Holly allows us to see the ways we have duped ourselves about our own motivations and emotional needs. If, after all, love is the greatest and most creative emotion, then the lack of it is our greatest failure and motivates our most destructive behavior.

This being the case, perhaps it is time that we all begin to reconsider our need for the remedy Holly, so we can truly reevaluate the actual amount of creativity we bring to our life.

# 8

# Considering the Fifth Mood:
# The Need to Control

Bach refers to this mood as "over concern for the welfare of others." But I find that to be a bit overly polite. I think that the common bond among the remedies listed here is a need to control. That need may be borne within, and the remedy type will hold himself or herself up to powerful self judgment and high standards in life. More often than not, however, the need for control will spill out into the lives of others, with the remedy type issuing a series of lectures on how life should be led. At best, the remedy types listed here are nosy and annoying to those around them. At worst, they are as destructive in their way as any other remedy type, and can wreak havoc in the lives of others.

The types listed here, therefore, tend to be rather aggressive to some extent and in some manner. They are extroverts, at least in the way they carry their "good news" to the world or in the advice that they offer, whether it is wanted or not. All of these five distinct types share a tendency to reach out emotionally and/or intellectually to others. This places them in sharp contrast to the types gathered under the concept of doubt, which is a group of rather shy and introverted types.

The remedies and the types described here, therefore, stand in direct opposition to those who doubt. (Often those with control issues might do well to develop a healthy sense of doubt when it comes to their almost supreme sense of self.) Each type in this group shares a tendency toward pronouncement, either shouted out loud or issued *sotto voce*.

When we take upon ourselves any of the patterns listed here, we act in ways that allow us to avoid living our own lives and actually taking responsibility for what we do in life. Instead we become overly interested in the actions and lives of others.[1] This

---

1. This, for me, is the supreme irony of this mood. Just as each of the remedies listed here would think of responsibility and self-control as two of the greatest virtues of mankind, each is lacking in these things. The more they seek to control others around them, the more they tend to be out of balance emotionally and out of control themselves.

mood—this emotional pitfall—is such a strong hindrance to spiritual growth that Bach made it one of his largest and most diverse groups of remedies.

Those who are in need of one or more of these remedies tend to not see the "log in their own eye," while seeing all too clearly the mote in the eyes of others.

> This mood—this emotional pitfall—is such a strong hindrance to spiritual growth that Bach made it one of his largest and most diverse groups of remedies.

My experience has taught me that this is perhaps the most cohesive group of remedies, with the remedies for fear coming a close second. I have also noticed that patients who need any one of these remedies on a constitutional basis are very likely to need it in combination with one or more of the other remedies in this group, at least for part of the time.

Because the remedies in this chapter suggest a patient that has a greater degree of will and confidence than average, I have found they are less likely to need any of these remedies in combination with the remedies for doubt, since the emotion of doubt stands in direct opposition with the emotional states listed here.

In the same way, it is less likely that any constitutional type described here will need a remedy for indifference in combination with their constitutional remedy.

On the other hand, in my experience, the remedies listed here have a deep affinity with the remedies listed for those who are in despair. The two groups of remedies share a level of energy—many are strong personality types, and are forceful with their personalities and energy—and an outlook on life. Also both of these groups, as well as the remedies for those who are overly sensitive, contain remedies for passionate types. These are our aggressive types, our "hot" remedies, if you will. Further, these groups all contain remedy types that display some very negative and even destructive traits that can support each other in bringing about healing. These traits tend to be worn on the remedy type's sleeve—by which I mean that they are obvious to all, even to the patient himself, even if he will not admit it. This places them in opposition to, say, the remedy group for those who are in a state of indifference. This emotional state is often carried more deeply within and may be hidden, even from the patient himself. Again, this makes it less likely that the remedies for control and those for indifference would be used in tandem (with the exception of the Chestnut remedies, which, like wildcards, mix well with everything else).

I say these things with the caveat that anything and any combination is possible, when dealing with Bach remedies.

One final note: I would put Crab Apple in this grouping, instead of in among the "Remedies for those who Despair" where Bach placed it, if I were grouping Bach's thirty-eight remedies into their seven groups or "moods."

I believe that not only is Crab Apple a remedy that displays a range of control issues, but that it is perhaps *the* remedy for those with control issues.

I note this here, so you will also read and consider that remedy as well if you are reading this section in the hopes of finding the best remedy for a patient who exhibits issues with control.

## Control and the Homeopathic Pharmacy

The homeopathic repertory does not have a mental or emotional rubric that lists the remedies for those with control issues. Instead, these issues crowd the pages in smaller, more specific rubrics.

Among the remedy types that display a strong need for or sense of control are: Arsenicum, who is perhaps the homeopathic type with the strongest need to control their environment and those within it; Natrum Muriaticum, who can be perfectionist in their outlook, most especially when it comes to the cleanliness of their personal environment and the behavior and speech of the children; Calcarea Carbonica, who can display rigid behaviors and demands of all sorts; Causticum, who can be highly passionate in their quest for what they perceive as justice for all; and Sepia, who brings a weighty and rigid concept of control to their world, especially to their work environment.

The remedies in Bach's group of those who are controlling (like the homeopathic remedies that share this outlook) tend to be surprisingly conservative in their outlooks. They are very slow to change because they themselves are often convinced that what they are saying, thinking, and doing is quite right and for the benefit of all. In fact, the process of change can be just as hard for this group as it is for those in despair (especially Oak, but also Crab Apple, Elm, and Willow). Change can be the most stressful event in a controller's life, since it always involves a loss of control to some extent. Therefore, look for any of the patient types listed in this chapter to take a change of address, job, or even the change of political party in charge after an election very seriously, and to be much stressed as a result. Look for them to display physical complaints during these times of stress, especially allergies and digestive complaints.

## REMEDIES FOR THOSE WHO ARE CONTROLLING

- **Chicory**—for those who are possessive
- **Beech**—for those who are intolerant
- **Rock Water**—for those who are rigid
- **Vervain**—for those who are excitable
- **Vine**—for those who are willful

## CHICORY · THE REMEDY FOR THOSE WHO ARE POSSESSIVE

Bach notes that Chicory types are "those that are very mindful of the needs of others; they tend to be over-full of care for children, relatives, friends, always finding something that should be put right. They are continually correcting what they consider wrong, and enjoy doing so. They desire that those for whom they care should be near them."

• **While Chicory may be needed on an acute basis from time to time, it is primarily a constitutional remedy.**

• **Chicory is one of Bach's original remedies, the Twelve Healers.**

### Botanical Information

Chicory (*Chicorium Intybus*) is also known as endive. There are two types of endive, with common chicory being the flat-leaved. Its leaves resemble those of the dandelion. This plant is so common to roadsides, fields, and even to some gardens that we are all familiar with it, although we may have always considered it to be a weed.

Common chicory grows very tall, with many stalks and bright blue flowers. Its flowers are not long lasting. They will die as soon as they are picked, and flowers that bloom in the morning will fade by afternoon.

Chicory is eaten as a salad green. It can be highly invasive in the garden and has to be well tended.

### Chicory in General

When we think of the most typical example of the patient in a negative emotional state relating to the remedy Chicory, we think of the "Nosy Mother." She is the parent who intrudes into her adult children's lives, showing up at their door unannounced and uninvited, telling them how to clean their houses, cook their meals, and choose their appropriate mates.

This is the parent who mothers without any emotional boundaries and who will tolerate no back-talk or independent thought on the part of her children.

This mother rules her home, and her children's home, with an iron fist. But that fist is clothed in a velvet glove. And that soft, soft glove is this mother's idea of love.

The Chicory patient presents herself as a loving being, as a person who is motivated by love and by a desire to help those she loves. And, in "helping" the loved one, the Chicory inevitably controls them, all the while telling the loved one that what is being done to and for him is being done "for his own good."

Chicory is, therefore, another of our remedies who wears a mask. Just as Mimulus masks inner fear with the appearance of strength, Beech masks a judgmental nature with the appearance of tolerance, and Agrimony masks despair with false joy, Chicory wears the mask of unconditional love, while offering a kind of love that is anything but without conditions.

The Chicory state may also be played out as the "Wrathful Mother." This is an even more destructive emotional state, in which the Chicory moves beyond being intrusive and becomes an emotional tyrant.

The most notable character based upon this remedy type is Mother Rose in the musical *Gypsy*, who insists that everything is coming up roses, and is oblivious to her children's suffering. She is the mother who takes her children in hand and shapes them into what she herself wants them to be, ignoring their wants, and, in the case of Baby June, their chronological age. The only way the children can manage to have any say in their own lives is by running away and escaping from their mother's clutches.[2]

Bach compared the Chicory state to the archetype of the "Universal Mother," the nurturer that exists in every man or woman. In the negative Chicory state, this ability to nurture is lost. Chicorys are incapable of raising a child to be independent and strong. They are incapable of forming a love bond with another independent adult in adult love relationships with those who choose to share their lives. The idea of independence in any form is a terrible thing for negative Chicorys. For Chicory types, the love bond is a dependent, claustrophobic thing.

> Chicorys are incapable of raising a child to be independent and strong. They are incapable of forming a love bond with another independent adult. The idea of independence in any form is a terrible thing for negative Chicorys.

For the Chicory types, the natural flow of nurturing love that Bach refers to as coming from the "Universal Mother" is blocked, and the natural love that should flow freely and without restriction becomes both conditional and selfish. In other words, the "love" offered by Chicory types is not really love at all. It is a negative and highly destructive emotional tie based in selfishness and control. In this game of love, Chicorys are cruel taskmasters who control the objects of their love, crowd them, and use whatever tools are at hand—guilt and pity being the two most common—to keep the loved one bound to them.

Therefore, the Chicory type, like many of the other Bach types, takes a positive

2. The obvious archetype of this "Wrathful Mother" is Medea, the character in Greek mythology who slays her own children to have her revenge upon her husband. This is the most extreme example of Chicory love.

emotional bond and perverts it. What should be a creative impulse that nurtures the object of love and strengthens and inspires both parties becomes both negative and destructive. In the case of Chicory's negative state, the emotional bond that has been perverted is the strongest and purest possible, the bond of love.[3] And those who are the object of a Chicory's love will find themselves weakened and demeaned in receiving it.

For Chicory types, love must always be earned, by performing some action or deed. More important, love always means that they will be given all the attention they need whenever they need it, and for however long they need it.

Loved ones are being used by Chicorys to fill some inner void. As surely as Agrimonys will turn to alcohol to make them feel complete, Chicorys will turn to love and focus on an object of their love.

To be sure, this object need not be a single person, or, indeed a human being.

Most often, patients in a negative Chicory emotional state will focus on their child or children, or on a mate or boyfriend or girlfriend, with the full force of the selfish emotional bond they call love. But some Chicory types will focus instead upon the crowd and will seek to find in an audience what they lack in their life. Others will turn their attention to an animal, particularly a house pet like a cat or dog, to fill the emotional void in their lives. (This can often work out particularly well, because dogs are usually far more willing to do as they are told than children are. And, unlike children, dogs don't grow into adults who want to make their own choices in life and move out on their own.)

Chicory's behavior in supposed nurturing relationships—one that consistently sets his own wants and needs above those he supposedly loves—suggests an infantile idea of love, as do the methods the Chicory will resort to to get what he wants. The negative Chicory will turn to manipulation, to guilt, to deceit, even to breaking and entering (for his loved one's own good, of course) to achieve and maintain control in the relationship. And all of this suggests that the Chicory state involves some sort of emotional retrograde, like the Centaury or Cerato negative emotional states. Chicorys are frozen in a childlike emotional state in which they want what they want and they need what they need. They are, in this state, quite incapable of being reasonable on the subject of love or of loving in a mature and nurturing manner.

3. While the archetype of "Mother Love" is used to represent the idealized state existing between mother and child that the Chicory has twisted into a destructive emotional state for both parties, any true love bond can be twisted by Chicory's negative emotional state. The love bond between adults can be upset by the Chicory state, and the Chicory may respond to feelings of not being loved by becoming clingy or even by becoming a literal stalker of their loved one. In a parent-child bond it can be the child who is the Chicory, demanding obedience while proclaiming that what he or she wants is love.

Instead, the Chicorys' emotion of love is intertwined with the idea of self and self worth. In order to be gratified, they must be obeyed. And, in the words of Willy Loman,[4] "Attention must be paid."

In my experience, Chicory is more often needed as a constitutional remedy than it is as an acute medicine. And Chicory types fall among Willow and Crab Apple types as among the hardest to cure. Because they are convinced that they are totally motivated by love and refuse to see the destructive results of their behavior, they will often not see any reason to take any remedy of any sort, especially one associated with selfishness. No one (with the possible exception of Willow) is more defensive and more insulted by being presented with the notion that they are doing anything wrong. To them, their motivation is the loftiest of all—pure love. And they feel that they have it down pat— that they can love with one hand tied behind their back.

Things become trickier still in cases that require a combination of Crab Apple and Chicory. This patient not only presents herself as a loving mother, but as a perfect mother as well, with a clean house, dinner on the table, and tidy children who have already done their homework by dinnertime. This patient often has such a stranglehold on herself and her whole family that it is all but unthinkable to actually make any suggestion for change.

The results are equally difficult to bring into balance when a patient combines the need for Chicory with Willow. This patient will stress feelings of ingratitude any time she perceives a glimmer of independent thought on the part of her loved ones. As the Willow state involves bitterness, look for the Chicory/Willow to become increasingly angry and bitter any time he or she feels abandoned or ignored.

Whether it is needed by itself or in combination with other remedies, the need for Chicory is usually long term. Change can come slowly, as the Chicory type moves into emotional balance.

But this is not to say that Chicory is not useful in acute situations as well.

It is of special value to almost anyone at the point when the shock of losing a loved one begins to change into the deeper state of grief at the loss of a love bond. When the patient tries to hold on to the bond, perceives it as a physical thing, combine Chicory with Sweet Chestnut to help the patient let go of their partner and stand alone. This combination will not end the patient's grief, as grief is a natural and needed process, but it will allow them to stop being frozen, still clinging to their deceased love, and begin their healing process.

In daily life, think of Chicory as the remedy to take when you feel that you are not getting the attention you want or when you are tempted to feel self-pity. Whenever

---

4. Loman is the central character in Arthur Miller's play *Death of a Salesman*. The character is not a Chicory, but the quote is.

your ego feels damaged and you want to soothe it at the expense of others and their time, energy, and/or attention, take Chicory instead and get on with it.

### Negative Qualities of the Type

The negative Chicory state is one that dominates others, demands assigned behaviors, and feels that love must be earned. The negative Chicory will insist on the career that her child must have, and will even force good deeds upon others, telling them that it is simply for their own good. The irony is that she will also keep track of these "favors" that she has forced on others, at some point demanding that they repay her for her "good deeds." Chicorys are deeply manipulative people who will resort to emotional blackmail to force others to follow their will. Like Willows, Chicory types hold grudges for a lifetime and have great problems with forgiveness. Finally, Chicory types may also have bad tempers, and whether they are adults or children, they tend to have fits if they do not get their own way.

### Positive Qualities of the Type

In their most positive state, Chicory types can become the embodiment of Mother Love. The Chicory type is capable of loving truly and unconditionally. The patient who, in a negative state, controls and suffocates those he or she supposedly loves can, in a positive state, make their loved ones feel as if they can spread their wings and accomplish great things, sure of a steady flow of love and support.

The positive Chicory, male or female, may be called an Earth Mother, who provides security, safety, and nourishment. Who not only allows independence, but encourages it by offering a love that nurtures all creative possibilities.

### The Chicory Child

In many cases, the negative Chicory emotional state is born in childhood. There are many young Chicory types among us. These are the children who greet the guests at their parent's parties as if they were their own. They love to be the center of attention and will beam while drifting through the spotlight of attention.

They become angry when they are told at last that it is time for them to go to bed. By robbing them of the attention they crave, their parents are creating a situation in which Chicory children will turn to their ever-present Plan B. For Chicory children, Plan A is to always have full attention through charm and flattery. They will move through the party telling everyone how beautiful they are and how much they love them. In the same way, when they are alone with their parents, they will climb into their laps and tell them how beloved they are, and that they are the best parents in the world. And all is well, as long as their parents are willing to interrupt their own conversation and focus on them.

But when they are asked to leave the party, or when their parents are busy and cannot turn their full attention to them, Plan B goes into action.

In Plan B, very simply, Chicory children continue to be the center of attention by any means possible.

Chicory children come to the conclusion early on in life, just as Yoko Ono did, that negative attention is second to positive attention, and better than no attention at all.

Other children, when asked to leave the party after a brief appearance, say goodnight and go off to bed, or to the top of the stairs where they can continue to watch the adults unseen. Chicory children, however, become more and more agitated with each attempt to remove them from the room. They finally erupt into a full-scale tantrum and have to be physically removed.

But, even as they are being carried out, they are the center of attention.

Attention is what Chicory children want and it is what they will have, no matter what they must do to get it.

Because of this, Chicory children can be very difficult for their parents and can cause a great deal of stress in the marriage. Unless they are met with a firm hand, they will literally take over the household. In extreme cases, they can, in their utterly self-centered need for attention, present a danger of sorts to a new baby that is brought into the house, or a puppy that is adored by all. The loving little Chicorys, who so adore the new arrival while the parents are in the room, may give a sharp little pinch when they are left alone with their new sibling or pet.[5]

### The Chicory Adult

Often, the overriding issue motivating Chicory adults is abandonment. Whether they are aware of it or not, they have strong sense of abandonment based upon some past experience, and strong fears of being abandoned once more. This sense of abandonment makes them very wary on the subject of love, and very selfish in terms of love. Their seemingly loving behavior is a mask that allows them to manipulate the emotions and behavior of others.

Chicory types need to learn the lesson of true love. They need to risk all, present

---

5. One of my favorite old movies is *The Bad Seed*, which is made all the more amusing by the fact that it was written to be a very serious drama. In it, little Rhoda is seemingly the perfect child. She dresses well, and keeps telling everyone how much she loves her mother. Unfortunately, the mother finds out that her own parentage, which had been kept from her, includes some very bad blood. The movie, and the play from which it was taken, presents the question of which will dominate: bloodline or upbringing. As little Rhoda reveals her true colors and begins to set people on fire and drown her playmates, the question seems to be answered that blood will tell. Either way—blood or behavior modification—little Rhoda is a great example of Hollywood's idea of a Chicory child.

themselves as they truly are, extend their heart without manipulation or demands, and allow the other person to accept or reject their love. They will find a wonderful freedom within themselves to give and receive love once they have achieved this level of development.

Chicory is not a remedy type that is more common in one stage of life than it is at any other. As I have said, it is very common in childhood. It is also common in young adulthood, when the Chicory falls in love for the first time, but experiences this emotion as something he or she needs to control by controlling the other person.

You will also find Chicory types in adults of all ages. It can come on as a negative emotional state in adults moving toward middle age, who begin to fear that they will never be loved. As their desperation intertwines with their desire for love, they become more and more selfish in their approach to love relationships.

And seniors certainly fall into the trap of the Chicory state as well. Often, as we move into our senior years, this Chicory state is focused on our children. Children of Chicory elders are controlled by their parent's need for physical, emotional, and financial help as they enter the final years of their life, and also by their increasing needs for attention. Like Chicory children, these parents have decided that they would rather have attention for negative reasons—feigned illness, for example—than no attention at all.

Although it is not generally linked with one age group or stage of love over another, it would be tempting to say that it is gender linked since Chicory is considered to be a perversion of the purity of Mother Love. Certainly, we expect women to be more likely to enter into a Chicory state than men, and this is true to some extent. But do not make the mistake of thinking that men do not enter into the negative Chicory state. They do. They often will be more volatile in the Chicory state, however, and more prone to try to control the emotions of the loved one through force or the threat of force.

In other words, don't ever underestimate the need for Chicory for any patient, of any age or gender.

### The Chicory Animal

While this remedy does not have the depth of action that it does in humans, use it in cases when you know the animal was abandoned and for the animal that pines when left alone. It is also very helpful for the cat that won't stop rubbing up against your leg to get attention, or the dog that is apparently quite willing to do something that is sure to get it punished, because it will then get the attention it craves.

### Chicory in the Homeopathic Pharmacy

I consider the homeopathic remedy Sepia to be the closest to Chicory. For Sepia, too, love carries a task to be performed, a behavior to be enacted. Sepia fails to love the very one that she truly and deeply does love. For her, love is conflicted and trapped within.

### Issues that Suggest Chicory

Abandonment; aging; animal care; codependent behavior; diarrhea; fatigue; kidney troubles; mother issues; nail biting; numbness; rheumatism.

### In Conclusion

Two remedies among Bach's thirty-eight deal with the concept of love and the ways that the pure nurturing energy of love can be blocked or perverted into a destructive bond. The first is Holly, the second is Chicory. Holly and Chicory are similar remedies in some ways because both deal with the idea of love and how it is embodied in our primary relationships. They especially are most similar in the destructiveness of their behavioral patterns.

Both Holly and Chicory are quite capable of outbursts. The Holly type can descend into a rage for apparently no reason. The Chicory type will more likely have an emotional outburst or temper tantrum than rage, and will usually become upset when he either feels ignored (and is not the center of attention) or feels that he has not been sufficiently thanked or appreciated for his largess.

While Holly relates to the patient's feelings of separation from the emotion of love itself, and the Holly type cannot feel love even from those who offer it, the Chicory type presents a false loving face that seeks to disguise his genuine motivators, selfishness and greed. While no one can be as cold or cruel as a negative Holly, no one else can be as self-centered and clinging as a negative Chicory.

The behaviors of the two types may have similarities and both deal with issues relating to love, but Holly and Chicory represent two quite different types. One is cut off from love, and the other perverts the idea of love for the sake of his or her own selfish needs.

## BEECH · THE REMEDY FOR THOSE WHO ARE INTOLERANT

Bach insists that Beech is "for those who feel the need to see more good and beauty in all that surrounds them. And, although much appears to be wrong, to have the ability to see the good growing within. So as to be able to be more tolerant, lenient and understanding of the different way each individual and all things are working to their own final perfection."

- **Beech is both an acute and a constitutional remedy.**

## Botanical Information

The beech (*Fagus Sylvatica*) tree commonly grows to sixty feet in height and has a pyramidal shape. Because it tends to have a short trunk, its branches often touch the ground. Grass and other plants will not grow under the beech because of this.

The beech is a deciduous tree that is known for its bright red leaves in autumn. The beech has both male and female flowers on the same tree. The flowers bloom in early spring as the leaves are coming out.

The tree is native to Northern Europe and Great Britain, but now grows in temperate climates around the globe.

## Beech in General

Beech, like Chicory, the remedy that precedes it in these pages, wears a mask. The Chicory type presents himself as loving but in reality uses the love bond for selfish purposes. Beech, on the other hand, portrays himself as tolerant and very fair, while, in reality, he is judgmental and very close-minded.

In some cases, the Beech type can be an out-and-out hypocrite, in that he is aware of his true inner feelings and truly presents a false front to the world. This is common in our culture in circumstances in which, like it or not, our society has changed the mores and laws surrounding behavior. So, those who in the workplace once told jokes at the expense of a particular group or spoke of a certain type or person in a derogatory manner have learned to watch their words or keep their mouths shut without changing their inner opinions. This hidden intolerance speaks of a negative emotional state that is well treated by Beech.

In other cases, the Beech type carries his bias on a subconscious level and honestly believes that he is tolerant toward everyone. This, in my experience, is the more common type. Most often, the Beech type is liberal-minded and upholds and fights for political causes that would assure fair treatment and equal rights to all. But, while he struggles for the rights of all—racial, religious, and sexual minorities alike—and gives money to all the "right" charities, deep within is a belief that, while these minorities are to be championed at a distance, none belong next door.

So the difference between these two types—each standing at opposite sides of the continuum of Beech behavior—is only in the degree of their intolerance and level of self-awareness. Certainly, those among us who choose not to look at ourselves honestly can avoid all sorts of unpleasant truths.

And, to be sure, the Beech state is an unpleasant one for all concerned. Like any other negative emotional state built upon a lie, the Beech state can be destructive to the Beech himself and to all those close to him.

Even at its most benign, the Beech state sets up something of a war within the patient. He is, after all, dedicated to truth and justice for all on the one hand while on the other hand he is hiding his own inner intolerance. The moral fiber of the type demands that he be true to himself and allow himself to feel as he feels, but in this case it forbids him to be who he is and feel how he feels because he knows that his inner feelings contradict everything he stands for.

Let me be clear—the Beech type is not in a destructive emotional pattern because he is intolerant. In our culture we tend to agree that tolerance is good and intolerance is bad, and we pass laws that reinforce this particular judgment, but it is not for me to decide what forms of tolerance and intolerance are bad or good and whether, for instance, the moral judgment of a person with passionate religious beliefs that are in opposition to the secular law of the land should side with his faith or with the law. The issue here is not conservatism or liberalism, it is honesty.

The Beech type lives in a state of constant emotional stress because he is intolerant even with himself. Were he able to simply feel his feelings, good or bad, tolerant or intolerant, he would at least have a starting point from which he could change and grow. But as long as he denies his feelings because he intellectualizes them and judges them instead of just *feeling* them, he sets up an emotional pattern in which he can never escape his own self judgment.

Like all the other Bach types—especially those that are masked and present to the world a "self" that is counter to their true inner self—the Beech type must first admit the truth to himself before he can honestly judge himself and decide whether changes have to be made. Just as the Agrimony must admit that he is not happy (and take an honest look at possible substance abuse) and the Chicory must admit that she uses love in a manipulative manner, the Beech must admit that, for better or worse, his words just don't match his heart. Then the possibility for change exists.

Often, the Beech state does not just exist in individuals, but is found in whole groups or families. The Beech state of intolerance is one of the Bach negative emotional states that actually seem to be physically communicable. It spreads especially effectively from parents to children. It also spreads easily among children on the playground or in any other under-supervised arena of social contact.

When the individual in authority in any group—the teacher in school, the boss at work, or the minister in church—is a Beech, that individual's intolerance can spread like wildfire among those in subordinate positions. This is how the Beech state can be destructive to all those around the Beech.

Like the other remedies in this group, Beech types can be especially humorless. They can also be rather powerful and dominant personalities and are often extroverted.

They can also be very rigid in their personality traits, very pedantic with their families, and stern disciplinarians with their children. Beech types, like other types in this group, can be very rule conscious, and have very high standards as to what is acceptable for them. They want clean and tidy homes and children and dinner on the table when they get home. Like Crab Apple, they may strive for perfection when excellence is the better goal.

Because of this, Beech combines well with Crab Apple when perfectionism and intolerance are intertwined. It also combines well with Rock Water and Vine when the patient is especially rigid and demanding.

Finally—and this is important—some Beech types live their lives thinking they are presenting themselves in a manner that suggests honesty, but they are, all the while, simply fooling themselves. This is because we are, when dealing with the Beech's masked emotions, once again dealing with perception on the part of the Beech himself rather than the perceptions of those around him. Many Beech types, especially those that live and work in the public eye, believe they are presenting themselves as very fair and tolerant people, but they are not. While some Beech types are victims of "liberal guilt" and come across as well-educated,

> In the end, it is the sheer duplicity of the Beech that is the source of his negativity and stress. As Big Daddy rails in Tennessee Williams' *Cat on a Hot Tin Roof,* they are the chief purveyors of mendacity in our world today.

well-intended souls who are in denial of their inner intolerance, others are only fooling themselves with their razor-thin veneer of fairness and tolerance. We see face after face on our television screens that have smiles plastered on them, but whose eyes never seem to smile. Some Beech types wear their bias on their sleeves, but spend their days and nights thinking that the face they show to the camera convinces the world of their sincere intent.

In the end, it is the sheer duplicity of the Beech that is the source of his negativity and stress. As Big Daddy rails in Tennessee Williams' *Cat on a Hot Tin Roof*, they are the chief purveyors of mendacity in our world today.

Beech is one of the Bach remedies that may require extended use before the constitutional patient experiences relief. It also often works best when combined with other remedies.

Beech mixes well with Larch when the Beech type cannot reveal his inner intolerance because he lacks the moral fiber to do so. Larch's weak personality undermines Beech's strong determination.

Consider mixing Beech with Heather for patients who tend to be weathervanes in terms of their tolerances. These are the patients who will tend to go along with the crowd and raise their voices high for or against a particular cause once they are sure which opinion will yield them the best results personally.

Agrimony and Beech are a powerful combination as well. Together, they can be very helpful for the patient who is the ultimate false friend, who shows a broadly smiling face to those of whom he does not approve, only to betray them behind their backs.

The patient who shows the combined attributes of Beech and Agrimony is all but incapable of being honest about his feelings with anyone.

Beech is also a powerful tool for one aspect of physical healing. Because it is the remedy for those who are intolerant (which could be considered a sort of emotional "allergy"), it is very helpful for those who have physical allergies of any sort. Allergies are, after all, a state of physical intolerance based in an overactivity within the patient's immune system. And the remedy that can help the patient whose emotional "immune system"—his sense of judgment—is overly active can also help the patient whose physical immune system is overly active.

Therefore, try using Beech for seasonal allergies before you try an over-the-counter medication. It may be very helpful.[6]

In the acute context, consider using Beech for any situation in which you feel you are presenting yourself in the best light possible instead of presenting yourself with honesty, when you are overcompensating and tempted to be overly generous to mask your true feelings, or when you feign friendship or kindness that you do not feel.

## Negative Qualities of the Type

While it would be easy to say that those in a negative Beech state are simply those who are intolerant to people who are different from them—who have different colored skin or a different religion or a different sexual preference—the core issue is not one of opinions, good or bad, but that of living in a manner that is not consistent internally and externally. The problem is that Beech layers a false mask of behavior and language over an inner emotional self that is biased and intolerant. The fact that the Beech, to a greater or lesser extent, is aware of his real feelings as well as his false façade, creates an ongoing level of emotional stress that limits the Beech's ability to live, think, and feel with authenticity.

## Positive Qualities of the Type

I cannot say that the Beech type who has moved into a positive state votes as you wish he would, or agrees with you on your political beliefs. What I can say is that the positive Beech lives his life honestly and is able to examine and understand his own feelings and make changes where changes are due. The positive Beech type enjoys the strength of character that he once pretended he had. And this strength allows him to integrate all the diverse aspects of his character into a solid and harmonious whole.

And because of this, the positive Beech accepts the same need for integration of the diverse aspects of humanity and is able, at last, to truly tolerate the rights of all to exist and prosper.

6. Crab Apple is also very helpful for allergies, since it is the cleansing remedy. And either Crab Apple or Beech can be combined with Holly for allergies that are especially explosive.

### The Beech Child

I do not personally believe that the Beech state is ever inborn. It is a learned state of being, as, indeed, are most of the other Bach states as well.

As I have said before, I believe that the Beech negative emotional state is highly contagious. Certainly, it is rife in our culture, especially when we consider the subject of race. Instead of being a society that can be said to be fully tolerant of everyone, our culture, in reality, supports various levels of intolerance. And our children are the beneficiaries of our thoughts, words, and actions.

Our children learn the differences among people early on, and learn to exploit those differences for their own benefit. They learn to call names at a young age. As the Beech state deepens, they can also learn to become very upset if they feel that someone is approaching a task in the wrong way and will complain loudly about it. In time, their loudness will become sarcasm.

The Beech child who has learned his lessons of intolerance well can become one of the most difficult and uncontrollable adolescents.

### The Beech Adult

Beech is not a remedy that is linked with any particular stage or life, or with one gender more than another. In fact, it is an all-pervasive remedy that affects the vast majority of us, to one degree or another, at every stage of life.

Certainly, it has not been my experience that most of us become more open-minded as we grow older, so it is important to note that some seniors can move into a deep pattern of Beech behavior. In the elderly, Beech often blends with Willow to form a personality type that is both intolerant and bitter.

Many adults are silent when it comes to their Beech state. They will give an indication of their inner prejudices only when pressed. Most of the time, they try to avoid the subjects that touch on their hidden intolerance, because they are uncomfortable with their own feelings.

Some adult Beech types wrestle with feelings of inferiority, but they use these secret feelings to demean others and thus feel better about themselves. They cope with themselves by condemning others.

Also, the Beech is very sensitive to both physical and social environments. Because of this, they can be overly concerned with personal comfort and possessions.

### The Beech Animal

I have never found a really good application for this remedy with any of my animals. Other remedies, such as Holly, Vervain, and Vine work much better for aggressive animals or those that bully smaller animals.

Since I don't think that the human feelings of intolerance and bigotry are shared with the rest of the animal kingdom, I don't find a place for this remedy in a veterinary kit.

### Beech and the Homeopathic Pharmacy

The homeopathic remedy Platinum has much in common with the Beech type. Platinum works from ego, and from a judgmental state, often feeling as if "she is born of noble blood." The bearing in Platinum tells others that they are inferior and were simply placed in her way to be judged.

### Issues that Suggest Beech

Aging; allergies; immune dysfunction; menopause; mother issues; nail biting; rashes and other skin conditions; rheumatism; ringworm; sciatica; tinnitus; warts.

### In Conclusion

The need for Beech is sneaky. The moment you read this or any other material written about this remedy and think, "Well, I certainly don't need that," you had better start taking it.

The remedy Beech reminds us that we have to look at ourselves honestly at all times and judge our own motivations as honestly as we try to judge the motivations of others, if we are to be truly healthy. Just as I want to know who is paying for the medical research that will yield a specific result and net a particular company millions of dollars, I also want to know what aspect of my character "funded" a particular opinion, thought, or action, and what that aspect has to gain from it.

In the end, the remedy Beech is more about honesty than it is about intolerance. Certainly, the Beech type can be very flinty and rigid and deeply intolerant of the rights of others. But in reality one man's intolerance is another man's liberal largess. What matters in the end is that we embody the truth of our beliefs, and stand up and take responsibility for our actions, without masking our intent in honeyed words or false smiles.

## ROCK WATER · THE REMEDY FOR THOSE WHO ARE RIGID

Rock Water, writes Bach, is for "those who are very strict in their way of living; they deny themselves many of the joys and pleasures of life because they consider it might interfere with their work. They are hard masters to themselves. They wish to be well and strong and active, and will do anything which they believe will keep them so. They hope to be examples which will appeal to others who may then follow their ideas and be better as a result."

- **While Rock Water is primarily a constitutional remedy, it does have acute applications as well.**

### Botanical Information

Odd as it may seem, this "floral essence" is not made from any sort of plant material. Instead, it is made from the pure water of a mineral spring.

### Rock Water in General

Rock Water types are stern taskmasters and, often, perfectionists. But while our other perfectionist, the Crab Apple, extends his or her energetic need for organization and cleanliness on others, the Rock Water is hardest on himself. The Rock Water type is a stoic. He believes that he is making himself purer, cleaner and healthier by denying himself the things he particularly enjoys in life.

> The Rock Water type lives by the Old Testament. For him, all that is accomplished in life must be accomplished through sacrifice and hard work. The New Testament concept of grace, as it relates to accomplishment or personal growth, is unknown to him.

As is always the case with our negative emotional states, the Rock Water takes a virtue and warps it into a destructive practice by placing it out of balance with life's other virtues. In this case the Rock Water type takes the virtue of discipline and makes it such a dominant trait in his character that this clarion virtue becomes a hindrance.

The Rock Water type lives by the Old Testament. For him, all that is accomplished in life must be accomplished through sacrifice and hard work. Anything that is pleasant but does not help the Rock Water move toward his goal (which is quite often health related), put food on the table, or serve some other specific purpose must be removed from his life, cut out like a surgeon removes a tumor. The New Testament concept of grace, as it relates to accomplishment or personal growth, is unknown to him.

In fact, the Rock Water tends to be very suspicious of anything that he feels comes too easily. In general, the Rock Water type is suspicious of anything that seems too easy or too "soft." It is perhaps this trait of the Rock Water type that most suggests the source of the remedy. Rock Water types can be as rigid and hard in their behaviors, in their manners, and, indeed, in their bodies, as the rocks over which the water flows in the springs that are the source of the remedy itself.

But while Rock Water types tend to be suspicious, they can be very vulnerable to anything that appeals to their desire for personal growth and, especially, physical health. They therefore can become medical junkies, moving from doctor to doctor in an attempt to "get better." They are especially sensitive to anything that they see as "scientific." Rock Water types tend to educate themselves thoroughly on any or all subjects related to their own personal health, and to the health of those they love. They tend to be up-to-date on any or all new scientific studies that relate to their own health.

Rock Water types also tend to always be in on the latest health craze. They eat the "right" breakfast cereal and make sure they buy only the purest organic vegetables.

Surely all of this is very good if it is kept in balance. But, remember, the Rock Water state suggests that the patient is in imbalance. The Rock Water type may have begun his journey by wanting to better himself and be healthier, but, over time, that positive impulse controls him to a greater and greater extent and he can become compulsive in his habits and behavior.

But unlike the other remedy types in this category, the Rock Water type does not force others to do anything they do not want to do. Instead, he feels that if he lives his life perfectly—if he can demonstrate the success of his lifestyle to others firsthand—then they will be drawn to him and emulate him. It is the hope of the Rock Water type that others will recognize the wisdom of the Rock Water "Way of Life" and begin to live as he does.

In this way, Rock Water mirrors the intensity and zeal of two other remedies in this group, Vine and Vervain. When it comes to his rather joyless approach to life, Rock Water combines the willful intensity of Vine and the tidal wave of confidence that is Vervain with the rigidity and exhausting demands of Crab Apple's perfectionism. For the Rock Water, there is no rest for the weary. There is always more that he can do to make himself stronger, healthier, more spiritually evolved. There is always more work he can do to become a worthy example for others to follow.

In the end, the fact that Rock Water chooses to lead by example and not by hectoring on street corners makes little difference. With his strict dietary needs, his demanding schedule, and his rather brisk superior attitude, the Rock Water can be a trial to be around.

Like Mussolini, Rock Water types can be counted on to make sure that the trains run on time. They are fervent followers of schedules and make sure that each aspect of their daily schedule occurs on time every day. They do not tolerate tardiness in others and never allow themselves to be late for anything. If anything, the Rock Water is five minutes early and puzzled that everyone else isn't there to meet him.

This rigidity of purpose extends to all parts of the Rock Water's life. He desires, above all else, to attain and maintain his highest level of mental, physical, and spiritual functionality and awareness. He will sacrifice any possession, any relationship, to achieve this goal. Rock Water types often feel that their daily "schedule of events" is more important than their career—indeed, it can easily become their career—so they tend to work at surprisingly low-level jobs that allow them enough money to continue with their real work and enough freedom to indulge their needs. The Rock Water type may be obviously intelligent and quite capable of attaining a higher level of work, but he settles instead for work that does not interfere with his personal research and training.

And training is an excellent word for the Rock Water approach to life. At their worst, Rock Waters drive themselves as if they were athletes preparing for the Olympics. Only the Olympics are always ahead of them. There is no off-season—no period of time during which they can relax their harsh rules for living.

The Rock Water is usually fixated upon the idea of personal health (and can be quite a hypochondriac as well), but the rigidity of the type can focus on other areas as well. The Rock Water may be the person at work who will not leave until the job is done, who acts as if his or her life depended upon meeting every deadline, no matter how small. The Rock Water tends to be the martyr in every group, the one whose attitude says, "If I don't do it, it won't get done." While this Rock Water type avoids ever speaking his or her mind, the rolling of his eyes or her loud sighs drive the point home. "I am dedicated to this work and you are not." Or, "Why can't you be more like me?"

Like the Vine or the Crab Apple, the Rock Water type is supremely assured that what he is doing is right. And that word "right" is very, very important to him.[7] In fact, it is all he's got, given that he has subsumed every other desire to achieve his far-reaching goals. If the Rock Water became convinced that he was on the wrong path, his entire world would collapse under him.

For Rock Water types, especially those who focus on religion as their avenue of "expertise," this is a very serious thing. The Rock Water who rigidly adheres to a specific religious belief or ritual can experience untold agony when their belief system is shaken or found faulty. This is a calamity that shakes the Rock Water to his very core, leaving him to question everything in his life.

Like the Crab Apple, the Rock Water would do well to learn spontaneity and fluidity, and to replace his goal of perfection with one for excellence. In striving for excellence, he can bring back into balance the other aspects of life—especially his emotional life—that he had ignored. He can finally understand that perfection, if it exists on Earth, is a gift of God and not the product of human labor.

---

7. The Rock Water lives in a negative emotional state in which he would rather be right than be happy. And being right means that the Rock Water cannot allow himself to deviate from his path for any reason. He must also deny any thoughts that run counter to his plan, any doubts that enter his head. And, as is always the case, this denial of legitimate feelings makes the Rock Water weaker in the long run, and becomes a source of continual stress in his life. In most cases, the Rock Water hides his insecurities even though he feels them from time to time. Rock Waters can have a fear deep inside that they might be wrong, that they might have dedicated their lives to something foolish or something that they never can accomplish no matter how hard they try. If the Rock Water can face his fears, he can learn to make the changes that will bring him back into balance. Because of this issue of fear, adding Mimulus to Rock Water can often be the key to finding the remedy that will help him learn to live in the moment and take life as it comes.

Because of the emotional, mental, and spiritual rigidity of the type, the Rock Water tends to be beset with physical rigidity as well. The Rock Water type tends to suffer from all sorts of symptoms involving stiffness and pain. He may suffer from chronic back pain, joint pain, or, especially, neck and shoulder pain. His muscles tend to always be tense, making him an easy target for injury when he overexercises or over-lifts. And, as many Rock Water types tend to exercise with the same diligence that they do everything else, you will often see them running with bandages or working out while in obvious pain.

Like the other Bach remedies that are primarily used in the treatment of chronic emotional states, the Rock Water type may need to take the remedy for some time before its impact is felt. And, like some of our other more compulsive types, the Rock Water may feel that there is nothing wrong with him that needs treatment. Since he is likely to already be taking everything he has researched and feels he needs to be healthy and strong, he may see not the need for any sort of flower remedy. This can make him very hard to treat.

Rock Water does, however, blend well with a number of other remedies that can help the patient find a gentler path in life. As I have mentioned, Mimulus, Vervain, Vine, and Crab Apple all blend especially well with Rock Water.

Water Violet is perhaps the best blend of all. Use these two remedies together for the patient who feels that he is able to spiritually move beyond the level of humanity through self-denial and a withdrawal from the hustle-and-bustle of life. The Rock Water/Water Violet type will want to breathe pure air and to live an ascetic lifestyle that sets him above the common man.

Also think of Wild Oat in combination with Rock Water for the patient who latches on to an artificial path in place of a natural purpose in life. This combination is excellent for patients who become attracted to cults and other communities that offer them a rigid set of rules and a lifestyle of self-denial that they use as a substitute for their own unique life's path.

In its acute use, think of Rock Water for those times when you find yourself being excessive in your self-discipline. It can be a brilliant remedy for those times when we tend to overthink a situation and our plan for dealing with it. When planning and thinking leads us nowhere and no plan seems good enough to achieve our goals, and we end up spinning our wheels. We should also think of Rock Water when we become compulsive in our efforts. When we diet too strictly, or overexercise. It can also be very helpful when we get obsessive about meeting a given deadline. It can particularly help students who are studying for their exams, so they can balance their actual physical needs with their overriding need to prepare for the testing. It can help all of us in the same way, so we will work effectively but not obsessively when we are struggling to meet any sort of work deadline.

## Negative Qualities of the Type

The keynote of the Rock Water state is rigidity. Rock Water types, in their desire to excel mentally, emotionally and spiritually, become rigid in their behaviors and habits. Ironically, over time, their need for personal perfection actually undermines their achievements as it drains them of both their personal energy and their enjoyment of accomplishment. This same drive toward perfection will also undermine the Rock Water type's ability to achieve his ultimate goal. The Rock Water wishes, above all else, to be an excellent example to others. But as others increasingly perceive the Rock Water as humorless and driven, they are less and less likely to want to be like him.

Rock Water types can easily become trapped in patterns of self-denial. They refuse to let themselves enjoy anything—because enjoyment, like everything else, must be earned.

And the very things they do to become healthier—their special diets and exercise programs, for instance—often undermine their health and weaken rather than strengthen their physical body. Rock Waters may look into a mirror and see themselves as wonderfully healthy beings, but others may see them as gaunt and tense, and, again, will be highly unlikely to want to emulate them.[8]

Finally, the Rock Water type is often haunted by the feeling that his life has no real purpose, no center—that he has no real personality of his own, only a long list of rules. Rock Water types may suspect, over time, that their lives are made up only of compulsive behaviors, and that they are too open to the ideas of others—the specific experts who write books on diet or health care and who set out life plans, which Rock Waters can't resist trying. At the same time, they are absolutely closed to the possibility of doing things in any way other than the way their experts have told them, or that they, through their own research, have decided things should be done. This dynamic of almost total sureness undermined by a suspicion of doubt creates a great deal of stress and further weakens Rock Water types.

And yet, they remain rigid and stoic, unwilling to take any small pleasure in life that is not consistent with their goals. They, for instance, are totally unwilling to eat a piece of birthday cake.

## Positive Qualities of the Type

There is much that is positive about Rock Water, even when they are in a negative emotional state. Like Oak, this is a Bach remedy type that we can discuss in terms of

---

8. Because of these deep issues with food and diet, Rock Water types, like Crab Apple types, may fall prey to anorexia, bulimia, or other eating disorders. The Crab Apple will fall into eating disorders as a form of control, while the Rock Water will continually distill their list of allowable "healthy" foods until they are not eating a diet that can sustain their life.

positives, even superlatives, because the injuries that the Rock Water state causes tend to wound the Rock Water himself rather than others. Where other people may find the Rock Water to be dull, or may consider him to have a martyr complex, they do not find him particularly offensive, nor are they intimidated by him. In fact, they may quite enjoy the fact that the Rock Water, like the Oak, tends to be overly diligent and very reliable. They will happily lean on the Rock Water to meet a difficult deadline or to do the work of others while those others go out to play.

Rock Water types are considered benign because they tend to leave others alone and don't force their views on other people. Because they so want to lead by example, Rock Water types are easily ignored by those who do not want to be led.

But once Rock Water types attain a more positive emotional and behavioral state, they are at last capable of incorporating new thoughts into their old regimen. They can learn to be less protective of their health and lifestyle and can live life more spontaneously. They can learn to be adaptable, where once they were rigid.

And, perhaps most important, they can learn to communicate with others and exchange ideas. The Rock Water who once refused to spell out his life's philosophy to others, expecting them to garner what they could from his exemplary life, now can give some very valuable information to others and let them decide whether they act on it. And the Rock Water, with his new fluid mindset, is now open to new information and new methods by which he can live life more fully.

### The Rock Water Child

Don't expect a wild sense of humor in a Rock Water child. Instead, the typical Rock Water child, like the adult, is self-motivated and very self-disciplined. Since the Rock Water state is a learned behavior that is rather slow to develop, children tend not to display the full range of Rock Water behaviors. Even those who have been thoroughly indoctrinated in the concept of stoicism show only the beginnings of what will, if left untreated, become a pattern of self-denial.

Children left in their natural state tend to be attracted to humor, excitement, and discovery. Usually children showing a tendency toward Rock Water behaviors regain their natural joy in life quite quickly with just a dose or two of the remedy.

Use Rock Water with children who tend to take things too much to heart, try too hard to please, and are too willing to listen to anyone they perceive as being in authority.

### The Rock Water Adult

As adults, Rock Water types tend to have a strong affinity with the past. In fact, they may seem older than they are. They often have ideas about how to live that are based in ancient philosophies of health or religion. They tend to revere and study history. Rock

Water types also seem to be very future-directed. They always focus on goals that are still ahead, no matter how long they have already struggled toward them. Therefore it is only the present moment that they ignore. They are mired in the past and directed toward the future, but out of touch with the moment in which they live. It is perhaps because of this that the typical Rock Water type is incapable of being spontaneous and simply living "in the moment."

They also tend to be attracted to simple clothes, food, and surroundings. Since they have absolutely no interest in being on the cutting edge of fashion, their clothes also seem old fashioned and their hairstyle will tend to emphasize practicality over style.

In the same way, Rock Water types will not spend a lot of money on a big house or a new car. Possessions are looked upon with the same eye toward practicality as everything else. If a Rock Water is going to spend a lot of money, it will be on books, education, or a top-of-the-line computer with which they can get more work done.[9]

Many Rock Water types find their way into the health field, which often proves a natural fit after their lifetime of compulsive research in the subject. You will especially find them in the areas of nutrition and exercise. They have all the facts at their fingertips and will be happy to motivate you to perfection if you ask them to do it.

They also are motivated to work in some aspect of religion, even if their own spiritual rigidity has moved them from a place of true spirituality toward an obsessive adherence of dogma.

Many Rock Water types can be found among our elderly, since the untreated Rock Water state only deepens over a long period of time. These Rock Water types use their time in retirement to enhance their studies and their slavish dedication to perfection.

### The Rock Water Animal

While many animals like to have their daily milestones occur at the same time and in the same way day after day, I do not find any constitutional need for this remedy in animals. Instead, it can be helpful if your dog's dinner is late or if its schedule is affected by an upset in yours. A dose of Rock Water can help soothe it and help it to adapt to changes that occur.

### Rock Water and the Homeopathic Pharmacy

It seems too easy to say that Arsenicum and Rock Water parallel each other, but they certainly do. Both are obsessed with good health and both are virtually insane on the topic of diet, but no Arsenicum can really live and let live. They have no poker faces

9. As author Christopher Isherwood wrote in his journal during the stage of his life when he retreated into a strict religious community, "No more toys, only tools."

when it comes to the failings of others. They make faces every time they see someone eating a cheeseburger.

The Rock Water type also reminds me of the Apis type, the task-oriented busy bee, who spends all day every day in flight, improving her hive. Rock Water can also be as protective of his lifestyle and environment as the bee is of her territory. In both cases, the only time that either the Rock Water or the bee gets really angry is when their territory is intruded upon in a way that makes them feel threatened.

### Issues that Suggest Rock Water

Accidents; asthma and other breathing disorders; chronic back pain; digestive disorders; eating disorders; father issues; ileitis; insomnia; neck and shoulder pain.

### In Conclusion

Rock Water is a complete anomaly among Bach's pharmacy of floral essences. It alone is not an herbal-based remedy, but is the product of pure mineral-enriched water instead.

Because of the nature of its material origin, Rock Water stands as a link between Bach's flower remedies and other forms of alternative medicine and other philosophies of treatment.

Rock Water links Bach's treatments to the so-called gem elixirs, which are healing essences based on the properties of specific mineral crystals. Rock Water also suggests the viability of the cell salts, which are the products of a homeopath named Schuessler. Like Bach, Schuessler stepped away from the practice of pure homeopathy to simplify their treatments and direct them within a specific sphere of action. Bach took his treatments into the realm of psyche and spirit, while Schuessler took his into the physical body alone. He ignored the emotional symptoms of the patient as Bach came to ignore the physical symptoms.

The existence of Rock Water among Bach's flower essences suggests that Bach was, perhaps, not totally dedicated to the notion that true healing can only come about through the use of benign, nonmedicinal herbal essences. It suggests that Bach himself must have been open to the idea of using sources beyond the herbal for his remedies, and makes us wonder at what other remedies he might have developed if he had lived long enough to continue his work. The presence of Rock Water also confuses the purity of Bach's philosophy of healing, however, because in his writings, he is very insistent that his herbal remedies stand head and shoulders above any other form of treatment, in that they are utterly benign and able to touch upon the true (spiritual) cause of disease.

With Bach's death, we were left with many of the same questions that remained when Hahnemann died. We can only conjecture as to the path Bach might have taken had he lived longer, and how his thinking might have evolved as his experience with his own treatments grew.

We are left with the question mark that the remedy Rock Water represents. On the one hand, it remains a steadfast tool for healing when the patient's mood matches the remedy's action. On the other hand, we are left asking a simple question: "Where's the flower in this flower remedy?"

## VERVAIN · THE REMEDY FOR THOSE WHO ARE EXCITABLE

Vervain, writes Bach, is for "those with fixed principles and ideas, which they are confident are right, and which they very rarely change. They have a great wish to convert all around them to their own views of life. They are strong of will and have much courage when they are convinced of those things that they wish to teach. In illness they struggle on long after many would have given up their duties."

- Vervain is excellent as both a constitutional and an acute remedy.
- Vervain is one of Bach's original remedies, the Twelve Healers.

### Botanical Information

Vervain is usually referred to botanically as Verbena (*Verbena Officinalis*). It is also known as the "herb of the cross," or the "herb of grace." European verbena is native to Northern Europe and Great Britain, but now grows extensively throughout the world.

The verbena plant is often thought of as a weed. It can be highly invasive, and can grow in the worst soils and in hot, dry places like beside roads and empty lots. This is a sturdy plant that grows very upright, with a deep and strong root system.

Verbena flowers in late summer and early autumn. It has light lilac flowers. Both the flowers and the leaves of the verbena plant are used medicinally. Verbena is a sedative, used in cases of nervous exhaustion and melancholia. It is not to be taken by pregnant women.

### Vervain in General

The negative emotional state reflected in the remedy Vervain is the very embodiment of the yang principle. The Vervain types' attention, emotions, and very life force are all directed outward: they are the very definition of the word "extrovert." They are always in motion and forever restless in mind, body, and spirit. Like Barbra Streisand's character in *The Way We Were*, they go from cause to cause, preaching, hectoring, doing everything in their power to convince others that their message—whatever it is and whatever its content—is absolutely right and should be embraced by all. They are natural salesmen and the embodiment of the "hard sell."

Now, the fact that they are restless by nature and brimming over with energy does not mean that this restlessness applies to their thoughts and their causes. Perhaps surprisingly, the Vervain type has a "fixed" mentality. Like the other remedies of this group, especially Rock Water (which precedes Vervain in these pages), Vervain locks in on a specific topic or cause and lives and dies by that cause and the spreading of it. They are the natural evangelists, no matter whether their cause is political, health-related, moral, or religious. Like Rock Water, Vervain has stumbled onto something that has changed his life, but, unlike Vervain, he has no interest in leading by example. Instead, the Vervain type is brimming over with excitement when it comes to sharing his discoveries, insights, and "road-to-Damascus" experiences with you.[10]

What is fluid about the Vervain are the words that come out of his mouth—Vervain types tend to be very quick-witted and, like Impatiens types, prone to speak rapidly and at great length—and these are the techniques that he will use to get and keep your attention. The Vervain type who is on fire about his topic will use theatrics, emotional blackmail, intimidation—anything to keep his audience alert. In fact one Vervain-founded self-help cult once refused to let the audience members leave the hall during lectures for any reason, including bathroom breaks.

> If you have ever experienced a moment when you were dealing with another person who seemed to be coming at you from all sides at once, who threw you off balance and made you feel that you were being interrogated and each aspect of your life judged, you likely have had an encounter with a Vervain.

Since Vervain as a remedy type belongs to this category of controlling personalities, it is riddled with control issues. But where Rock Water and Crab Apple (which has so much in common with, and I think belongs in, this group of remedies) mostly turn their need for control inward and torment themselves, Vervain turns these issues outward and seeks to control and subsume the will of others.

Granted, this is not always an unpleasant experience. In fact, many Vervain types are extremely charming and charismatic individuals, whether they are in a negative or positive emotional state. How they use their natural charm, however, is determined by their own internal motivations. Where the positive Vervain will use his charisma in a creative manner—many of our best performers, actors, singers, and dancers are Vervain

---

10. Often this is the only sure way to tell the need for Rock Water from the need for Vervain. Both may be obsessed with their diet and the state of their health, and both may fixate over every mouthful of food they take in. But the Vervain will literally trap you into a corner so he can explain the virtues of his lifestyle choices, while Rock Water will display himself as an example of just what can be achieved through careful dieting.

types, who are capable of exuding a personal charisma[11] that can touch each individual in a crowded theater and make them feel as if they were communicating directly with the Vervain. The negative Vervain, however, uses his gifts for one purpose only—control. Few other types are as grasping or as power-hungry as the Vervain. Elm may have powerful ambition and a wide reach when it comes to success and prestige, and Vine may dedicate his life to the acquisition of money and power, but what Vervain lacks in hard work and will they more than make up for with personal energy and drive.

If you have ever experienced a moment when you were dealing with another person who seemed to be coming at you from all sides at once, who threw you off balance with the sheer force of his personality and made you feel that you were being interrogated and each aspect of your life judged, you likely have had a one-on-one encounter with a Vervain. Or you might have had a more pleasant contact with a Vervain, during which you felt that the other person's eyes could look directly into your soul, and you have never felt so understood on so many levels at once—and afterward found that you have donated money or bought a new car without being fully aware of it.

Along with their charisma, Vervain types are also extremely confident. They are confident of their own strengths and abilities, and supremely confident that they are right in all that they are saying. Because of this many negative Vervain types lack what I think of as a "seven second delay button."[12] They are confident in themselves—perhaps overly confident—so they will say whatever comes to their mind. They are sure their charm will override the content if what they have to say is too strong or salty.

Of course, this is not always the case. Vervain types can be very hurtful with their language, and they may even be considered to be verbally abusive.

The Vervain will tend not to notice when his language injures others or any of the other mistakes he is making, or the people he is hurting or alienating with his language and hyperactivity. His full attention and energy are directed outward, and the Vervain type has little time or energy to spare on self-examination. If the Vervain uses his critical facilities at all, he directs them toward others and not toward himself.

In fact, the Vervain will not do anything that will undermine his sense of confi-

11. This is not to say that the highly opinionated, verbose Vervain cannot come across as being a loudmouth or a bore who forces his thoughts on others. Believe me, he can. In the same way, he can seem like an egotistical jerk. But none of this changes the fact that, when he wants to, he can also be very charming.

12. All live-radio shows have a seven-second delay button, which allows the producer to prevent coughs, sneezes, and foul language from getting on the air. Most of us have what I think of as an inner seven-second delay button, which allows us to edit ourselves as we speak. Vervain types either don't have these buttons, or choose not to use them. They say pretty much whatever comes into their minds.

dence, perhaps because he suspects that he would not be able to continue on his selected path if he were to stop and examine himself and his actions, words, and motivations. If there is a physical image I can give you of a Vervain, it is of a person running on a treadmill. Like the rabbit selling batteries on television, they keep going and going and going.

The seemingly endless energy Vervain types exude can make them quite a handful, especially when they are young. (This will be described in greater length below.) Often the word "hyperactive" will be applied to Vervain types, and children in a negative Vervain state are often treated with powerfully toxic allopathic medications when they could find a good deal of help with the remedy Vervain.

So the Vervain is charismatic and confident, but one last word remains to fully describe this type: relentless. Like a standup comic with sweat flowing on his face, whose jokes are bombing again and again, the Vervain type is unable to leave the spotlight until he has brought the crowd back to his side. Vervain types thrive on attention and honestly prefer negative attention to no attention at all. They are those entertainers who are always happy to see their names in print, no matter the context, and always happy to see their photos in magazines, even if they are on the "worst dressed list."

Vervain types are always "on," always spontaneous, always impulsive. They tend to act or speak before they think, and, as a result, say and do a great many things that they are forced to regret later on. Often, they will break things without meaning to or appear very awkward, even drunk, because they move without thinking and are unaware of their physical position and the distribution of their body weight. So Vervains may literally come "crashing down" as they trip and fall, or they can figuratively crash through their words or actions. Either way, their lives are a juggling act, one in which they attempt to keep all the juggled objects under control and in the air simultaneously.

This juggling act as well as his constant running on a treadmill (it is not for nothing that physical movement always seems to play into imagery of Vervain's emotional state) create a good deal of stress for the Vervain.

Perhaps first and foremost, Vervain is physically beset with self-inflicted injuries of all sorts. When he cooks, he cuts or burns himself. When he walks, he trips. When he plays with toys, he breaks them, and harms himself in doing so.[13]

Vervain types also tend to have very stiff and sore muscles. Their necks and shoulders can be particularly tight. Many Vervain types can suffer chronically from what is called "wry neck," a condition in which neck muscles spasm and the patient cannot

---

13. Somehow, when the Vervain is in the spotlight, he is much less likely to hurt himself. The Vervain type who seems very awkward in his own home can be very graceful when in public. Perhaps the Vervain's supreme focus on the topic of his presentation, during which his mind will not wander from his topic, allows him a physical grace as well.

turn his neck in any direction. Vervain types can also suffer from repetitive stress conditions like carpal tunnel syndrome and from chronic mouth and jaw pain.[14]

Vervain types, like Elm and Oak types, can fall prey to overwork and wear their bodies down into any number of chronic diseases over time. Heart disease and hypertension are common.

Vervain types also have a tendency toward emotional breakdowns, and can have a very rough time during midlife. This will be especially true if the cause to which they have dedicated years of their life is not moving forward into the public consciousness as they feel it should. In their middle years Vervain types, who usually avoid introspection at all costs, may be forced by health issues or economic troubles to reevaluate their goals and decide whether or not their zeal had been well placed. This can be a time of extreme emotional stress for Vervain types, as can any time of serious illness that leaves them bedridden. Vervain types, used to being in constant motion, make perhaps the worst patients possible when they are forced to do the one thing they do not wish to do: rest.

Vervain types are youthful and may appear younger than their years, both physically and emotionally. And they typically remain interested in education all their lives, and enjoy new ideas and new things, especially innovative electronics. They are especially interested in learning anything new that directly applies to their area of expertise, although they will be highly critical of anything they judge to be inferior.

Vervain types can fall prey to any number of ailments associated with issues of immunity, as they tend to tax their immune systems through the stress of their daily lives.

While Vervain is a powerful constitutional remedy, it is also a vibrant medicine for use in acute circumstances. It is, in fact, the remedy from this group that is most useful for acute treatments. Think of Vervain as your "Christmas Eve" remedy: use it in those circumstances when you are too wound up to sleep (it blends well with White Chestnut for insomnia) or when you feel that you are overexcited or too caught up in present events. Vervain is especially useful for children and animals with a natural curiosity and an overdeveloped sense of excitement.

Vervain can act as a calmative when you feel nervous. Think of it also when you really, really want to be heard and are being overly forceful in getting across your opinion. In fact, any situation in which anyone is being opinionated is a situation that suggests Vervain. It is also helpful when anyone is forming preconceptions of others and then acting upon those instantaneous judgments.

Vervain is another of our truly "universal" remedies that is needed by each and

---

14. Note that a combination of Vervain and Impatiens—an altogether excellent mixture for many patients of various needs—can be strongly indicated for patients with these pains.

every one of us, to a greater or lesser degree, more or less often. It belongs among the remedies contained in your home kit.

## Negative Qualities of the Type

The patient locked into a negative Vervain pattern of thought and behavior combines a seemingly overbearing and relentless nature with an apparently endless amount of energy. As such, they are people that most of us will avoid if possible. After all, no one wants to be pushed into a corner, and this tends to be Vervain's way of dealing with those they feel are not listening. He must be heard and he must be agreed with. There simply is no other option.

With their drive to make their audience understand and agree with their zeal as their motivation, Vervain types simply tend to be too intense for others to bear for long. They feel things too strongly and express these strong feelings too often and too forcefully. Other people with strong personalities of their own simply get burned out on the Vervain passion and, instead of becoming their followers, they close their minds to whatever Vervain is saying, right or wrong. But those with a weak sense of self or a weak concept of what they can accomplish in life will easily fall prey to the Vervain type and sign up for a life in service to them and their causes.

American politics and religion are filled with Vervain types. Often we are told by pollsters that they are "polarizers," and that they are the politicians who are either loved or hated. Vervains are controversial in the same way when they stand behind the pulpit. They express their religious views as strongly and candidly as they do any other views. In doing so they often build congregations made up of slavish followers while their church is reviled by many others.

Vervain types seem always to be embroiled in some sort of controversy, and they are people who are not easily forgotten. Vervain's zeal can have tremendous impact in a world that often seems boring and bland. While they exhibit many negative traits, they are never—especially on first viewing—dull.

## Positive Qualities of the Type

Truthfully, even negative Vervain types have some positive qualities, especially if they can emphasize their natural charm over their egomaniacal tendencies. But Vervain must learn to balance the various aspects of his personality and accept the fact that every person on Earth has an equal right to praise and attention as well as an equal right to their opinion.

Once the Vervain type accepts these simple realities, he is often able to pause and reflect upon himself, his actions, and most important, his true motivations. The Vervain, who works his wonders for the sake of power or fame when he is in a negative emotional state, can learn to "use his power for good" when he moves into a more positive state.

The Vervain who works from honest and altruistic motivations can literally move mountains. He can use his charisma to build movements and to change the world.

Further, the positive Vervain has come to understand that the truth that he speaks is his own form of truth, and that it may not represent a workable reality for other people. This Vervain is more than willing to have each person find his own way to enlightenment and can, in fact, be an excellent motivator who can help others identify and achieve his or her goals.

### The Vervain Child

Very often, Vervain children are labeled as hyperactive. They tend to go at things with too much energy and often break things unintentionally. They may also be tattlers, who find the behavior of others to be unfair and feel they must report it. Along with this, they are honest and loyal children to both parents and friends. They feel that there is a value system that transcends the needs of the individual and that must always be followed. This is the child who will question the parent if the parent's behavior seems different than their verbal instruction. And who will take any responsibilities given to them very seriously and will do their very best to please all concerned with the results. The Vervain child wants to please and achieve and may put a great deal of emphasis on winning and on his or her achievements.

### The Vervain Adult

Vervain adults tend to be tense, both in body and in mind. They may have trouble quieting down at night or allowing themselves to get the amount of rest they actually need. Often, they have trouble sleeping if they have not made their point well enough or accomplished enough that day. They are driven by a deep desire to share their insights. They believe in the principle of transformation, but often are locked on a fixed notion of how and when that transformation should take place.

The Vervain personality mixes overconfidence with charisma and a certain relentlessness of character. They tend to have a large amount of dedication as well. This personality can form very early in life, and children can begin to exhibit Vervain traits from a very young age. In the same way, the Vervain state can be lifelong, and we likely have as many older Vervain types as younger ones in our society.

Two stages of life stand out for the Vervain type. In young adulthood, the Vervain is likely to spend some time searching for his or her cause in life. In college, they tend to be very politically involved and try out a number of different causes, each with equal amounts of dedication and zeal. Once they find the cause or philosophy that "speaks to them," the Vervain type tends to become very fixated in his ideas and behaviors—a pattern that can remain until the next time of special intensity for the Vervain.

In midlife, many Vervain types are forced by circumstances—personal health and economics are the most common, although divorce certainly comes into play—to reassess their lives and decide whether or not their efforts have been worthwhile. Therefore, you will often see Vervain types making sudden and drastic changes in their life at this time. They will suddenly feel their life has been without purpose and suddenly become restless while they seemed quite sure of their path before. They may suddenly quit their job or end their marriage, or suddenly move. The Vervain is not the type to be happy with a new car; only a new cause, a new reason to get up in the morning will satisfy him.

### The Vervain Animal

This remedy quite literally saved us when we adopted our new dog, Django. Django came to us from the streets of Brooklyn. Our great old dog, K.D., had recently died at age fourteen, and, accustomed as I was to her slow, complaining ways, I was not prepared for the cannonball that was Django. He seemed always to be a blur of motion. We would joke that he was able to teleport himself around the house, but we soon grew tired of him leaping into our laps without warning, knocking things off tables with his tail, and frightening our guests with the force of his welcome. The last straw came when the cleaning lady quit because he kept leaping on her from behind when she vacuumed.

Had it not been for Vervain I might have given up on Django. With the help of this remedy, he quickly acclimated to our home and became calm enough that we could begin to work with him and train him. Now he sits on command and manages to bring himself back under control, except in times of thunderstorms, but we're working on that (yes, we have put Mimulus in his mixture because of his fear of thunder).

Try Vervain for any sort of hyperactive pet, any animal that flies out of control or has unpredictable, even dangerous behavior, and for any animal that you feel you just can't trust even if they are well behaved most of the time. It will help slow the animal down and calm and center it. It is not a cure-all, but it will help bring it to a place where you can start training and bonding with it. It combines well with the fear remedies—Mimulus and Aspen—and with Sweet Chestnut and Impatiens for animals that fly out of control or act without thinking, always to their later regret.

### Vervain and the Homeopathic Pharmacy

Here we have the homeopathic Causticum state, along with other remedies of the Tubercular Miasm. Like Causticum, Vervain has some insight, some secret that can bring about a wonderful transformation in all who come to understand it. Both will embody aches and pains like rheumatism and carpal tunnel syndrome that will literally force them to stop pushing.

### Issues that Suggest Vervain

Broken bones; carpal tunnel syndrome; chronic laryngitis; digestive troubles; eye tics and twitches; heart disease; hypertension; jaw pain; immune dysfunction; infections and inflammations of all sorts; injuries; insomnia; mouth pain; neck pain; nerve pain; nervous breakdowns; nightmares; rheumatism; rheumatoid arthritis; sciatica; stress.

### In Conclusion

Until now, I have only briefly alluded to one of the other important aspects of the Vervain type's personality. That is dedication. No other type is as willing to make the sacrifices the Vervain zealot will make for the sake of his cause or his goal in life. Time, energy, health, relationships—all mean nothing when they are weighed against the Vervain's intense zeal for that which the Vervain has stumbled upon as his central interest. Whether that interest is politics, religion, or show business—or any other fixation, from business to law to feeding the poor—the Vervain will attack all issues involved with equal zeal.

Even those Vervains locked in a deeply negative emotional pattern and those motivated in their work by all the wrong things display a dedication to their task that is impressive to say the least.

## VINE · THE REMEDY FOR THOSE WHO ARE WILLFUL

According to Bach, Vine types are "very capable people, certain of their own ability, confident of success. Being so assured, they think that it would be for the benefit of others if they could be persuaded to do things as they themselves do, or as they are certain is right. Even in illness they will direct their attendants. They may be of great value in an emergency."

• **More often than not, Vine is a constitutional remedy, but it can be used acutely as well.**

### Botanical Information

The common grapevine (*Vitis Vinifera*) is a woody perennial that is cultivated across the world for its fruit, grapes. There are many different varieties of the plant grown across the world. While it is impossible to know exactly where it was first cultivated, it was likely in an area of Central Europe. The plant, growing naturally, is native to Asia Minor.

The grapevine is cultivated not only as a source of food, but also as a medicinal plant. The sap of the grapevine is used medically in the treatment of tumors and cancer, and as a tonic.

Grapevines can require a good deal of work to grow successfully. They prefer warm climates, hot sun, and dry heat.

The flowers of the vine are small, green, and very fragrant. They bloom in early to late spring, depending upon the climate.

### Vine in General

In his musical *Lady in the Dark*, Kurt Weill wrote a song about a woman named Jenny, who, as Weill puts it, "always would make up her mind," often with disastrous results. As a child, Jenny decides on Christmas Eve to trim the family Christmas tree and manages to burn down the house. Again, as Weill puts it, "Jenny was an orphan on Christmas Day." As an adult, Jenny decides to write a memoir, and wives shoot their husbands all across America as a result. Yet Jenny is never deterred from making up her mind. She is confident in her decisions, no matter how many times she leaves disaster in her wake.

Jenny is, of course, a Vine type. She is willful, confident, and, once she has made up her mind to something, completely determined. Once her will is locked onto a goal (Vine, like the other remedies in this group, tends to "lock onto" goals, ideas, or faiths, and then has trouble letting go. They are like terriers that have bones in their mouths.) She is not to be swayed, discouraged, or beaten.

Vine types, therefore, can be highly destructive to those they perceive as "getting in their way," or those that they feel are trying to undermine them by disagreeing with them regarding any aspect of their goal.

On the positive side, however, stand next to a Vine if you ever find yourself in a crisis—if your airplane is going down, or the cruise ship you are on is capsized by an errant wave. No one is better than a Vine in an emergency.

We tend to revere Vine types in our culture, especially female Vine types. Often, they are the characters in fiction that we either love or love to hate. Scarlett O'Hara and Joan Collins's character Alexis on *Dynasty* are both Vine types. They will stop at nothing to get their way and reach their goal—even if that goal is revenge.[15] Like these characters, Vine types are at their very best during a crisis. Their quick minds focus on solving the crisis at hand, with amazingly detailed plans of action. They remain calm and focused, and, as long as their orders are followed precisely and to the letter, no one gets hurt.

---

15. The patient who needs both Vine and Willow can seem like an angel of vengeance, so determined is he to mete out punishment on those who have harmed him.

But the Vine type tends to approach daily life, when there is no crisis at hand, with the same hammerlock of will that he uses when he deals with a life-and-death struggle. Like the other remedies in this group, the Vine type is "locked in." In this case, he is locked in by an overabundance of willpower that all too often deceives him as to just how much force of will is required in a given situation. That can make the Vine type behave in a manner that others think of as "bossy" in some situations and downright tyrannical in others.

The Vine type can display the personality of a run-away train—as if humanity were transformed into machinery. They are goal-orientated, success-orien-tated people, who allow themselves to be hated, but

> The Vine type can display the personality of a runaway train.

never circumvented or disobeyed, to achieve their goals. They are people of force, of anger, and, potentially, of violence.

Because of their intense natures, it can be confusing to tell the difference between the Vine type and the Vervain type at times. Both are confident that what they are thinking and/or doing is correct. But where the Vervain type's efforts are centered in offering his opinion on nearly everything or spreading the good news of his particular insights, the Vine type's domination of others is more far-reaching and all pervasive. In short, it comes down to the difference between being pushy (Vervain) and being bossy (Vine). The Vine is locked-in, fixated upon the idea of "What We Should Do." He is willful and dominating. The Vervain type is opinionated and zealous, but less inclined to take control of all aspects of the lives of others and less willing to use others to achieve his ends. Where Vervain uses his innate charm to manipulate others, Vine sim-ply dominates them.

Often, you will find that particular patients combine the need for Vine and the need for Vervain. The two remedies work so well together that they almost may be thought of as being one remedy in some cases. For the patient who is absolutely com-mitted to his own way of thinking and taking action, and who is completely intolerant of the ideas of others and to any form of criticism, blend Vine and Vervain for an excel-lent result.

Not only is the Vine type bossy, but he tends to be fussy and rather petty as well. He may have an enemies list all his own, in a Richard Nixon sort of way. Like the bit-ter Willow, the Vine type who is locked into a negative emotional pattern tends to be deeply suspicious of others and their motivations (perhaps because he is so deeply aware of his own motivations). The Vine type is quick to take offense, quick to ask, "What do you mean by that?" when he hears any words other than praise. He is, above all else, capable of being stubborn. He finds disorder or chaos in any form intolerable, like a Crab Apple. He demands that everything within his environment is to his lik-ing. No detail is too small for him to comment upon. Again, like Crab Apple (which, obviously, is another remedy that combines very well with Vine), when the Vine type walks into a room his first words will often be a statement of what is wrong with the room or the people in it. He will say, "It's hot in here," or "Where did they get this crowd?"

The Vine type makes the absolute worst patient, bar none. Pity the poor physician who must treat him. The Vine will direct his own medical treatment and berate the doctor, who he feels is not as skilled as he should be. In the same way, the Vine is slow to praise any professional person and quick to find faults with their efforts. He is a very demanding customer, and a very difficult, faultfinding boss. He is also, for the record, very slow to pay.

Vine types can make overbearing parents, who tend to tell their children exactly what they should do at every moment in their lives. They will ask their children if they have finished a given task, even if the deadline is still far away. They will often actually finish tasks for their children (and for others, employees, hired-help and the like) before they even give them a chance to do it themselves. The person to whom an assignment was given—and Vine types are very good at giving assignments—may walk into the room to find the Vine busily completing the task that was just assigned.

Vine is one of our personality types, like Impatiens, for whom time seems to go too slowly. Thus they, like Impatiens types, are always looking at their watches wondering why it is taking everyone else so long to do what they themselves could do so much faster, and with so much better results.

Vine types will physically invade the personal space of others. In the same way, they invade the territory of others and think nothing of looking through their personal effects. The Vine, of course, will be highly protective of his own space and possessions, but will not apply these strict expectations of conduct to himself in the same way that he does to others.

In this way, and in so many others, the Vine type displays a wide dichotomy of acceptable behaviors. While he operates by one set of rules ("for the good of all"), everyone else finds that they have a much narrower range of allowable alternatives or actions. Thus, the Vine is something of a hypocrite, just like the other types in this group of remedies with control issues.

Finally, there is one aspect of the Vine personality that has not been explored, and that is Vine's behavior when order is maintained and everyone is doing as they were told. Under these circumstances, the Vine type can be surprisingly easy to get along with. He can even seem quite charming. When the Vine type perceives that all is well in his universe, he can relax completely and even display a surprising sense of humor. A Vine type can often display an almost completely unexpected sense of humor—one that can be very dry and quite witty. Even when they are very tense or highly agitated, they are capable of a gallows humor that catches everyone else off guard. On the subject of humor, it is also interesting that Vine types very often highly prize humor in others. They will tend to ignore the apparent faults of those who make them laugh and will want to reward humorists with special privileges. The intense Vine type can be surprisingly at ease when he perceives himself to be victorious.

Anything, however, that overturns the applecart of peace and prosperity can create an abrupt change in the Vine's behavior. Where only moments before he was in a state of bliss, he now focuses on the source of his dismay. And the Vine very quickly—much to the surprise and tense shock of those around him—returns to type.

Often new employees or potential allies will find that the Vine is the essence of charm itself on first meeting him. It is only when they first cross him, perhaps by disagreeing with something that he has said, that they will see his true colors.

Vine types like to let others figure out the rules for themselves, often by punishing them when they step out of line. They will let new acquaintances walk into their traps of expectation or behavior and punish them abruptly when they walk, unsuspectingly, into the minefield.

Vine blends well with the other remedies in this group, especially with Vervain and Crab Apple (which I believe belongs in this group). It also mixes well with Willow (when bitterness and willfulness combine into the most dreadful of parents, like Bette Davis' mother in *Now Voyager*) and with Holly (when rage and willfulness collide).

Consider combining Vine with Beech when the intolerant patient puts aside his mask of fairness and replaces it with an iron will. And with Rock Water, when Vine's will turns outward Rock Water's interior sense of stoicism. The resulting patient is the strictest of people, demanding not only obeisance, but also perfection from others.

We all need Vine as an acute remedy from time to time, for those moments when we are being stubborn, faultfinding, or demanding. When we lock our will, even for no good reason. Most of all, turn to this remedy immediately when you are acting as a know-it-all. In those moments when you realize that it has not even occurred to you that what you are saying, thinking, or doing could, in actuality, be completely off base, reach for Vine.

### Negative Qualities of the Type

The negative Vine is, in many respects, the only remedy type capable of nearly matching the bitter Willow type for sheer negativity. In his endless list of rules and demands, his ongoing monologue of criticism, and his overwhelming willpower, the Vine type wears down all others until they tend to simply give him his way. Further, the Vine type is a person literally possessed with the notion that he is right, in all things and all ways. In order to be right, Vines are quite capable of underhanded tricks. Vine types will grasp after power, they will bully, whine, and fight. As power itself is often their ultimate goal, all other aspects of the human experience are secondary in importance and tend to fall by the wayside. They demand obedience from others and can be harsh, ruthless, and cruel. Other people can even lose their status as humans in the eyes of Vine, and become obstacles to be removed.[16]

### Positive Qualities of the Type

When the really negative types, like Vine or Willow or Holly, manage to transform themselves into a more positive state, they are capable of accomplishing great things.

As natural leaders, the positive Vine types will also be willing servants. Vine types can learn to know when they should lead and when it is better for them to follow. They will happily humble themselves for the sake of love and of those they love. Further, positive Vine types not only have learned that they have strengths and weaknesses, but they have learned that they are sometimes right and sometimes wrong. It is now more important to them that the right opinion and idea prevail, not that their opinion or idea be perceived as right.

Positive Vine types are among our finest teachers, and they will teach with love and gentleness. They can also be balanced and compassionate leaders on all levels of our society. Perhaps most important, they are also capable of strong and compassionate parenting.

### The Vine Child

I have heard that some children just seem to be born willful, but I have never seen such a child myself. I have been told of children who refused to yield to any will other than their own, and that, from the very first time their eyes met their parents', it was obvious that behind that baby's eyes was a mind that would not be swayed by reason, discipline, or force.

This may be true, but, hopefully, such children are rare.

---

16. It is perhaps too facile to use the example of Hitler and his Nazis when discussing the Vine type. The sheer horror of what this most bitterly negative of all Vine types accomplished is beyond the pale in a book that most often uses literary or movie references to discuss various patients. But Nazi Germany is our best example of what a deeply negative, deeply and truly evil Vine type can do, and how they can pervert the thinking of others, and even the masses, often by convincing them that it is quite all right to hurt a particular group or individual, because they are not really quite human. Deeply afflicted Vine types are quite capable of using bigotry as a tool to achieve their own goals.

Note that most often in human history—again, Germany between the World Wars is a prime example—populations turn to Vine types during times of great crisis, just as individuals turn to Vine types when crisis erupts. Most often, the Vine will be more than willing to lead and more than likely to take advantage of the crisis to grab as much personal power as he can. In this way, the negative Vine leader almost always ultimately betrays his own people.

More often than not, the Vine state is not one that is seen in young children. Instead, it begins to form during adolescence. Often, a child who was quiet and obedient will, seemingly overnight, change into a rebelling, belligerent young adult. And parent and child begin a long battle of locked wills.

I have no easy solution to this very difficult situation, other than to suggest that when the child will not cooperate even to the extent of taking Bach remedies, it is very helpful if the parents remember to take the remedies themselves.

### The Vine Adult

While there is no specific stage in life that suggests the need for Vine more than any other, it is perhaps needed slightly more often for young adults and for adults through middle age. The intensity of the Vine constitutional emotional state suggests that younger people are simply more capable than older ones of sustaining it. This is not to say that you will not find a constitutional need for Vine in the elderly. You most certainly will. But often the patient who was a Vine type in youth will move from the dominating Vine into the bitter Willow state as they age, if they have not had any form of treatment to bring them back into emotional balance. I have found that these two remedies and the types of patients who need them have much in common. Many patients will need a combination of the two remedies, and others will move from one type to the other.

In the same way, while both genders certainly need the remedy Vine, my experience suggests that men have a slight edge when it comes to the constitutional need for the remedy. Part of this may certainly be because we culturally tend to think of male Vine types as villains while we think of female Vines as heroines or strong women (again, think of Scarlett O'Hara)—as if the willful and determined emotional state in men leads them to destructive acts, while the same state in women leads them to greater success and higher achievements. I am not going to sidetrack into a discussion of the truth or falsehood of these assumptions, but I note that it often seems as if men are more quickly assessed as needing Vine than women. Often women Vines are not considered to be in a negative emotional state as quickly and easily as men. So don't underestimate the need for this remedy in female patients, and don't underestimate the impact it can have in their lives.

### The Vine Animal

This is a great remedy for animals—in my experience it is an excellent remedy particularly for dogs—that are very territorial. Think of this remedy for the dog that will growl or snap, even at his master, if it feels that its territory is threatened.

This is a great remedy for animals that behave in a dominant manner with other, weaker animals, or refuse to allow a new animal to enter their pack.

### Vine and the Homeopathic Pharmacy

Certainly, the remedy Lycopodium comes to mind as a possible parallel remedy for Vine. But while Vine completely sure of himself and of his position, Lycopodium, with its central issue of lack of self-confidence, lacks confidence and overcompensates for his inadequacies through aggression.

Nux Vomica, another remedy that suggests forceful behavior patterns, comes much closer to Vine. Nux can be as driven as Vine and as dominating a presence.

But perhaps the remedy Veratrum Album, a homeopathic constitutional type that often feels that he is delivering a message from God, is closer still. Veratrum types, like Vine types, feel enlightened and become self-righteous in their knowledge. Like Vine types, they are forceful in their approach and willing to win their way by almost any means.

### Issues that Suggest Vine

Abuse; ambition; circulatory troubles; constipation and other digestive complaints; earaches; father issues; irritable bowel syndrome; jaw or mouth pain; headache; heart troubles; hypertension; infections; lockjaw; sore throats.

### In Conclusion

When we consider the remedy Vine, we must remember that the remedy itself, like those who need it, has something of a stigma attached. So, when we consider Vine we must, as always, remind ourselves that Bach felt that we *all* need all of his remedies at one time or another. The emotional states they suggest are common to all humans from time to time or on a more continual basis. It can be difficult to admit the need for a given remedy when we treat ourselves and others. And Vine, along with Willow and Holly, are certainly remedy types that most of us don't want to think we need.

But the need for Vine does not suggest a cruel killer any more than the need for Chestnut Bud suggests a stupid fool. We often have to deal with the most extreme examples of the type when we study the remedies, and we sometimes don't consider the day-to-day implications as we do so. Vine is needed far more often by individuals who are depending upon their willpower instead of finding balance in their full range of emotions. These individuals begin to feel great stress as they pour their will into achieving a goal and, as a result, become more negative and irritable. They tend to lash out in a manner that others perceive as threatening and dominating.

Now, I do not suggest that this is a good pattern. The Vine state is, like every other emotional state described in these pages, destructive. But it is nothing more than any other emotional pattern—the particular behavior a given patient uses to survive and achieve his or her goals. As such, it is no different than the other thirty-seven.

Each Bach type describes a behavior pattern a given patient uses to move forward as best he or she can. But each is, in reality, a block of some sort that holds the patient back from actual achievement, which can only come about through emotional balance and an honest understanding of self as well as the situation at hand. The Bach remedies, used singly or in combination, can offer just such a balanced state of mind and heart.

When we use Vine, or any other of the remedies we must avoid value judgments and help the patient to do the same, no matter what we think of the types each describes. We each need all the remedies, and we each have all the types within us. We must let our compassion for ourselves and others override our sense of judgment when we select and use the remedies.

# 9

# Considering the Sixth Mood:
# The Curse of Indifference

There is a denial of reality, or, at least, of present circumstances, implicit in the mood that Bach describes as the "lack of sufficient interest in present circumstances," and that I simply call indifference. Those sharing this mood also share a certain unwillingness, either an unwillingness to deal with situations the patient feels were thrust upon him, or an unwillingness to exert the physical or emotional energy it would take to transform those situations for the better. Either way, those sharing this mood find themselves in a state of stasis, as if they were not wholly present within their bodies, and they seek to find a way to escape the present situation.

The survival strategies adapted by each of these remedy types involve indifference. Each is a variation of a theme in which the remedy type shows little interest in their surroundings and in the needs and wants of others. Some, like Wild Rose, have all but totally given up on the idea of change and transformation and have settled instead in a mindset that is resigned to fate as it is perceived and shows no interest in life as a result. To a lesser degree, Clematis and Honeysuckle share this sense of resignation. Clematis escapes into a dream state and Honeysuckle escapes into the past, which is seen as a better place and time. Mustard and Olive share a sense of weight and exhaustion. Mustard carries the weight of emotional exhaustion and clinical depression. Olive struggles with an actual physical state of depletion and exhaustion.

> Those sharing this mood also share a certain unwillingness, either an unwillingness to deal with situations the patient feels were thrust upon him, or an unwillingness to exert the physical or emotional energy it would take to transform those situations for the better.

And then there are the Chestnuts. Two of our three obsessive-patterned Chestnut-based remedies are part of this group. White Chestnut loses interest in the present moment because his thoughts are locked on one specific topic, perhaps a slight, perhaps an all-consuming philosophy. But, whatever the specific direction of his thinking, his obsession of thought takes him away from his surroundings and life in this moment.

Chestnut Bud is likewise obsessed, but he is obsessed with behavior rather than with thought. In severe cases, the Chestnut Bud can be truly compulsive in his behaviors. He may have to regularly count the number of stairs to his doorway, or turn a light switch on and off an established number of times before he can proceed. Or, as in more common cases, the Chestnut Bud may be a prisoner of his habits, especially of bad habits, like smoking or eating before bed. Some Chestnut Buds are cyclical in their obsessive behaviors. Others are not, but have bouts of obsessive behavior from time to time or are utterly unpredictable in their bad habits. But, either way, they are as removed from their life in the present moment by their habits as the White Chestnut is by his thoughts.

Those who find themselves constitutionally locked into this mood are often prisoners of their own imaginations as well, finding a contentment in the invisible world that eludes them on the physical plane. Therefore, you will find Clematis with his daydreams and Honeysuckle with her photographs, each substituting an alternate reality for the one at hand.

With the exception of White Chestnut, the remedy types listed here tend to be rather passive types, who tend to lack either the passion or strength to get involved in causes, activities, or, often, with the world around them.

And each of these types is disconnected with life in the present moment. When we are living in the healthiest manner possible, we have a balanced perspective of time and the passing of time in our lives. Therefore, we are able to "edit" our past—learning from what we can, holding on to the memory of what we should, and letting go of the rest—and work toward the future while we live in the present moment of our lives. We must be present in our lives, in body, mind, and spirit, to live them effectively. To drive safely on the highway, we must be focused not only on our location, but also upon the actions we must perform to travel safely. And yet our minds tend to drift even in this situation (which we know to be dangerous and statistics tell us is likely the most dangerous thing we do on a regular basis) when we hear a song we like on the radio, or our attention is distracted by putting on make-up or talking on a cell phone.

The remedies in this group remind us that we must be present in our own lives—that we must be aware, not only of ourselves, but also of those around us. That we must balance our needs with a compassion for the needs of others. To live this way—so that we can not only be our brother's keeper, but our own as well—we must keep our attention on the present moment and remind ourselves that "sufficient unto the day is the evil thereof."

These remedies can help us do just that, to stay aware that if we simply make today all it can be then we have done a great deal to shape tomorrow.

Back in the early 1970s, when I was a child, I can remember my older sister reading a huge paperback philosophy book with a psychedelic cover by Baba Ram Dass called

*Be Here Now.* At the time, I was more attracted to the blue and orange of the letters, but now I can appreciate the concept as well. If we are to live fully and completely, we have to come to terms with where we are in time and space. We have to be fully integrated in our bodies, minds, spirits, and environment. We must also be integrated in our communities of work and home life and with our families and friends. Only then can we live complete lives. The remedies listed here have been created for just that purpose, so we can fully integrate ourselves within our world.

When considering remedy mixtures, remember that the remedies in this group work particularly well with those listed as remedies for those who Doubt and for those with Fear. Those remedy types often share a sense of limitation and depletion with the remedies listed here.

## Indifference and the Homeopathic Pharmacy

Whole books have been written that study the effect of indifference on our mental and physical health. Some suggest, and Bach would agree, I think, that the state of indifference suggests some form of denial of reality, an inner shifting or censoring of external realities. Sometimes this takes shape as a denial of self or self-want, such as with the homeopathic remedy Natrum Muriaticum, a type that tends to refuse to allow himself or, more commonly, herself the very things she wants most. Interestingly, the Natrum Mur type often embodies this emotional state by becoming allergic to the very thing she desires. A Natrum Mur type may, for instance, adopt a pet she adores, a pet that fills a deep emotional void in her life, only to develop a terrible allergy to the cat over a period of time and ultimately has to give it away. In the same way, Natrum Mur types become allergic to the foods they love, or to the sun and sand of the beach, which they also tend to adore.

The homeopathic repertory is filled with rubrics that relate to the subject of indifference. The topic of indifference itself lists thousands of remedies over a number of pages. Leading remedies in the homeopathic pharmacy for those who are indifferent include Phosphorus, which often masks indifference with a sleepy and somewhat withdrawn demeanor as will Clematis; Staphysagria, usually thought of as a very active, passionate type, but who is also capable of long periods of withdrawn indifference to the very things that he or she is most passionate about, commonly a depressive state similar to that of Mustard; and Gelsemium, a remedy thought of in acute situations as a remedy for those with flu or lingering, debilitating diseases (in a constitutional context it is used as a treatment for those with multiple sclerosis, among many other things), often presents a patient type who is too exhausted to care, which parallels Bach's Olive.

The repertory's rubrics break down the concept of indifference into many different categories, mindsets, and behaviors. For those who are indifferent to everything, a state similar to the Wild Rose mindset, a leading remedy is Carbo Vegetabilis. This remedy type is known for its willingness to simply sit and let the world go by. Under the interesting rubric "indifferent to pleasure," one remedy stands out: the highly emotional Pulsatilla, who usually is considered a patient type interested in everything. Since the opposite intensity is also present in any remedy type clearly displaying a specific intensity, one Pulsatilla type may show passionate interest in anything that brings her pleasure, fattening foods chief among them, while another may have just as strong a disinterest in the things she once loved.

The group of remedies in this chapter all play out the concept of indifference in their own unique way, just like the homeopathic remedy types described above. The Bach types present two sides of the coin just as the homeopathic types do. Some will ride a roller coaster, showing great interest in the things and people around them at times and retiring into a haze of disinterest at other times, instead of simply presenting a constant and consistent lack of interest. This lack of consistency can be troubling to those around them at best. At worst—often when the indifferent type is a parent—their inconsistent emotional behavior can be devastating to those who depend upon or care about them.

The quality of indifference is often thought of as being a lesser thing, more acceptable than the more aggressive emotional states. Perhaps this is because it tends to be a quiet state in which the patient pulls inward and does not push his thoughts and suspicions upon others, as we have seen with the overly sensitive in an earlier chapter. But it is not, as we will see in the pages ahead. The state of indifference is a cool state, where the overly sensitive state is hot. Indifference is the source of cancer, as the state of over sensitivity is the breeding ground of heart and circulatory disease. While indifference is quiet, it is as destructive as any of Bach's other six negative emotional states. And it can be harder to diagnose and harder to treat than the other states, because it is an emotional state that can be buried deep inside. This makes it even more important that the remedies listed here—which are, in my opinion, the most underprescribed of all of Bach's remedies (especially Chestnut Bud)—are fully understood and considered in any combination of Bach remedies.

## REMEDIES FOR THOSE WHO ARE INDIFFERENT

- **Clematis**—for those who are vague
- **Honeysuckle**—for those who are nostalgic
- **Mustard**—for those who are in depression
- **Olive**—for those who are exhausted
- **Wild Rose**—for those who are indifferent

- **White Chestnut**—for those who have obsessive thoughts
- **Chestnut Bud**—for those who have obsessive behavior

## CLEMATIS · THE REMEDY FOR THOSE WHO ARE VAGUE

Bach tells us that Clematis types are "those who are dreamy, drowsy, not fully awake, with no great interest in life. Quiet people, not really happy in their present circumstances, living more in the future than in the present; living hopes of happier times when their ideals may come true."

- **Clematis is both an acute and a constitutional remedy.**
- **Clematis is a component of Rescue Remedy.**
- **Clematis is one of Bach's original remedies, the Twelve Healers.**

### Botanical Information

Also known as "traveler's joy" and "old man's beard," Clematis (*Clematis Vitalba*) is a very fast growing deciduous climbing plant. It is capable of covering entire areas of woodland in a single season. Each plant can produce up to 100,000 seeds, which are spread by wind or water, in a single season.

Clematis is native to central and southern Europe and now grows in gardens, by roadsides, riverbeds, and on the edges of forests in temperate climates worldwide.

Clematis blooms in late summer and into early autumn. The flowers are light-colored, usually white, and fragrant. After the flowering the plant displays feathery seed heads from autumn through spring. These seed heads give the plant its common name, "old man's beard."

### Clematis in General

It's a toss up in my opinion as to which remedy type is more pleasant, the Agrimony or the Clematis. Both present faces that contain humor and goodwill to all. And where Agrimony has Elwood P. Dowd, who sees giant invisible rabbits as its literary icon, Clematis has James Thurber's Walter Mitty, who can turn his humdrum everyday life into an exciting adventure by escaping into a world of daydreams as often as possible. Both are kind and gentle souls, and, like them, Agrimony and Clematis types can be so nice that you hate to give them a remedy. Rest assured, however, that neither will have to yield their virtues through Bach treatments. They will simply be able to apply them to their lives instead of having to escape into a bottle, as the Agrimony will tend to, or into his own world of imagination, as the Clematis does.

The negative emotional state projected by the Clematis type does not necessarily seem negative to others—he is not aggressive or destructive like a Holly or Willow type. In fact, he is quite the opposite, mild and very easygoing. The negativity of the type is slowly revealed to others in his vagueness and almost total indifference, even to issues of considerable import.

When asked what he wants for dinner, the Clematis type will respond that he doesn't care. And he will be telling the truth. He will happily eat whatever is put before him, whether it is homemade or delivered in a box. Just so long as he is not called upon to decide what will be made.[1]

Asked what he wants to watch on television, he will reply that he doesn't care. Asked what he wants for Christmas, he doesn't care. Ultimately, the Clematis type will honestly not care what happens to him and will limit his own life experience through sheer apathy, forcing the responsibility for his own existence onto others.

This, of course, is a rather extreme example of the type, but it is one that has been examined by one of America's greatest authors. In 1853, Herman Melville wrote a short story called *Bartleby the Scrivener, A Story of Wall Street*. In this story, a mild-mannered man named Bartleby is hired by a firm to work as a notary. At first, everything seems fine. Bartleby is well liked and does his work as directed. One day, when asked to perform a set task, Bartleby says, "I would prefer not to." In the Clematis way, he remains polite, if vague, in that he can give no reason for his preference. But he also remains firm. He would prefer not to.

His politely-stated preference to not work snowballs through the story until Bartleby's "I would prefer not to" extends to every aspect of his life. The man who hired him takes on more and more of Bartleby's responsibilities out of concern for him. In the end, Bartleby dies, apparently because he ultimately simply loses the will to live.

This is the progression of the Clematis state, not that it has ever been, in my experience, fatal. Like our other negative emotional states the Clematis state is a continuum, progressing from the simple acute state of daydreaming in a history class that bores the patient to a chronic state in which the patient ultimately loses all touch with reality and retreats into a fantasy realm. In the physical context, the Clematis state is represented acutely by a fainting episode and constitutionally by a coma state. It is because of this physical loss of consciousness that Bach made Clematis a part of his Rescue Remedy blend.

The key to understanding this type lies in understanding the link each of us has to the objective reality of the world around us. Each of us filters that reality through our

---

1. He will also be quite happy to help make the dinner, as long as someone tells him what to do. Clematis types tend to not like to take the initiative for anything, even something as small as deciding what's for dinner. They tend to drift off, waiting for someone else to make the decision and tell them what their part will be. Even when they find themselves in positions of authority, Clematis types will tend to shy away from taking the initiative, preferring to take orders rather than give them.

senses as well as our mind. We interpret reality every second of every day. Just as the cameraman and the editor shape the content of what appears on our television screen—the degree to which the projected picture represents the actual event being depicted depends upon both the skill and the intent of those involved—our eyes and ears, working in tandem with our brains, determine just how closely our perceived reality parallels our world's objective reality.

Clematis is the remedy that relates to our link with the reality of our lives and the world around us, and how dependable that link is. As Bach so importantly notes in the quotation that opened this section, Clematis types are "those who are dreamy, drowsy, not fully awake, with no great interest in life. Quiet people, not really happy in their present circumstances . . ."

That final phrase gives us the root cause of the Clematis state. The Clematis type is not happy with his life, at least not his present set of circumstances. And since he lacks both the drive and the know-how to break free of those circumstances, he adopts an emotional pattern of exaggeration and creative editing of his situation instead. Clematis, therefore, is the perfect remedy for the lonely child who invents an imaginary playmate. For the bored worker who drifts off into daydreams, leaving his work and his cubicle behind. For all those who, when the cameras of their eyes and the microphones of their ears begin to record unpleasant events, begin to tinker with their perception of reality instead of changing those events. When objective events begin to be colored by a subjective haze.

> Clematis is the remedy that relates to our link with the reality of our lives and the world around us, and how dependable that link is.

Just like all of Bach's other remedies, Clematis represents an emotional state we have all experienced at one time or another. We have all employed the Clematis strategy of survival at one time or another to avoid difficult situations. We have all played a musical tune in our head while some professor droned on and on from behind a lectern or while someone in authority criticized our efforts. In acute circumstances it can represent a method by which we can rather pleasantly avoid an unpleasant reality. In the constitutional context, however, the Clematis state represents creativity used in a destructive manner. It is, therefore, another perversion of a positive attribute. Well used, this sense of creativity and imagination we all possess can be used to actually shape a new reality, whether as a work of art or as a visionary step forward in technology or cultural achievement. Negatively employed, this same creative imagination can become an undertow that drags the patient down deeper and deeper, further and further away from reality.

The constitutional Clematis type will not only manage to trip over his own two feet simply because he is not paying enough attention to what he is doing to walk safely (or to safely walk across the street without being run over by a car he didn't notice), he will also lose valuable time on a daily basis, time lost from work and study to day-dreaming.[2]

Like the Honeysuckle and the Impatiens types, the Clematis type is out of sync with time. Not only does he have trouble melding his perceived reality with the objective reality around him, he has trouble keeping his attention in the moment at hand. But where the Honeysuckle type is solidly linked with the past and is disinterested in the present, and the Impatiens type is rushing toward the future and ignoring the past, the Clematis is as vague about his time-sense as he is about his sense of reality. A Clematis type may be more interested in the past, especially if he feels that his life in the past was more pleasant than it is now (note that the Clematis will be more wistful for the past than the Honeysuckle, who will be deeply nostalgic for all things passed by). Or the Clematis may be focused on the future, if he becomes convinced that the future holds hopes that the present does not (many Clematis types are great science fiction and fantasy literature fans and will seem more conversant about the world of Star Trek or Star Wars than they are about their own). Or the Clematis type may simply seem out of sync with the present moment, as if he was drifting along outside the passage of time.

However a given Clematis type displays his lack of understanding of time, look for him to be chronically late. He will underestimate the amount of time that a task will take or overestimate by many hours the amount he can actually do in a single day. He will fail to consider travel time in his plans and, in doing so, may end up arriving an hour early or a day late, either way with a slightly puzzled look on his face.

And expect to see that slightly puzzled look a great deal. The Clematis type, who is anchored neither by time nor by the real world, tends to always be a bit puzzled. He can react like a person who has been shaken awake from sleep when spoken to. He is, in his constitutional state, a sleepwalker who wanders through life, depending upon the kindness of strangers to keep him safe.

The vagueness of the type links this remedy type to Aspen, who shares his tenuous hold on reality. But the Aspen type, who also tends to misunderstand and to misinterpret the passage of time, is anxious, while the Clematis type, through his drowsy haze, is more trusting. When he falls, he fully expects someone will catch him. The patient who feels anxiety coupled with vagueness will greatly benefit from the combination of

---

2. Modern electronics offer Clematis types many tempting ways to avoid reality for many hours on end. Expect Clematis types to find great comfort not only in their televisions, but also in their video games—especially fantasy games—and in the Internet, the computer and the iPod. Clematis types of generations past had to read a fantasy book and then daydream about what they had read, but modern technology offers many more direct routes into fantasy.

Clematis and Aspen. This combination is so harmonious and potent that I have almost considered the two remedies to be one in many cases, at least as far as the needs of specific patients are concerned.

Two other remedies that combine very well with Clematis are Honeysuckle and Scleranthus. As I have noted, the Honeysuckle type will have strong ties to the past and will be very nostalgic for what he feels was a better time. The patient who needs Honeysuckle and Clematis in combination is even more strongly linked to the past, to the extent that he has trouble functioning in the present moment. And the patient needing Clematis and Scleranthus will have his vague tendency toward indifference coupled with indecision, leaving him helpless when he is asked to choose between the chicken and the fish.

Clematis is valuable for those moments in our daily lives when we are less alert than we should be, when our attention drifts away from the world and into our inner being. For patients who lock onto their inner dialogue to the point that they disconnect from the world, the combination of Clematis and White Chestnut is very helpful. As I noted earlier, Clematis is valuable if the patient feels faint or if there is a loss of consciousness in cases of physical trauma. Even in cases of serious trauma or long-term serious illness, Clematis can help if the patient seems to be slipping away or if the patient is perceived to have lost the will to live. If the patient has been worn down by illness and has developed a death wish, consider combining Clematis with Gorse and/or Olive.

## Negative Qualities of the Type

Clematis types are nearly always lost in thought. They are absentminded, forgetful. But often there is a clear purpose to this forgetfulness. Clematis will forget to tell someone bad news, or information that will make them look bad. They will spend their days daydreaming, and will spend more and more time daydreaming as they fall behind in their work because they were daydreaming to begin with. So Clematis types will withdraw more and more into themselves as they feel challenged or threatened. And, more and more, they will forget to tell other people—whether coworkers or mate—the things they need to know in order to achieve their life goals.

This makes the Clematis type a very difficult partner of any sort. Those who work with or live with a Clematis have to learn to deal with the fact that, for the Clematis, information is control, and memory, or lack thereof, is the method of choice by which the Clematis retains control. They will not pay the bills on time or be home in time to eat the dinner that was prepared for them. To their partner, the Clematis will sometimes seem like an overgrown child or a very large weight they have to drag along. Indeed, the Clematis type will often display many behaviors that would be termed passive-aggressive, linking this negative emotional state with that of Centaury, who is also very passive-aggressive. Clematis and Centaury are often given in combination for this reason, and it can be highly effective for those patients who become a burden on those who live and work with them.

### Positive Qualities of the Type

The positive Clematis is the visionary—one that the world needs. This Clematis type is a romantic pragmatist who balances reality with the possibility for transformational change. The Clematis who has moved into an emotionally balanced state is able to differentiate between reality and fantasy and able to use his creative imagination to shape reality. The positive Clematis is fully in tune with reality, with time, and with the details of life that once bored or threatened him. In his state of full awareness, he is able to achieve great things.

### The Clematis Child

Clematis children are wistful dreamers. They tend to physically need much more sleep than other children and daydream for much of the time they are awake. They are quiet children, obedient children, and are quite willing to do as they are told. If they don't want to do what you tell them to, they will either forget[3] to do it, or do it very slowly, as if in a dreamlike trance.

Clematis children will usually have an imaginary friend. This is not because they do not have real friends, but because they learn early in life that they are more comfortable within themselves than they are in the world. For the young Clematis child, like the young Aspen, the world of make-believe and the world of reality are very closely aligned. The young Clematis type, like the Aspen child, will hear voices, talk to toys or plants as if they were answering him, and show discomfort or fear around anything unpleasant or threatening. He often has difficulty with any sort of discord in the house and withdraws from any confrontation.

There is no shier child than the Clematis, or one who needs his parents more to help him come into the world and channel his wonderful imagination. The Clematis child needs a gentle anchor to the world around him. Pets can often help. A Clematis type will be a gentle companion for a dog or cat, and the living, breathing animal will teach him about the real world in a way that a stuffed animal cannot.

Many teens move through a Clematis phase as they approach adulthood. They will sleep for many, many hours at a stretch, and will show little interest in the world around

---

3. Clematis types have a wonderfully selective memory at any age. They can instantly forget any information they do not wish to retain—deadlines, details like the amount of money they have in the bank, and worrying things like taxes being chief among them—while they can display a wonderfully keen memory for pleasant things or things that catch their attention or imagination.

them. Instead they become glassy-eyed from boredom or from inner flights of fantasy. These young adults will have a strong tendency toward drugs or alcohol, because they enhance the Clematis dream state. Creative young Clematis types have a special affinity for marijuana and parents need to be very careful to protect these children from themselves. Their vulnerability to this and other drugs can become a long-term habit, because young Clematis types lack the inner stability to balance their desire for exploration with a core sense of direction.

Young Clematis types can often be helped by combining Clematis with either or both Wild Oat or Walnut. Walnut can give them an inner sense of stability and Wild Oat can help them find their path in life. The three remedies combine extremely well for young adults who are "in crisis" due to a lack of proper channels for their creative energy.

### The Clematis Adult

Just as Clematis is often needed by those who are on the doorstep of adulthood, it is also commonly needed by the elderly. The Clematis state often comes to the fore as a patient faces the last stage of life, when a patient chooses to live within dreams and memories rather than deal with the details of real life any longer. In these cases, it will often seem as if there is not a complete link between the patient's body and his soul— as if, from time to time, that soul was floating up out of the body, traveling to other times and places, and then finding its way back home. Elderly Clematis adults tend to feel as if they have outlived their usefulness in life, outstayed their welcome. They are unhappy with the fact that they are still alive, especially if they have been taken out of their own homes and put into medical facilities. They drift, waiting for the end to come.

Although I have found that the need for Clematis is especially strong in young adulthood, at the same time that Wild Oat is often indicated, and during the last stage of life, it is also needed by patients at every stage of adulthood. It is commonly needed by those who are not challenged by their life's work, or, ironically, by those who find themselves too challenged by their work, who retreat into daydreams to avoid tasks they are unable to tackle (combining Clematis with Elm often helps these patients).

The state of disinterest represented by Clematis can occur at any time and at any stage of life. Clematis can help us to restore our natural interest in life whenever we lose our full attention for life and turn inward instead.

### The Clematis Animal

Perhaps the most important use of this remedy for animals is physical, not emotional. Use Clematis for animals that have been unconscious or are losing consciousness. It is especially helpful for animals that have been ill for a long time and have waning life energy (combine with Olive or Gorse), or for older animals that are slipping away.

Clematis can also be helpful for animals that spend the day alone and are bored and lonely. (It combines well with Hornbeam or White Chestnut in these circumstances.)

### Clematis and the Homeopathic Pharmacy

The homeopathic remedy that comes closest to the Clematis state is Opium. Like the drug, the homeopathic remedy speaks to the comalike opium state, where the drugged move into a twilight area, sluggish and blissful.

### Issues that Suggest Clematis

Aging; asthma; awkwardness; curvature of the spine; dementia; hypoglycemia; learning disabilities; lung problems; narcolepsy; pancreas troubles; psoriasis; sleepwalking; slurring speech; stress; trauma; unconsciousness.

### In Conclusion

As noted above, the Clematis type is an editor of reality. Clematis types who manage to function within the "real" world of business and school demands and adult responsibilities will mix a degree of attention to reality with a tendency to "tune out" life's more boring or stressful details. Clematis types who lack the innate intelligence or drive to remain strongly linked with reality and balance their real and imaginary lives tend to keep their finger more fixed on the edit button, however. Often they will turn to either drugs or technology to help them avoid reality. At their worst, Clematis types seem to be a constant source of confusion, disappointment, and stress for those who love them or depend upon them in any way. The very fact that they are loved and/or depended upon may be enough to make them withdraw further into fantasy. This leads to even greater stress and confusion for those who do not understand the dynamics of the Clematis types' emotional structure.

Thus, the Clematis, who originally finds a happy escape from stressful reality within the realm of his own mind, ultimately visits reality less and less as his survival strategy causes more stress for those around him and results in a progressively more negative and stressful "real world" environment. As is often the case with constitutional Bach types, the Clematis ultimately creates or enhances the very thing that he originally meant to escape with his negative pattern of thought and behavior.

## HONEYSUCKLE · THE REMEDY FOR THOSE WHO ARE NOSTALGIC

Bach instructs that Honeysuckle types are "those who live much in the past, perhaps a time of great happiness, or memories of a lost friend, or ambitions which have not come true. They do not expect further happiness such as they have had."

• **Honeysuckle is both an acute and a constitutional remedy.**

### Botanical Information

The honeysuckle (*Lonicera Caprifolium*) vine is cherished, both for its highly fragrant and very beautiful flowers that bloom in May and June, which are red on the outside and white inside, and for the fiery orange berries the plant produces in September and October. Honeysuckle is common to gardens in temperate regions worldwide. It is a hearty climber, and is often used to cover pergolas and gateways.

In natural settings, it is found in woodlands and on the edges of forests. It is said to be found naturally growing in the Scottish heath.

Honeysuckle is native to Southern Europe. Its common name is "Italian woodbine."

### Honeysuckle in General

There is a tendency in the Honeysuckle constitutional type to want to cover every-thing in amber, to preserve and protect the past, and to resist change, above all else. It is a constitutional type that often develops in old age, when the past becomes a refuge for those who are fearful of the future and challenged by the present. Or in middle age, when the children are grown and gone and the pets have passed away. When the house seems large and empty, filled only with memories.

> There is a hollowness within the heart of the Honeysuckle type, a hollowness that the patient believes can only be filled by memories of the past.

It is often the remedy for the widow who wants to remember a happier time, or for the parent who refuses to change anything in a child's room after the child has moved on to college. These are people who live in a state of wishful regret—not a regret of any specific thing that was done or not done, but regret that time has moved on and that happy times are now in the past.

There is a hollowness within the heart of the Honeysuckle type, a hollowness that the patient believes can only be filled by memories of the past. The Honeysuckle has lost his path in life and his ties to the future. For him, life holds no future promise, no excitement yet to come. The best parts of life are in the past, and these parts need to be preserved and cherished.

The Honeysuckle type, then, is one of our remedy types out of his proper place in time. He has lost a sense of who he is and how he appropriately fits into the passage of time. Just as the Impatiens type ignores the past and focuses completely on the future (even if that "future" is only seconds or minutes away), the Honeysuckle type ignores the future and turns his full attention backward. Like the Impatiens type, the Honeysuckle fails to live in the moment at hand. In doing so, he limits his ability to experience life and achieve all that is set before him to achieve.[4]

While the Honeysuckle type will not necessarily tend to run late and fail to turn up for appointments on time like the other remedies with a poor sense of time, the Honeysuckle will often find himself or herself walking through life with little or no interest in it. He goes to the doctor's appointment simply because it has been made or because it is expected of him. She shows up on time for a meeting simply because it is something to do. What interests the Honeysuckle is memory—specifically, the memory of better times, better places.

The word that best describes the Honeysuckle, therefore, is nostalgic.

Nostalgia can be defined as "a wistful longing for the past, typically for a time or place with pleasant associations." This definition tells us why Bach placed the remedy Honeysuckle in the group of remedies for those who are indifferent. Like Clematis, the Honeysuckle type becomes indifferent to their life because they are unhappy with the present state of affairs. Just as the Clematis type retreats from reality into a fantasy world, the Honeysuckle type retreats from an unpleasant reality into a very pleasant memory, perhaps to a time of wicker rockers and lemonade on the front porch, or to a summer of love.

As the Honeysuckle type retreats from reality, he becomes more and more indifferent to his surroundings and to the details of his life in the present moment. His very indifference to his surroundings and to his present-day existence reveals the Honeysuckle to be in a state of emotional and mental disorder. He lacks interest in what should be of great interest to him—his own life, and the details and decisions that will not only shape his future health and comfort, but also determine whether or not he accomplishes all in life that he might. The Walnut type stands at a crossroad and does not know which way to walk, and the Wild Oat type struggles hard to find his path. The Honeysuckle type knows his path, but abandons it because he finds no value in it and no promise in the future. Like the Gentian, the Honeysuckle abandons his proper path and costs himself the rewards of the journey in doing so. Where the Gentian type

4. Clematis, the remedy listed before Honeysuckle in these pages, also lacks a sense of time and the present moment. Since the Clematis type can be fixated on either the past or the future, his time sense can be seen as something of a combination of the Honeysuckle type and the constitutional Impatiens type.

stops his journey because he is too easily discouraged by any setback, the Honeysuckle stops moving forward in his journey, abandons his goals, and actually seeks to turn back because he is hoping against hope that he might be able to walk backward in time as well as space.

No simple discouragement creates the Honeysuckle emotional state. Only a deep emotional wound can cause a patient to yearn so strongly for the past that he or she becomes indifferent to the present. Many widows, after a period of overt emotional distress, turn to a state of quiet grief that may be described as a Honeysuckle emotional state.[5]

To enter into a Honeysuckle emotional state, a given patient must first conclude that he is deeply unhappy, on some profound level, with his present circumstances. Patients do not simply choose to fixate on the past. They are driven into the past by a deep sense of displeasure and/or discomfort. In a moment of sorrow or stress or trauma, something within reminds them, through an association with some sense or memory, that they were happier at another time, or in another place. And a deep sense of nostalgia begins to take shape deep within.

Certainly, we all have need for this remedy at some time or another. No matter how happy our lives, no matter how good our choices, we all have moments when we look back with a sense of dull ache for what has been lost. On some level and to one degree or another, we all ache for lost loves, for happy times past. The difference between the simple acute state, where our longing passes and the alarm clock rings and we turn our attention to the new day, and the deeper, far more complex constitutional state is that, for the patient in chronic need of the remedy, each new day is faced with a sense of dread or with a hollow sense of indifference. The only happy notes in the life of a constitutional Honeysuckle are those that are struck in memory.

The fact that the Honeysuckle type is indifferent to his present and his future is a crippling thing. It weakens his ability to function and to thrive. It robs him of his appropriate joy of life in this moment, and of all possibility of future achievement. In doing so, it not only cuts away the patient's potential in all things, but also his ability to feel and receive love from those around him. As with many other Bach remedy types, the true issue for the Honeysuckle is one of perception. Because he perceives that all the best that his life had to offer is now in the past, the Honeysuckle type will fail to see what life is offering now and will offer in the future. It is as if he has blindfolded himself to the world around him and turned his sense of sight inward and backward to his past.

---

5. This is often a remedy for those who grieve, as is Water Violet, who withdraws into a lonely state of aloof grief. The two remedies can have much in common. But Water Violet often does not even consider clinging to the past and will show no interest in photos or antiques, which Honeysuckle will greatly value. The two remedies work well together in combination, especially in cases of deep grief.

In focusing on the supposedly better past (and, of course, the Honeysuckle must be sure to keep the past covered in gold dust, and never think about the realities of past challenges and difficulties, or the faults of loved ones now gone), the Honeysuckle type blinds himself to the beauty that still exists. So even if the Honeysuckle type himself or herself is a benign being to a great extent, Honeysuckle must be considered a highly negative emotional state. Unless his memory is intruded upon or besmirched in any way, the Honeysuckle type is very easy to deal with. All is well as long as others play along with their roles in the Honeysuckle type's memory plays.

But that does not mean that all is truly well or that the Honeysuckle is emotionally healthy while he is locked in his haze of memory.

Among the remedies that combine best with Honeysuckle are Water Violet and Chicory. Since all three of these remedies relate to the idea of lost love, they may be used as needed in any combination for patients who are in grief. Typically, Chicory (often combined with Sweet Chestnut) is an important remedy for the first stages of grief, when the patient may have sudden emotional swings or erratic actions, while Water Violet and Honeysuckle are more commonly needed as grief becomes a more or less chronic emotional state and the patient quiets into a state of withdrawal. But all are important and should be considered, in combination or separately, to help those who have lost loved ones move through their process of grieving.

Honeysuckle also commonly combines with Mustard, another remedy in this group of remedies for those who are indifferent, in cases in which a sense of nostalgia for the past is linked with depression, and with Olive when a patient is exhausted and depleted by his or her loss and only finds solace in the past.

Honeysuckle is often combined with two other remedies from this group, Chestnut Bud and White Chestnut.[6] In both cases, the Chestnut obsession—obsessive behaviors in the case of the Chestnut Bud (a combination that yields an easily distracted or even confused patient) and obsessive thoughts in the case of the White Chestnut—lends intensity to the Honeysuckle type's nostalgia.

Finally, consider the combination of Honeysuckle and Star of Bethlehem. Use this mixture when a patient has retreated into the past as an escape from some specific trauma or loss in the present. It is also important to note that this is a great combination for patients haunted by past trauma or deeply buried memories they cannot quite bear to look at but at the same time are unable to release. Many victims of abuse in

---

6. If you're getting the idea that the remedies for indifference combine better with other remedies in the same group than they do with others, you are likely right. Certainly, the remedies in this group tend to enhance each other and help strengthen a patient's resolve to find new interest in life and new passions in the world around him.

childhood need the combination of Honeysuckle and Star of Bethlehem later in life to release their memories of abuse and move forward in their lives. Typically, these patients will insist that their childhoods were rich with happy memories and will be greatly resistant to having these memories examined.

## Negative Qualities of the Type

The Honeysuckle carries an emotional weight with them every day of their lives by not wanting to let go of the past, of both sweet and bitter memories. They glorify the past by clinging to it, glorify past joys and past triumphs. They refuse to look at the present moment or at the future because they fear both. They are, as a result, homesick. No matter that they are in their own homes, they are homesick. Homesick for a place that does not exist any longer, that has passed away. (Perhaps metaphorically, Honeysuckle may be our best acute remedy for homesickness in travelers.) When Honeysuckle types cling to the past, they are willfully refusing to let what is behind them pass away as it should. They cling to what is gone, try to make what is intangible tangible. In trying to do the impossible—bring the dead back to life, reestablish a way of life that is gone—they create an emotional burden not only for themselves, but also for those around them. The determined and passionate Honeysuckle will not hear anything that is less than encouraging of their position or that they feel in any way intrudes upon or upsets their glorified sense of the past.

The negative Honeysuckle can be a very demanding type. To enter their world is to agree to live with them in the past and to further agree never to let reality—of the past, present, or future—cause upset in any way. This is a great deal to ask of self, but even more to ask of others. Many families are deeply disrupted by the presence of a negative Honeysuckle type.

## Positive Qualities of the Type

A Honeysuckle type who has moved into a positive emotional state is quite capable of learning from life as they live it in the present day. They store up experiences, and their gathered personal history makes them a living encyclopedia of knowledge. Instead of being trapped in a cycle of memories of the past, the positive Honeysuckle is able to move fluidly from past to present and into the future.

Often they are graduates of the school of hard knocks, but they are people without regret who have gained true wisdom during the unfolding of their lives. They are uniquely gifted with the ability to transform the future by living in the present and learning from the past. As the adage states, those who do not learn from the past are doomed to repeat it. The positive Honeysuckle type has indeed learned all he needs to from the past, and is able to release it and move on.

### The Honeysuckle Child

Since children tend to live in the moment and are quite busy, especially in their early years, gathering new sensations and new experiences from moment to moment, there are very few children who will need this remedy. It is, however, a valuable remedy for children who have faced a trauma that has sent them searching in their small library of memories for comfort. The chief use of this remedy is for the child who has lost a parent or grandparent or some other loved one through death or divorce and who cannot move forward from grief. (See above for other remedies to be used in combination with Honeysuckle for these circumstances.)

### The Honeysuckle Adult

Each passing year increases our potential need for Honeysuckle, as each brings us a greater number of memories, good and bad; a greater number of battles won and lost; illnesses conquered or not; and relationships that continue or end. Most often, it is a remedy that is constitutionally needed by those who are middle-aged or older. It is typically only needed in younger adults who have sustained a specific loss that has left them in a state of depletion and grief.

For those of us who have passed midlife, the desire to relive our lives, especially our youth, can be more potent than our desire to actually live them in the present. This is especially true for those who have lost a mate or parent, or sometimes even more traumatic, a home. The loss of anything that offers us stability in the present can be enough to send us searching for that same sense of stability in our past, and, in doing so, can encourage the negative Honeysuckle emotional state.

### The Honeysuckle Animal

While it can be impossible to tell whether an animal feels nostalgic or not, this remedy can have some valuable uses. For instance, I have found it very helpful for animals that are taken on vacation with their owners but are not adjusting well to the new surroundings. Just as Honeysuckle can help humans who are homesick when traveling, it can also help pets cope better while on vacation.

In the same way, think about this remedy (perhaps in combination with Walnut) for animals that have been adopted recently and are brought into a new home, but are not adapting well to their new surroundings. It can be especially helpful for older animals that have been rescued but have unknown old habits and schedules.

### Honeysuckle and the Homeopathic Pharmacy

The Natrums, a rather large group of remedies based upon the substance sodium, and particularly Natrum Muriaticum, which is made from sodium chloride or table salt, have much in common with Honeysuckle. In fact, Natrum Mur tends to retain memory as it does everything else and uses happy memories as a balm for present day hurts.

Another remedy, Capsicum, matches Honeysuckle's yearning for the past and for home. Capsicum's keynote symptom of "regret and sorrows of the past" and its deep yearning for all that is past strongly parallels Honeysuckle's homesickness.

### Issues that Suggest Honeysuckle

Aging; divorce; grief; homesickness; hypoglycemia; insomnia; lung problems; memory loss; menopause problems; myopia; overweight; senility; tumors.

### In Conclusion

While Honeysuckle belongs to a group of remedies in which each expresses the concept of indifference in a different way, it also belongs to another interrelated group of remedies pertaining to inertia. Along with Gentian and Walnut and Wild Oat, Honeysuckle is a remedy type lacking in forward motion. Indeed, like a snowball rolling downhill, all the energy in the Honeysuckle type's emotional life involves a backward and downward motion, racing toward the past.

The Honeysuckle type has stopped all forward movement, all exploration of their present world or of the potential new realm the future represents. So they, along with other passive types such as Centaury and Clematis, yield much of their rightful responsibility for their own life to others, allowing those who take responsibility for them to do so with a free hand.

## MUSTARD · THE REMEDY FOR THOSE WHO ARE IN DEPRESSION

Bach comments that Mustard types are "those who are liable to times of gloom, or even despair, as though a cold dark cloud overshadowed them and hid the light and the joy of life. It may not be possible to give any reason or explanation for such attacks. Under these conditions it is almost impossible to appear happy or cheerful."

• **Mustard is most often used constitutionally, although it can be used acutely when needed.**

### Botanical Information

Known as "charlock mustard" or wild mustard, this plant (*Sinapsis Arvensis*) is considered by some to be an herbal, and by others to be a noxious weed. Wild mustard grows quickly and easily, thrives in almost any condition, and can be found in gardens, by roadsides, in fields, and in waste areas all across the globe.

Wild mustard is native to Great Britain, and today grows nearly everywhere, from Africa to Siberia. The wild mustard plant has small yellow flowers that cluster at the top of the stem. The stem itself is known for its many bristles. It flowers from May to July.

As an herbal treatment it is said to infuse a sense of joy and vitality. Since it had been used as an herbal remedy, it is somewhat unusual that Bach included mustard among his pharmacy, because he attempted to avoid including any plants that had a history of medicinal use.

### Mustard in General

Patients who experience the sense of depression common to the Mustard type will usually describe it in the same way: a black cloud has descended upon them, without warning. Or that they suddenly feel as if they were in a cave, again without warning. During these times, these patients will feel that all light has been blocked, and, with it, all hope. The darkness comes suddenly and leaves suddenly, without warning in either direction. The gloom is so intense during these times of depression that the Mustard type feels life is totally out of his control, as if he were a passive participant in his own life. He may even feel as if a possession of sorts were taking place, in that the depression seems to have a mentality of its own. Further, the Mustard type's depression almost seems to be imposed upon him, as if some outside force had forced it upon him. The Mustard type experiences the state of depression as if something external, that is not a part of him, is blocking him from his own experience of life and the world around him, interfering with his senses, and placing an invisible barrier between him and the rest of the world.

> Mustard is Bach's remedy for those who are depressed, and it can be used to treat a continuum of emotional states, from a sudden acute state for melancholia or a "bad mood" to a long-term state of clinical depression.

In many cases, this sense of depression, although very real, is apparently without cause. The Mustard patient will be unable to identify the source of his negative emotional state or give any clue as to a reason for his depression. The Mustard type may have been leading a happy and balanced life before the onset of his emotional symptoms, but that emotional sense of balance has been suddenly upended by a sudden sense of negativity and a weight of gloom.

Mustard is Bach's remedy for those who are depressed, and it can be used to treat a continuum of emotional states, from a sudden acute state for melancholia or a "bad mood" to a long-term state of clinical depression. This sense of depression is accompanied by a sense of lethargy and weight, and often of exhaustion (Hornbeam, Bach's remedy for those who are emotionally exhausted, is often linked to and used in combination with Mustard). The Mustard patient also has a sense of darkness and feels cut off, certainly emotionally if not physically, from the world and from those around him. Along with these sensations is a sense of apathy and indifference that links Mustard with the other remedies in this group. Like these other remedy types, the Mustard type will show little interest in the world around him and the details of life. Unlike some of the other remedy types, however, inside the Mustard type (although it may be buried very deep) there is a person who desperately wants to be interested, even passionate about life, but who has lost his ability to spontaneously interact with others. Something has ruptured his ability to feel passionately about anything and has left him cut off, from the world, from those that he cares most about, even from his own feelings.

The Mustard negative emotional state is unusual within Bach's pharmacy because the Mustard state of depression is something that almost seems to be visited upon the patient rather than the patient's own survival strategy that has taken him out of a state of emotional balance. The negative emotional states described by almost every other remedy type involve situations where the patient himself, based on personal experience or strong messages received from authority figures like parents, has made a decision or a number of decisions as to how he should act. He has formulated a pattern of behavior that has become destructive over time, even if it was once successful. Therefore, most of the negative emotional states treated by the Bach remedies are destructive patterns that we have visited upon ourselves.

But with the Mustard state, it is impossible to determine the cause, impossible to assess responsibility.[7] Perhaps it is caused by a particular mixture of chemicals within the patient's system. Perhaps by a negative thought, or a series of negative thoughts that go unnoticed by the patient himself. Perhaps it is genetic. Perhaps the cause of this remedy state is something we will never be able to define or pin down.

Now, this is not to say that Mustard cannot be used in cases where the patient is aware of the cause of his depression. As Bach puts it, "It may not be possible to give any reason or explanation for such attacks." In other words, it also may be possible that he can. And if that patient is also experiencing the sensations of weight, of darkness, and of indifference that are common to the type, Mustard will still be very helpful in returning the patient to a state of emotional balance. Note, however, that often, when the patient is depressed and the cause of the depression is known—most especially if the cause involves a business setback or a crisis in the patient's personal life—the remedy

---

7. This makes Mustard one of the few remedies that does not, by its very nature, suggest that it would blend naturally and well with Chestnut Bud. Since Chestnut Bud is the remedy for those who tend to make the same mistakes over and over again, it is a valuable remedy in combination with any other remedy that is based in misperception on the part of the patient in the forming of his or her negative emotional state. Since the Mustard state is seemingly without fixed cause, Chestnut Bud is not usually called for as an adjunct remedy.

Gentian, used singly or in combination with Mustard and other remedies, can be very valuable. (Some consider that Gentian and Mustard are like Aspen and Mimulus: Gentian is the remedy for depressions from known causes, while Mustard is for depressions from unknown causes. I personally don't think that the two remedies break down quite so neatly, but there is a great deal of overlap with the two remedies and they combine beautifully.)

Just as Holly is used to treat a wide range of aggressive behaviors and emotional states ranging from irritated to enraged, Mustard may be used in the treatment of a wide range of emotional states related to depression. In day-to-day life, it is most commonly used to treat simple bad moods, when we feel out of sorts for no good reason. It is also used in the treatment of sorrow or dejection. Also within Mustard's range of treatment are pessimism, joylessness, melancholia, lack of humor, dark moods, introversion, negativity, a tendency to take things too seriously or to literally, simple depression, and clinical depression. It may be called upon in all situations in which the basic keynotes of the Mustard type are present: a sudden or rapid onset of symptoms, a sense of darkness and/or weight and burden, and, often, an unknown reason for the symptoms.

Mustard combines well with a number of other remedies, most especially with Gentian, as noted above. It often is combined with Olive and Gorse. Consider the combination of Olive and Mustard for the patient whose depression seems linked to a state of physical exhaustion. Mix Gorse and Mustard (and possibly Olive as well) for the patient whose depression is linked to a long-term health struggle and whose depression is linked to that struggle, which seems hopeless to the patient. An emotional state that blends depression and hopelessness can be brought into balance with Mustard and Gorse.

Mustard mixes well with Scleranthus for patients who have wild mood swings and combines with Aspen for patients who are anxious and overwrought in their depression.

Mustard can be used with either Elm or Oak in cases where the patient has moved into depression as a result of overwork. The patient who needs Elm and Mustard together is probably working in a fast-paced industry, a patient who is young and moving up the ladder of success. Often this patient will feel he is in over his head at work and that things will soon come crashing down. He may feel inferior, that he will soon be discovered as the phony that he is. This is likely someone who is working long hours and feeling overwhelmed as a result. When these feelings combine with feelings of depression, of being cut off emotionally from coworkers and family members, the combination of Elm and Mustard is called for.

Since the Oak type tends to be more stoic, the patient needing Oak combined with Mustard will often suffer in silence. Very often, this patient can be deeply depressed for a long period of time until he either admits it or it is noticed. The Oak/Mustard type will not want others to know that he is in deep emotional distress, that he feels as if he has reached his breaking point. Most of the time, he will exhibit physical symptoms that drive him to the doctor's office before he will admit that he also needs emotional help and support.

Finally, keep in mind the combination of Mustard and Wild Oat. I have found it to be of special value again and again. The patient will experience a free-form depression, in which he questions his own existence and the existence of God. For those times in life when all of life seems to have little or no meaning, when we are wandering in the desert waiting for our manna, the combination of Mustard and Wild Oat can be very helpful.

Remember, depression can be a very serious emotional state and can lead to serious consequences. I am in no way suggesting that lay persons are fully capable of treating serious depression without the help of medical professionals by providing descriptions of a handful of Bach remedies that can be used in its treatment. As Bach himself intended, these remedies can be used in the home for acute emotional states—the treatment of day-to-day depressions. Seeking medical help is strongly advised for depressions that are deep and long lasting or involve thoughts of suicide.

## Negative Qualities of the Type

Perhaps the most difficult aspect of the Mustard state is that it separates the patient, segregates him from the rest of the world around him. That world, teeming with life and conflict, all but ceases to exist while the patient is in his depression. The patient, experiencing the indifference common to the type, feels no connection with others, no interest in their lives, their thoughts, or their problems. While the patient may yearn to connect, he cannot. Something, some external thing, has moved between him and the rest of the world.[8]

There often is a terrible struggle taking place within the patient who needs Mustard. Because the depressive state feels as if it were imposed upon the patient and not of his own creation, a Mustard type will struggle against his depression in a way that most other types will not. Most of our negative emotional states are of our own development, and develop over a period of time, so they seem comfortable to us, even if they cause us harm. They are old friends, familiar things. Often this is not the case for those in a Mustard state. The depression seems to be a terrible thing, a mysterious burden that suddenly appears. The patient can only struggle against it or stoically endure it until it passes.

---

8. Certainly, this feeling is common to those who are experiencing long-term illness, especially chronic pain, as well as to those who are depressed. And there is a strong link between depression and chronic illness, and those who are seriously ill often become seriously depressed as well. Therefore, the remedies Olive, Gorse, and Mustard are often all needed in cases of constitutional treatment. Just as our emotional lives often parallel our physical bodies, the remedies Olive and Mustard run parallel in their actions. As Olive is to the physical body, Mustard is for the emotional self. And the remedy Gorse works well with either or both when the struggle back to health seems totally hopeless.

For the patient who has experienced multiple bouts of depression, you will find that after the depression lifts, the patient lives in fear of the next "attack." For this reason, the remedy Mimulus may be required once the depression has lifted to fully restore the patient to a state of emotional balance.

### Positive Qualities of the Type

As Bach puts it, "This remedy dispels gloom, and brings joy into life." Mustard, in my experience, is perhaps the most exciting remedy to observe at work. Sometimes, right before your eyes, you will see the light return to the patient's eyes and witness the return of his old vitality and interest in life.

Those who have struggled with deep depression and who have been brought back to a positive emotional state know the true value of life. Just as surely as those who were chronically ill physically and then become able to move freely, those who were emotionally crippled by depression and then become well are truly, sensationally well. Their minds and hearts run free. Just as those who had physical pain and are released from that prison of pain are free to totally immerse themselves in the physical aspects of life once denied them, those separated from emotional communion with others joyously reunite with loved ones when depression passes.

Perhaps no other type surpasses the positive Mustard when it comes to the excitement he feels in the free exchange of ideas and emotions. No other type experiences such deep pleasure at the sight of his dining room table covered with platters of good food and surrounded by those he loves.

### The Mustard Child

While Mustard is not often needed in very young children, it is a very important remedy for teenagers who experience deep depression. During young adulthood, many of us question who we are and whether or not we are good enough to fit into our society. Often the children who are most at risk for serious depression are those who find themselves ostracized at school. Certainly young adults who question their sexuality are at very high risk of depression.

Often young adults who are struggling with their sexual identity will feel a great deal of guilt and can be helped by the combination of Mustard and Pine. In moments of great distress, when the young patient fears that he will take drastic action because of his deep distress, perhaps even commit suicide, the combination of Mustard and Sweet Chestnut can help, as can the combination of Mustard and Star of Bethlehem. Any depression that seems to have begun or be based upon a specific emotional trauma suggests the combination of Mustard and Star of Bethlehem, or even Mustard and Rescue Remedy.

### The Mustard Adult

The use of Mustard as a treatment for depression is no more common in one stage of adulthood than it is at any other. Depression can descend at any time, with or without apparent cause.

Certainly, however, depression plays a major factor in the last stages of life, when a patient, especially one who has struggled with a long-term illness or multiple illnesses of any sort, must face his or her own demise. This patient, and those who love and/or care for him, must often wrestle with deep depression as death approaches. Therefore, Mustard is among the most common remedies used for those in the final stages of life, and it is often needed not only by the elderly patient, but also by those around him. Often it can be used in combination with Star of Bethlehem to offer comfort and emotional support as death approaches.

### The Mustard Animal

I have never found a use for this remedy with my animals, but a homeopathic vet once told me that it can be very helpful for birds in cages, especially if they begin to remove their own feathers.

### Mustard and the Homeopathic Pharmacy

The homeopathic remedy that comes to mind here, not perhaps as a "depression remedy" but in the way it moves in and takes over, is Chamomile, which comes on quickly and without warning. Its pains take over the person, defining a new personality that controls them until the pain leaves.

Other remedies have this same pattern of sudden onset or onset without warning symptoms. These include Belladonna (which has the added parallel that the patient is unable to bear light and needs to move into a dark room) and Aconite, which carries with it a fear of death.

Many homeopathic remedies can be used in the treatment of depression. Perhaps the most important or commonly used is Aurum Metallicum, which is a remedy made from the metal gold. Aurum patients will experience deep depressions and suicidal thoughts, and their depressions will often be linked to their business or career. In this way, the action of the remedy Aurum parallels the combination of Mustard with Oak or Elm.

The combination of Mustard with Olive and/or Gorse is paralleled best by the remedy Gelsemium, a homeopathic remedy state that combines depression and physical exhaustion.

And the free-form depression based on a sense of randomness and meaninglessness is best paralleled by the remedy Sulphur. The Sulphur type will often suffer deep depressions in which he questions the meaning of life.

Other homeopathic remedies used in the treatment of patients suffering from depression include: Ignatia, for patients who have depression and grief; Lycopodium, for patients who feel depressed and inadequate; Sepia, for depressions that carry an emotional and physical sensation of weight; and Pulsatilla, for depressions that have wild mood swings (parallel to the Mustard/Scleranthus combination).

### Issues that Suggest Mustard

Adolescence; aging; death and dying; depression; fatal or long-term disease; manic depression; mood swings.

### In Conclusion

One last note: experience has taught me that there is a strong bond between the remedy Mustard and the remedy Wild Rose. Where the Mustard type is depressed, the Wild Rose type is resigned. This sense of heavy burden that accompanies the emotional resignation of the Wild Rose suggests that the depression the Mustard type experiences will lead into the Wild Rose type's deeper despair, if left untreated over time. A despair that leaves the Wild Rose patient concluding that they must accept their sorrowful lot in life, because there is nothing they can do to change it.

Another logical outcome of the Mustard type's depression is the Willow type's bitterness. Often the Mustard type whose long struggle with depression has gone unaided or even unrecognized will move into a deeper state in time—also quite resigned, in its way—in which the patient becomes embittered by what they perceive as their sad fate. This is especially common in elderly patients. The patient will tend to do nothing to change the circumstances of life that make him unhappy, but, unlike the Wild Rose who is rather stoic about his fate, the Willow type will become vengeful.

Either way, if the Mustard state goes untreated, the patient will move into a deeper state over time in which his bouts of depression become the norm. The Mustard type stops struggling against his depression and, instead, becomes quite resigned to it. The depression that once seemed inflicted upon him by some external source, and against which he struggled, finally becomes internalized. The depression is perceived as being a natural part of the patient and not an invader. At this point, depression yields to resignation, and the patient shifts from one remedy type to another. And with this shift, treatment becomes all the more difficult.[9]

9. I have found, again and again, that the more a patient identifies with his negative emotional state, the harder it is to bring it back into balance. Often the language the patient uses will give an indication of his internal struggle with the emotional state or his resignation to it. For example, if a patient tells you, "I have depression," he is telling you that he is carrying the experience, but is not resigned to it. He "has" it, but he is not living it. If, however, the patient says, "I am depressed," with the use of the simple word "am" he is identifying with the condition on a far more fundamental level. And, as a result, treatment will take longer and be more difficult. I have found this very simple trick of language to be true both in homeopathic and in Bach treatments.

## OLIVE · THE REMEDY FOR THOSE WHO ARE EXHAUSTED

Bach writes of the Olive type, "Those who have suffered much mentally or physically and are so exhausted and weary that they feel they have no more strength to make any effort. Daily life is hard for them, without pleasure."

• Olive is both an acute and a constitutional remedy.

• Even in acute uses Olive may be needed for a longer period of time than most other acute remedies.

### Botanical Information

The Latin name of the olive (*Olea Europaea*) tree gives us the information that it is, indeed, native to southern Europe. It also is native to India. It is also known as the "black olive," the "green olive," and the "King-of-trees."

The olive tree is long-lived and heat tolerant. It grows up to thirty feet tall. It is considered an ornamental tree in many gardens because of the unique beauty of its trunk. The olive tree is an evergreen that produces clusters of small white or pale yellow flowers in the early spring.

Note that many people are allergic to the pollen of olive trees and, especially, to contact with the leaves of the tree. For this reason, only sterile olive trees are available for sale in some parts of this country.

The olive tree has been a source of herbal treatments throughout history. For instance, olive leaf extract is used both as a tonic and an immune system booster.

### Olive in General

Olive is perhaps foremost among the Bach remedies for which we consider vitality—or the lack of it—to be the key. The patient who needs Olive is depleted, either mentally, physically, or both, and struggles with a literal lack of stamina that may manifest itself in myriad ways. Thus the emotional states associated with the remedy Olive include any that may be associated with exhaustion. This suggests that Olive is best used in combination with other remedies that speak to specific emotional issues often linked with exhaustion and depletion. Therefore, Olive is commonly used with Mustard, Wild Rose, Gorse, Hornbeam, Clematis, Elm, and Oak. Since few of us experience exhaustion without also experiencing other negative emotional symptoms, Olive is perhaps the Bach remedy that is least often used alone, and almost always requires a combination of other remedies to help it bring things back into balance.

Also, Olive is one of our few Bach remedies (Crab Apple being another) that suggest physical issues as well as emotional upsets. Olive can deal with the physical ramifications of exhaustion and can be used in the treatment of physical conditions such as chronic fatigue. It also can be used for patients experiencing anemia, weakness associated with a poor diet, and heart or circulatory conditions. Any exhausting or "wasting" condition can suggest the need for Olive. And since the need for Olive suggests overexertion on some level, Olive can be very helpful in soothing chronic injuries that have been brought on by overexertion on a physical level, such as strain from lifting. It can be helpful, therefore, for chronic back pain, shoulder pain, and chronic knee and ankle injuries, especially those that seem to recur again and again.

Because it is somewhat difficult to simply list the emotional states that Olive suggests, it can be difficult to identify the need for Olive on first sight as opposed to a number of other Bach remedies. For instance, it can seem confusing to tell the difference between Olive and Hornbeam at first. Both are in a state of chronic fatigue. But remember, Hornbeam is exhausted, but the exhaustion is an emotional state. If you can make the patient laugh, or interest him in a project, his exhaustion ends and his old vitality returns. Olive, however, is physically exhausted. He has no more energy to give. Unlike the Hornbeam state, in which the patient is emotionally separated from his natural vitality, there are quite literally no energy reserves left in the Olive state.

Also, it often can be very difficult to separate the need for Olive from the need for Mustard, the remedy that precedes it in this chapter. And, like Hornbeam, Mustard is quite commonly combined with Olive for the treatment of patients. Both the Olive and the Mustard type share a sense of weight. Both may seem to be exhausted, and certainly both may be depressed as well. But, where the Mustard often senses his depression as an external thing imposed upon him, and very likely has no understanding of its cause, the Olive type will feel his depression as a result of his struggles, as a result of the process that has so weakened him. He will be very much in touch with the cause of his depression and able to describe it in great detail. (Note, however, that both the Mustard type and the Olive type will want to withdraw into sleep and will want to sleep a great deal. This can be a point of confusion for those trying to decide which type a patient is.)

The Wild Rose type can also seem a lot like the Olive type. In fact, it is my belief that the two can be deeply intertwined. The Olive type (and the Mustard type along with him) who does not receive help for the exhaustion that he is experiencing, may well, over time, become a Wild Rose type.[10]

---

10. The Wild Rose emotional state is, in my experience, one of two that I consider to be "end states." By this I mean that they are the states patients move into slowly, over time, and in which they tend to stay. The Wild Rose state is one of resignation. The patient, who once fought against the emotional or physical health issues or life situation that plague him, has now become resigned to all such negative states and accepts them as his fate. This is a deep, long-lasting state and can be hard to treat. The other end state is Willow, in which the patient also becomes resigned to his "fate" but is embittered by it. Both Wild Rose and Willow are deeply negative states and serve as yin and yang to each other.

Again, both the Wild Rose and the Olive type will be exhausted; both will seem lacking in vitality and in fight. But the Wild Rose state is deeper, and more deeply negative than the Olive state. And the Wild Rose sense of resignation is wider ranged, and may well have multiple causes, some physical, some emotional or spiritual, and some formed by the patient's relationships and life situation. The Olive state, on the other hand, is more commonly caused by a single struggle, most often a struggle brought on by acute or chronic overexertion.

Olive can be confused with Oak in cases where the overly-responsible Oak type, in his need to achieve, wears himself down into a state of chronic illness from overwork. The fact that both Oak and Olive types tend toward heart conditions or develop heart conditions as a result of overwork makes the confusion of these types and the need for a combination of these remedies more likely. Olive can also be confused with Elm. But remember, the Elm type feels overwhelmed as a simple emotional state, while the Olive type feels overextended mentally, emotionally, and physically.

Finally, Olive may also be confused with Gorse, especially if a sense of hopelessness intermingles with a sense of exhaustion. And certainly these two remedies are very often used in combination for patients who struggle against an illness that will very likely prove fatal in the end. But where the Olive type is exhausted, he need not be fatalistic as well. Many Olive types, while depleted, continue to believe that things will turn around for the better, and many Gorse types, who are experiencing the hopelessness common to the type, are actually in a far better state of health physically than Olive types. In the end, with Olive and Gorse and all the other Bach remedies, it is a matter of perception that defines the patient's emotional being. Objective reality plays little part in the treatment of our chronically negative emotional states.

Now, while Olive may be said to come into its full glory as a remedy when it is used in the treatment of those who are chronically exhausted or depleted, it has important acute uses as well. Think of Olive as the best remedy for those times when our responsibilities in life force us to deplete our physical, mental, and emotional resources. Think of Olive when the weeks of effort and little sleep involved in finishing a term paper or a PowerPoint report have left us exhausted. In the same way, think of Olive as a remedy not only for the patient, but also for the caregiver, in cases involving a long struggle with illness or a long convalescence. And, by all means, think of Olive as an important remedy to give or take after the death of a loved one, especially if the process of dying was a slow one. The guilt and pain and loneliness of survival in the face of death always suggests Olive, most often in combination with other remedies such as Mustard, Pine, Sweet Chestnut, and Chicory.

## Negative Qualities of the Type

The idea of defining the "negative attributes of the Olive type" isn't easy. Olive is unique among the Bach types in that it doesn't really describe a negative state, certainly not one that has been created by or selected by the patient. It is, instead, often the result of the existence of other emotional states, like fear, depression, and despair, but it does not describe a negative emotional state in and of itself. Ironically, it often seems to suggest the passing of a negative state—physical illness or death—and the state of recovery that exists afterward.

Certainly, Olive suggests sorrow and depression. This is why it is so often linked with Mustard that it seems unlikely at times that Olive would ever be used without Mustard. And it suggests the emotional exhaustion and apathy common to Hornbeam, with which it is also often combined.

Remember that Olive, like Wild Rose (which follows it in this chapter) and Mustard (which precedes it), is part of the group of remedies that Bach identified as treating indifference. But the indifference experienced by the Olive type is not completely an emotional thing, unlike the other remedies in the group. It is also a physical experience, or, at least, the result of a physical struggle that has passed.

Certainly, the emotional aspects of the exhaustion may dominate. Olive can be very helpful to those who have undergone near-death experiences—close calls on the highway or plane crashes—and have survived, but are depleted as a result. In these cases, it is often needed in combination with Pine if survivor's guilt becomes an issue.

If there is a central issue that can be identified as the Olive type's most identifiable negative attribute, it would be that he simply has had enough. The negative Olive type has depleted every ounce of his energy, given all that he has to give to his struggle, his cause, his good works, and now he just wants to lie down. The Olive, like the Hornbeam, is not interested in anything and does not want to be enticed into any more work or conversation. Like the Mustard, he wants to sleep and withdraw from anyone or anything that he perceives will require anything from him. He wants to sleep. He does not want to talk. He is totally and completely indifferent to the needs or wants of anyone else, at least until he is given the opportunity to rest and recharge. The Olive type knows he has nothing left to give but tears if everyone else doesn't get off his back and leave him alone to rest. The only phrase that those who intrude upon his rest are likely to hear is, "What do you want now?"

Finally, for those who are in a chronic Olive state, there is always a lesson to be learned. As Mechthild Scheffer puts it in the excellent book *Bach Flower Therapy: Theory and Practice*, "The Olive state is always a call to humility, and at the same time a challenge to learn to deal properly with our vital energy, which is after all divine energy. Olive people find this difficult, for the physical warning system used by the higher self to signal that we are overdoing it physically, mentally or spiritually, is no longer functioning very well." So, while the Olive state does not itself reveal a negative emotional state like the other Bach remedies do, it does reveal a fundamental lack of knowledge of our minds and bodies and the limits of our strength. In the same way, it suggests a state of hubris, in which we think that we are the source of our own strength, and a need for a lesson in humility.

### Positive Qualities of the Type

When in a positive state, Olive types are filled with energy, strength and vitality. And they have become wise enough to know how to parse out their efforts so they will not become depleted again. They realize their strength is limited and live within their limits when they are under great stress. They have learned the lesson that they themselves are not the source of all good things for others.

Further, the positive Olive type is endlessly flexible; he is willing and able to change methods when changes are needed. And he is careful with personal resources,[11] maintaining a flow of all energy throughout his life.

### The Olive Child

For the younger patient, it is perhaps best to think of Olive as an acute remedy for overwork. For the times when the child has worked hard to complete a school project or when there has been illness in the family that has been a drain on every member of the family. This remedy is also useful for the period of recovery when the child is coming out of a serious illness. (Periods of convalescence can also suggest the remedy Wild Rose, especially when the patient seems resigned to his or her illness, or Gorse, for situations that seem hopeless. Any or all of these remedies combine well for young patients who are or have been seriously ill.)

### The Olive Adult

While there is no one stage of life that suggests the need for Olive, it is a simple rule of thumb that the older you get, the more likely you need the remedy Olive. Youth brings strength and vigor all its own. As we get older, we need a longer time to recover from any illness and more and more understanding of our physical, mental, and emotional limitations. This is especially true for those who struggle with chronic disease or who suffer from more than one disease at a time. As our recovery time becomes longer and our struggle with disease takes a greater part of our daily lives, our need for Olive becomes more and more important—both for ourselves and for those who care for us. Therefore, the remedy Olive belongs in every home that contains adults.

---

11. And while considering resources, let's not ignore money. The patient who overextends himself financially, especially when the money spent was for health services related to chronic illness, will experience emotional agonies that are in line with the Olive type's other struggles. Financial overexertion, therefore, should be listed along with the mental, emotional, and physical overexertion common to the type.

## The Olive Animal

While there is no simple emotional state that suggests Olive for animals, think of this remedy as one to use for any animal struggling with recovery from any serious illness or injury. It is also, by the way, said to be very helpful for any animal coming out of hibernation.

## Olive and the Homeopathic Pharmacy

Among the thousands of homeopathic remedies, the handful made from various acids are known to be of particular value to patients who are exhausted or depleted. Among these are Phosphoric and Sulphuric Acid, both of which share a sense of weight and exhaustion with Olive. But the homeopathic remedy known as Picricum Acidum, made from Picric Acid, shares many of the physical and emotional features of the constitutional Olive state. Among the homeopathic remedies, only Picric Acid has the symptom of total exhaustion that reaches to the level of mental and physical paralysis.

## Issues that Suggest Olive

Alcoholism; anemia; body aches and pains; chronic fatigue; chronic pain from injury; depression; exhaustion; heart disease; insomnia; lack of sleep; kidney disease; mouth pain; neck pain; midlife crisis; nervous breakdown; poor diet; upper or lower back pain.

## In Conclusion

Finally, one last consideration: in my experience, the very existence of the sort of exhaustion consistent with the Olive negative emotional state suggests that any patient in this state should seek medical assistance as well as use Bach remedies to support his sense of well-being. The Olive state can suggest a number of underlying physical complaints, some as simple to shift as a poor diet, others as serious as heart disease. It is important, therefore, that anyone who experiences Olive's exhaustion take it seriously enough to explore all possible causes. In cases in which the exhaustion is the result of or coupled with specific physical complaints, supportive medical measures may also be needed before the patient can be restored to health.

## WILD ROSE · THE REMEDY FOR THOSE WHO ARE INDIFFERENT

Bach identifies Wild Rose types as "those who without apparently sufficient reason have become resigned to all that happens, and just glide through life, take it as it is, without any effort to improve things and find some joy. They have surrendered to the struggle of life without complaint."

• **Wild Rose is most often used as a constitutional remedy, but it can be surprisingly effective as an acute remedy.**

### Botanical Information

The wild rose (*Rosa Canina*), also known as the "dog rose," is a deciduous perennial shrub that grows in temperate regions all across the globe. It is common to gardens and perennial hedges, as it is easy to grow and thrives in most types of soil. It is native to Asia Minor and Europe.

The wild rose produces fragrant flat flowers with five petals in late June or July. After the flowers fade, the plant produces red hips in their place in autumn. These are rose hips that are used in herbal treatments and teas. Rose hips are an excellent source of vitamin C.

### Wild Rose in General

In the Wild Rose type, we find a sense of resignation, as if the Wild Rose type's present situation is fated and that, in the words of many a science fiction movie, "resistance is futile," as well as an almost total lack of motivation on the part of the patient. He lacks motivation for either hope or change because he believes[12] there is nothing he can do to change his lot in life.

Because of the sheer negativity of the Wild Rose state, and because it is often associated with chronic illness or abusive relationships or issues of death and dying, it is often assumed to be a constitutional remedy, only useful in situations involving long-term issues. But this isn't the case. Wild Rose can also be an important acute remedy. I have seen it work almost instantaneously when a patient needed to get in touch with his sense of enthusiasm once more, or needed an extra dose of will power. Therefore, Wild Rose, which can be associated with perhaps our most negative emotional state of resignation, can be an incredibly helpful tool in keeping us on our diet when we are just dying for a donut or for any other of the myriad circumstances when we are tempted to yield to things we know are harmful for us; when we feel that because we will ultimately yield, why bother postponing the inevitable.

> Wild Rose can rewrite what is or is not inevitable, what is or is not fated in our lives. It can allow us the option to change when we feel we do not have such an option. As such, it is an incredibly important remedy, and one that is among our most underrated and underused.

---

12. As always, perception is a key component to any negative emotional state. The patient needing Wild Rose may believe that his situation is set in stone when, in truth, it could easily be changed for the better.

Wild Rose can rewrite what is or is not inevitable, what is or is not fated in our lives. It can allow us the option to change when we feel we do not have such an option. As such, it is an incredibly important remedy, and one that (along with Chestnut Bud) is among our most underrated and underused.

Make no mistake, the constitutional Wild Rose state is incredibly negative and incredibly hard to move. It is like a boulder that rests upon our shoulders, crushing us below its weight.

In fact, that which I call a negative emotional state may not, in all honesty, be considered an emotional state at all. The Wild Rose state is the opposite of emotion, because resignation represents a lack of emotion, a state of complete indifference. For this reason, it is not only logical that Bach placed Wild Rose among his remedies for those who are indifferent, but it must be considered that Wild Rose gives us the archetype for indifference: the patient who is devoid of yearning, or any emotion good or bad; who has yielded to what he perceives as his lot in life; who does not complain, but quietly, stoically accepts what he thinks is his fate. This is the patient who is lacking in emotion, in struggle, in motivation, who is, therefore, perhaps our hardest patient to treat. After all, the Wild Rose state represents a state that is one step lower and more negative even than the Gorse state, in which the patient wrestles with feelings of hopelessness. The Wild Rose patient has ceased to be concerned about this, or, indeed, any other issue. His resignation—which the Wild Rose type often ironically sees as a positive or even freeing thing, making him even harder to treat—is all that is left to him. For this reason, he tends to lack interest in Bach flower remedies or any other treatments. After all, if his fate is sealed, why should he attempt any form of treatment?

Because of their mindset, Wild Rose types often have to count on the fact that someone loves them enough to give them this remedy. They usually will not seek treatment themselves because they fully accept their situation and have given up on fighting back. They are somewhat sluggish, and completely unwilling to even consider that they can change their lives: the condition they are in is the condition they have always been in and always will be in, so why waste energy trying to do something about it? It is as if they were living in Seattle, a place where the weather is always cold and gray and damp. And it never occurs to them, as that gray weather makes them sadder and sadder and more and more weary, to just move to Los Angeles.

I consider Wild Rose to be one of two "end point" remedies because of its sheer negativity and complete lack of motivation. By this I mean that the Wild Rose state is one that many patients enter after they have passed through one or more other constitutional states, commonly Mustard or Gorse, in a downward spiral of negativity. It is an end point because once patients enter into a constitutional Wild Rose state they are likely to stay in it for the rest of their lives. The other "end point" remedy is Willow, which shares the Wild Rose type's deep negativity and sense of resignation, but Willow is aggressive (yang) while Wild Rose is accepting (yin) of his fate.

I have found again and again that Willow and Wild Rose types are the hardest to restore to a sense of creative freedom because of their joint negativity and sense of fate. Each gives you so little to work with in terms of emotional availability or cooperation. But the situation is not hopeless in either case. Both types can be helped—if they can be persuaded to take their remedy (and if they honestly continue to take it and do not simply tell you they are when in truth they threw it away the moment your back was turned[13]).

Wild Rose is often used in combination with one or more other Bach remedies. Most often it is combined with Hornbeam or Elm, either or both of which will help the patient who is overwhelmed with work and stressed as a result, but feels unable to rectify his situation.

It is also blended with Mustard and Olive, two other remedies from this group of remedies for those who are indifferent. When blended with Mustard, Wild Rose is used to treat patients who suffer from long-term depression, and who are resigned to their negative state. In the same way, Wild Rose lends a feeling of resignation to those in the state of physical exhaustion typified by the remedy type Olive. (On a more or less acute note, Olive and Wild Rose in combination can be helpful for any sort of recovery process that has left the patient exhausted. This combination can lift a patient's feelings and strengthen his belief that he will be well one day.)

Gorse, too, is an important remedy to use in combination with Wild Rose. The Gorse type feels hopeless in his current situation and the Wild Rose is resigned to a negative state of affairs, so this combination speaks to a particularly negative emotional state in which the patient feels there is altogether no point in struggling against his symptoms or situation, as that situation is hopeless and was hopeless from the start. Patients needing this combination often castigate themselves and others for attempting any sort of treatment or plan of action, as such things are doomed to fail. (In more acute terms, think of Gorse and Wild Rose together for patients in recovery who have recently experienced a setback, however small. This combination can help strengthen the patient's faith and let him withstand setbacks without falling into despair or giving up the recovery process. Gentian may be needed in this combination as well, or may be used singly if the setback was not severe.)

Gentian is an important remedy to be used in conjunction with Wild Rose. The Gentian type has both hope and faith, but these desert him quickly when he is tested. Like Mustard, it is another remedy type that erodes into a Wild Rose state over time, if

13. Be careful of Wild Rose types. They will tell you whatever they think you want to hear to get you off their back. This is especially true of elderly Wild Rose types.

it is left untreated. Therefore, Gentian and Wild Rose are something of a natural combination. They can strengthen a patient's resolve and his ability to understand that all healing is a process that it is usually cyclical in nature and never, as we always hope, linear. Therefore, this combination can help a patient withstand the ups and downs of the healing process and stay on his healing path even when his faith and hope are tested.

Perhaps the most difficult patient of all to treat is one who is resigned to his circumstances and also believes that the universe itself is a place of chaos and folly. This patient will not only lack motivation to make needed changes in his life, he will actually feel that, even if change were possible, it would be futile, as all things are ultimately futile.

This patient can benefit from the combination of Wild Rose and Wild Oat. Only this combination of remedies can reach the patient who not only is left without hope, but also exists without faith. The Wild Oat will sense that all existence is meaningless, that all attempts at understanding the nature of life or of change or of healing is pointless. He will therefore conclude that struggling against his circumstances is pointless, much as the Wild Rose will conclude that it is worthless. This is an important remedy combination as it reminds the patient that change is not only possible, but also that it is desirable.

Finally, consider Wild Rose and Chestnut Bud, another combination of two remedies taken from this very synergistic group of remedies.

Just as I consider these to be our two most underrated and underused remedies, I consider this to be a very valuable and very important combination. Wild Rose is for the patient who is resigned to a negative situation. Chestnut Bud is for the patient who does not learn from his own mistakes, who makes the same mistakes again and again. Therefore, in combination, they make a powerful dual remedy that can help any of us burst through the walls of habit, thought, and behavior we have imprisoned ourselves behind. Any bad habit, any negative cycle of thought or behavior can be ameliorated by this combination. Wild Rose adds motivation to Chestnut Bud's clarity of thought in identifying our weak areas, bad habits, and repeated mistakes, so together they can be a powerful engine for change—change for the good. They can help us eat better, stay on our diet, exercise as much as we should. They can help us take a clear and realistic look at the way we are living our lives, and the aspects of our lives that are ripe for change.

In fact, I have so much faith in this particular combination of remedies that I strongly suggest that you use it without adding any other remedies, at least at first. Since I think that each remedy has not only a particular message to bestow, but also a particular voice, I like to use as few remedies at one time as will be helpful. Therefore, I would give this combination a try first before adding other remedies, other voices, into the mix, so that the message will be received as clearly as possible by the patient. If these two don't get the whole job done, then add others as their need becomes clear. Add only one at a time, carefully noting any changes that take place.[14]

### Negative Qualities of the Type

We must be very careful with our definition of the word "negative" with this remedy. The Wild Rose type is not negative in the way that the Willow is, although the Wild Rose emotional state rivals Willow's for its depth of negativity. But the Wild Rose type, unlike the Willow type, is never overtly negative in his behavior, never aggressive in any way. In fact, it is keynote to the type that he does not complain, just as he does not struggle with what he considers to be his fate. Instead, he is devoid of emotion, absolutely apathetic. The Wild Rose type has moved beyond depression into a gray realm that is shapeless, formless, negative, and constant.

### Positive Qualities of the Type

Once Wild Rose types can begin to think and move in a more positive direction, once they begin to understand that life is a fluid thing and that we all have the ability to change and grow from our first breath to our last, they find within themselves the motivation that was once lacking. In fact, positive Wild Rose types are among our best motivators, not only for themselves but for others as well. They are natural motivational speakers, who are able to use their own lives and struggles as an example to help others find the strength and commitment within themselves to make the changes that need to be made. The positive Wild Rose type never resigns himself to the negative situation at hand, never settles for anything less than what is possible in terms of change.

The remarkable thing is that this remains true no matter the age or physical health of the positive Wild Rose. I have known Wild Rose types of advanced years who, once they have struggled through their resignation and depression, offered inspiration to all those around them, even from their hospital bed.

---

14. I know it's my homeopathic training that, at times like these, puts me in opposition with the many other writers who take the stand that Bach's remedies can be mixed and matched as you like. I find if I can start with only one or two remedies, and then add others that seem to be needed one at a time, I can be better aware of the actions of each of the remedies and can provide the cleanest and purest healing process possible. Therefore, I suggest that you use remedies singly or in pairs, especially when you are beginning a case or when you yourself are still learning about the remedies and their actions. If you use too many remedies at once, you will never know which remedy did what and which was effective and which was not. This is never dangerous in terms of Bach treatment, as it can be in other forms of medicine, but it is still sloppy and still makes the patient's healing process harder than it needs to be.

The positive Wild Rose lives every moment of his or her life, infuses it with passion and creativity. They also know the limits of their strength and energy.

### The Wild Rose Child

The presence of the negative Wild Rose state in children can lead us to fear that Wild Rose's negativity might be an inherited trait. While in my experience this negative emotional state is somewhat rare in children, there are some Wild Rose types who apparently have been Wild Rose types almost since birth. Like the adults of the same type, children who need Wild Rose never complain, nor do they ever struggle with the negative circumstances around them. Often, they are children who have chronic or life-threatening diseases, or have a family member whose health issues have colored the family's emotional dynamics. Sometimes, they are children born into families in deep conflict, into abusive homes, or into cultures that are in a state of upheaval or warfare. Often you will find a highly negative Wild Rose state in the child who is being sexually abused. They can appear rigid, emotionless, almost as if they were carved from stone. Young Wild Rose types invariably seem older than they are, and face the world without the usual curiosity, excitement, or humor of youth.

### The Wild Rose Adult

Like most of the remedies in this group, the Wild Rose negative state most often reveals itself in older patients. It seems that when we are young we are naturally interested in life, in all the new forms of stimuli that we can encounter on any given day. Only after we have lived a good number of years can we achieve a state of indifference to life in any of the ways embodied by this group of remedies.

Unless it is thrust upon us by extreme circumstances the Wild Rose negative state of resignation is one that takes years to develop. Usually, the patient will have moved through one or more other states, most commonly Hornbeam, Elm, Oak, Mustard, or Gentian, before reaching the Wild Rose state of full inertia.

Often patients of advanced years will move into a Wild Rose state, sometimes when they receive a diagnosis of fatal disease. Sometimes those who have lost a beloved spouse or a child will resign themselves to live out the rest of their days in hollow inertia. And sometimes when elderly patients have been taken out of their own home, especially if it is against their will, they will resign themselves and give up their fight for life.

While the Wild Rose state may come on suddenly as a result of a specific event or diagnosis (in such a case, combine Wild Rose with Star of Bethlehem for the emotional trauma), more commonly it is cumulative. It grows slowly, as the patient's life shrinks and his will to fight back and make important changes shrinks with it.

## The Wild Rose Animal

This is a remedy that can be helpful for elderly animals—especially elderly animals that find themselves suddenly without homes. It can be helpful for any animal that has been dumped into a shelter and, as a result, lacks a vital spark. It can also help any animal that is undergoing a long recovery from illness and seems disinterested in its food and surroundings.

## Wild Rose and the Homeopathic Pharmacy

The Graphities homeopathic type has much in common with Wild Rose. Both are stoically trudging through their lives, not even interested in dealing with situations that other people would quickly work to change or put to rest. In fact, Graphities types are sluggish in every way, mentally, emotionally, and physically. Like Wild Rose types, they tend to yield to their conditions and lack the ability to fight back or to move on toward health.

## Issues that Suggest Wild Rose

Blindness; bruises and injuries, especially chronic injuries; chronic illness of any sort; coma; deafness; hip pain; hypoglycemia; leg pain; lump in throat; psoriasis; senility.

## In Conclusion

I conclude this section with what is known as the "Serenity Prayer," because I think it speaks to the crux of the Wild Rose type's lack of motivation and lack in interest in bringing positive change into his own life. This brief prayer simply states: "God grant me the serenity to accept the things I cannot change, the courage to change the things I can, and the wisdom to know the difference."[15]

15. The so-called "Serenity Prayer" has long been associated with Alcoholics Anonymous. Bill W., the founder of A.A. reported that the prayer was first read in a meeting in 1942, and that it was originally found in an obituary in the New York Herald Tribune. It is believed that the prayer was originally a part of a sermon delivered by theologian Reinhold Neibuhr. It is important to us here, as it pretty much sums up both the positive and negative aspects of the Wild Rose state. I find it meaningful that the prayer's author chose the word "accept" when he states that there are things we must accept cannot be changed in each of our lives. For me, there is a fundamental difference between accepting situations and resigning ourselves to them. When we accept the aspects of our lives that seem "fated" to us, we allow that there are forces in the universe that determine the shape and outcome of our lives. We work within and alongside those forces to bring about the best result, not only for ourselves, but for those we love and for our community at large. When we resign ourselves, however, we move in a negative manner and stop working for the betterment of all. Instead, we fold inward and give up. The person who has accepted, for instance, the appearance of a chronic illness in his life has in no way given up fighting for the best and longest life possible. He is, in no way, indifferent, unlike the person who has resigned himself to illness.

The issue for Wild Rose types is that they lack the ability to understand just what aspects of life they can and cannot change while they remain locked in their negative emotional state. They can see no means by which they can change what is negative in their life, what they may, in all truth, hate but feel they must endure. Because of this they surrender their ability to change *any* aspect of life, and in doing so, abandon their ability to live.

The great irony of the Wild Rose state is that so many of those who enter into it think that they are yielding to God's will, that they are sanctified by their resignation. They are often stiff lipped and very willful on the subject. They believe they have moved into a place of acceptance, but they have not. True acceptance yields to a higher power but still strives to live a passionate and creative life. Instead, they have yielded all their ability to grow and change because of an overriding negative situation. Even those who are chronically ill and constantly in pain can enjoy positive aspects of existence. Wild Rose types, in their state of indifference, deny all that is good in life and stoically endure what they might, on some level or other, actually enjoy. They cut themselves off from others with their deep indifference, cut themselves off from loving and being loved. They cut themselves off from life itself, because one of life's great constants is change.

## WHITE CHESTNUT · THE REMEDY FOR THOSE WITH OBSESSIVE THOUGHTS

Bach comments that White Chestnut is "for those who cannot prevent thoughts, ideas, arguments which they do not desire from entering their minds. Usually at such times when the interest of the moment is not strong enough to keep the mind full. Thoughts which worry and will return, or if for a time thrown out, will return. They seem to circle round and round and cause mental torture. The presence of such unpleasant thoughts drives out peace and interferes with being able to think only of the work or pleasure of the day."

• **While White Chestnut may be used from time to time as an acute remedy, it is most often needed constitutionally.**

### Botanical Information

The remedy White Chestnut is made from the horse chestnut (*Aesculus Hippocastanum*) tree, which can grow to be between forty and sixty feet tall with a trunk that is between one and two feet in diameter. The tree is native to western Asia, in the region of Greece and Albania, from where it spread into all of Europe. It is now grown around the globe. It is a part of many gardens and is a familiar sight as a canopy tree in yards and in forests.

Horse chestnut trees are hermaphrodites, meaning that both male and female flowers appear on the same tree. The male flowers grow on top of what is called the tree's "candelabra," while the female flowers are produced lower down in the tree. The flowers bloom in May.

Parts of the plant, most commonly the seeds, have long been used as herbal medications. They are used both as an astringent and as a tonic to the circulatory system. They are said to be especially helpful for varicose veins.

### White Chestnut in General

Many Bach remedies have counterparts. By this I mean there are many remedies whose actions stand in opposition to another remedy. For every willful Vine state, there is also a weak-willed Centaury. Perhaps this is because so many of the emotional states treated by the Bach remedies represent emotional patterns that are out of balance, a swinging of the pendulum too far to the left or the right, creating a pattern of thought and behavior that is too aggressive or too passive.

> Instead of retreating into a warm safe place in his imagination, the White Chestnut patient becomes trapped within his own thoughts and cannot pull himself away. The White Chestnut may be pulled into a cycle of memory and regret typified by recurring thoughts of what he should have said, should have done.

Bach's remedy White Chestnut stands in counterbalance with Clematis, as the two remedies represent opposite ends of a pole. And both remedies deal directly with the mind and the power of thought, as opposed to true emotion. Indeed, both Clematis and White Chestnut tend to be cerebral types, people who lead with their minds and not with their hearts.

In the case of both emotional patterns, the patient retreats into a world of thought instead of staying "in the moment." The Clematis patient seeks refuge in his imagination, withdrawing from the world around him into a fantasy world. However briefly he makes his escape, the Clematis type finds solace within the territories of his imagination.

On the other hand, the White Chestnut type's mind is a prison of sorts. Instead of retreating into a warm safe place in his imagination, the White Chestnut patient becomes trapped within his own thoughts and cannot pull himself away. The White Chestnut may be pulled into a cycle of memory and regret typified by recurring thoughts of what he should have said, should have done, or he may become fixated upon what is to come, his future regrets, his future failures. In either case, the White Chestnut is tormented by his own thoughts.

Often, they will come upon him in moments of vulnerability, typically when he is drifting off to sleep. Sudden, and almost audibly, his thoughts intrude. Where the Clematis will all but fan the flames of his imagination to intentionally escape, the White Chestnut will put pillows over his ears to quiet the voices he hears inside his own head.

As Bach says, White Chestnut is the remedy "for those who cannot prevent thoughts, ideas, arguments which they do not desire from entering their minds." The key phrase here is "which they do not desire." The White Chestnut type cannot control his mental and emotional fixations. Nor can he quiet or control his thoughts. Instead, the White Chestnut will take on one or more of various behaviors to still his mind.

Some White Chestnuts will try to stay busy. They find that when they are focused within their conscious mind they are able to quiet their unconscious mind, or, at least, ignore it. Therefore, you will often find that White Chestnut types seem tense, rigid, and fixated. They tend to become so fixated on their work, or whatever has their attention at the moment that they will not hear people speaking to them, they will not notice an interruption, until they are startled by what is to them the sudden appearance of someone in their room. White Chestnut types startle easily. Because they tend to fixate mentally rather than flow freely with their thoughts, they are often less aware of the space around them than other types and often have the impression that others are "sneaking up on them." Like Clematis types they tend to move into an alternate reality within their mind and must be made aware of the presence of others from time to time. But the Clematis is like a person in a sweet dream, making their awakening a pleasant unfolding, while the White Chestnut is invariably given a rude awakening, in which he startles, shakes, and flails. No matter how many times it happens, it is never a pleasant event.

White Chestnut is one of three remedies based upon what is basically the same plant. White Chestnut, Red Chestnut, and Chestnut Bud (a remedy that shares White Chestnut's tendency toward indifference and appears next in these pages) all share a common trait: obsession. While the Red Chestnut is obsessed with the well-being of those that he or she loves and is therefore highly fearful and Chestnut Bud is trapped in a cycle of obsessive behaviors, White Chestnut is obsessive in his mind, with his thoughts. Both his conscious mind and his unconscious mind are fixated, cyclical, and obsessive in nature. In his unconscious mind, the White Chestnut plays the records of his memory over and over again, and this is not the sweetened, glorified memory of the Honeysuckle type. White Chestnut's memory fixates on failures, hurts, and injustices, which he can spontaneously recall many years after the fact and relive again and again in a cycle of unwanted, destructive memories. The White Chestnut type's memory tends to be just as flawed as that of the Honeysuckle type. But where the Honeysuckle type will make his memories just as sweet smelling as the flowers of the plant that gives the remedy its name, the White Chestnut type will, color his memories very darkly, especially when he is on the verge of slumber. Each memory has a nightmare quality to it that leaves the White Chestnut patient, when he can escape the cycle of memory, weakened and drained. The White Chestnut type's memory is a source of pain for him. It can leave him feeling flawed, damaged, or even—if he is religious and replaying his various sins—damned.

To keep his unconscious mind in tow, the White Chestnut type will keep his conscious mind very active. And, in doing this, he fixates with it as well. The White Chestnut must obsessively control his conscious thoughts so he can keep his obsessive unconscious mind under control. He fears that, if he allows his conscious mind to relax even for a moment, if he allows his imagination to take charge, as the Clematis so easily and happily does, then he will again be trapped by his own thoughts, and will return to his anxious cycle of memory and regret or his constant projection into what lies ahead. So he will focus very strongly on the task at hand to keep his own internal chatter down to a minimum. For this reason, White Chestnut types (who are often, by their very nature and restless intellect, in need of a source of focus) are often drawn into work that involves a great deal of focus. They can, for instance, work easily and diligently in the busiest newsroom and maintain focus while chaos whirls all about them.

Some White Chestnut types will also become obsessive in their physical habits as a means by which they can quiet their minds. Most of the time this takes the form of exercise. The White Chestnut discovers that, if they can only make their body tired enough, they can quiet their mind enough to sleep. And sleep is a great issue for the White Chestnut, as we shall see.

And so the White Chestnut begins a cycle of exercise. He lifts weights, he runs on the treadmill, he plays team sports—at which, unsurprisingly, he is very competitive—and finally he finds that he is tired enough to be able to sleep. And this begins a cycle of obsessive behavior that becomes a part of his daily pattern.

Other White Chestnut types will never turn to exercise. Instead, they substitute a pattern of overwork. They find that they will be able to sleep without disturbance if they work long and hard enough to exhaust both their body and their mind. And so they begin to work long into the night. They have their computers with them at all times. If, when they are ready for bed, they find that their mind is not quiet enough for them to sleep, they turn the computer back on (it is, invariably, in the bedroom with them, or close by) and go back to work. White Chestnut types are often comforted by the idea that, if they cannot sleep, at least they are accomplishing something with their time and not just wasting it by lying in the dark and trying to relax.

In time, this pattern becomes a trap of its own. The White Chestnut who decides that he will exhaust his mind by working often finds that his thoughts about his work become a prison of their own. He will, at any moment when his guard is down, become fixated and tormented by thoughts of work: all he has to do that he has not done, whether or not those in charge like what he is doing, a mistake he made at work twenty years ago that reverberates.

This idea of "letting your guard down" is key to understanding the White Chestnut. As always, the concept of obsession is all about control. The Chestnut Bud type becomes obsessive in his behaviors because he feels his life is out of control. So, instead of controlling his fate, he controls some aspect of behavior. In the same way, the White Chestnut feels out of control within himself. He feels separated from his own mind and feels that he cannot control his thoughts, and that these thoughts will cause him damage if he does not control them better. This gives the White Chestnut type continual anxiety, which is why this remedy is so often blended with Aspen. It is also often blended with Elm because of their common pattern of seeking blissful relaxation through overwork.

There is another frequent route of escape for the White Chestnut type. It is especially characteristic among those who have already stumbled upon either the idea of overexercise or overwork as a means of exhausted relaxation (and, remember, in the White Chestnut type's mind, only exhaustion offers a means of relaxation and quiet sleep). Often, the White Chestnut type who fails to find another means of relaxation will turn to alcohol or drugs as a means of escape. This is perhaps best typified in our popular literature by the character of Brick in Tennessee Williams' *Cat on a Hot Tin Roof*. Brick, fixated upon memories of a past tragedy, drinks until he hears an audible click. That click tells him that he has drunk enough for his mind to be quieted for a few hours and for him to relax.

It is the same with other White Chestnut types who drink or who take drugs. They use substances to quiet their minds in a way that they themselves cannot. And, in doing so, they invariably begin to fixate upon the drugs or the alcohol (let me note that White Chestnut types will gravitate toward drugs that quiet, often painkillers, and not toward substances that stimulate, like cocaine). White Chestnut types are, again like Chestnut Bud types, highly addictive personalities because they tend to fixate. Anything that brings them the result they desire once is something that they will surely try again and again to achieve the same result.[16]

Now, if there is one overriding issue for most White Chestnut types, it is insomnia. They tend to value sleep almost above all else, as it is their only time of relaxation. They tend to sleep little, and especially have trouble falling asleep. Like many other aspects of their lives, sleep is, for them, cyclical. By this I mean two things. First, White Chestnut types will typically have cycles for the possibility of sleep throughout the

---

16. In the same way, Chestnut types tend to also be believers in luck. They fixate upon anything they feel brings them luck. They will have lucky objects or pieces of apparel they feel can help them have success. Even if they never admit it, they are great believers in luck.

night. Each of these cycles is a window of opportunity. For instance, if they doze off in their chair in front of the television, once they awaken, get ready for bed, and get in bed they will have to wait another hour or two until they have the next opportunity to go to sleep. Usually, this will mean that they will get back up and work, or will turn on the television in their bedroom and watch a movie for a couple of hours. Other types may be able to drift off to sleep at any time, but not the White Chestnut type. Because he is a Chestnut, sleep has its own rituals, its own cycles, and its own rules.

The White Chestnut type's other sleep cycle involves a period of weeks or months. White Chestnut types will tend to have cycles in their life in which they can sleep and cycles in which they cannot. As much as they dread the intrusion of their own thoughts into their lives, they dread even more the sudden onset of insomnia that they know will last for many weeks once it arrives. During those weeks, the White Chestnut type will sit up most of the night, worrying, fussing, and roaming, while the rest of the house is quiet and still. Often the White Chestnut type will finally fall into a deep sleep just as the sun begins to rise, only to be awakened by his alarm shortly thereafter.

Certainly it must be noted that the very exhaustion the White Chestnut courts is a large part of the problem with his unruly mind. Because the White Chestnut exhausts himself and is further exhausted by the fact that his own mind will not quiet itself but chatters on, long into the night, the White Chestnut will find that he cannot think clearly the next day. So he must focus even more to function, and he will have even more trouble relaxing and sleeping that night because of his increased focus. Thus another cycle is formed, and another pattern of obsessive behavior is locked in.

Like most of Bach's other types, the White Chestnut patient's mental and emotional distress is largely self-created and self-sustained. Like the other types, he is out of balance within himself. He can seem to be very irritable and can be difficult for others to work with and to live with because of his ongoing sense of mental and emotional stress and tension. This is the type who, because he is often lost in the miasma of his own thoughts, can look at you as if he does not know you. Only for a split second, but in that second, you are quite aware that he is in a world of his own.

As White Chestnut is the remedy for mental obsession, it blends well with nearly every other remedy in Bach's pharmacy. (I wouldn't, however, think that you would be able to find anyone who needed Clematis and White Chestnut, at least not at the same time.) It can blend especially well with the very aggressive remedies, like Willow, for those who are obsessively vindictive; Holly, where it adds obsession to aggression; Vine, a combination in which the willfulness of Vine becomes fixated upon a subject or person; and Impatiens, a combination of obsession and mental irritation that yields a patient who is almost exquisitely driven and who, once they have targeted a goal, cannot be dissuaded from achieving it at any cost.

# The Riddle of the Chestnuts

Three of our Chestnut remedies are linked together by the quality of obsession: White Chestnut with obsessive thoughts that intrude into our lives, Red Chestnut with obsessive worry and concern for others, and Chestnut for obsessive behavior and chronic bad habits. This would be all well and good, if not for the fact that there is a fourth Chestnut remedy, Sweet Chestnut, which does not share the obsessive nature of the others. Sweet Chestnut can be very helpful to anyone in a moment of despair so it is most usually considered to be an acute remedy, since moments of true despair are usually a fleeting response to dire circumstances. But the acute nature of Sweet Chestnut keeps us from being able to tie up our study of the obsessive Chestnuts with a nice, neat ribbon.

The answer as to why Sweet Chestnut is so different from the others has to do with the plants from which the remedies are taken. Both Chestnut Bud and White Chestnut are taken from different parts of the same plant, the *Aesculus Hippocastanum*, or horse chestnut. Red Chestnut is taken from the *Aesculus Carnea*, a related plant.

Sweet Chestnut is taken from a completely unrelated plant, the Castanea Sativa. Although the plant's common name seems to suggest some relationship between it and other chestnuts, there is none. Sweet Chestnut has no more relationship to Red or White Chestnut than it does to any of the other plants in Bach's canon.

For this reason, the concept of obsession belongs solely to the trio of Chestnuts that are taken from the same family of plants.

White Chestnut can also be used in tandem with the more passive remedies for cases involving patients who are driven by their obsessive thoughts.

There are two remedies that I want to note, each with a particular virtue when used in tandem with White Chestnut. The first remedy is Mimulus. Since the White Chestnut type is obsessive in his thoughts, he is often riddled with very specific fears. Used together Mimulus and White Chestnut can melt way the patient's fears, quiet his mind, and give him a peaceful night's sleep.

The second remedy is Impatiens, which is of special value to the White Chestnut type with chronic insomnia. Since Impatiens is the other Bach remedy especially valuable to insomniacs, White Chestnut and Impatiens together can bring relief to even the most stubborn cases of insomnia. For patients who wrestle with insomnia, the two remedies should be taken together, with nothing else added, just before bedtime. If the patient needs other remedies, they can be taken at other times of day, with the mix of White Chestnut and Impatiens reserved for bedtime.

Acutely, White Chestnut can be used any time we hear the chatter of our own minds too loudly. For nights when we feel too wired to sleep, and for nightmares. White Chestnut soothes and comforts the mind, quiets our thoughts. I have always said that a dose of White Chestnut is like a weekend at the beach.

## Negative Qualities of the Type

White Chestnut types experience mental chatter, nearly audible voices running through their mind, interrupting their concentration and disrupting sleep on a regular basis. Because of this, many White Chestnut types experience a number of physical complaints, including chronic headaches and eye strain. (I noted earlier that White Chestnut types tend to focus strongly with their conscious minds. As a result, they tend to overfocus with their eyes, which causes vision issues, physical eye pain, and chronic dry eye.) They are also physically tense and driven in their behaviors, so they are given to chronic muscle pain, especially in the neck and shoulders, and to chronic mouth and jaw pain. They often will grind their teeth at night. Although they have very tight muscles, they often will not want to be touched, and will avoid massage that could help them.

White Chestnut types can be very difficult to live with. Because they tend to be "high strung" they may speak before they think. They tend to be honest, but may be ruthlessly so. They can be highly critical. For this reason, White Chestnut is often needed in combination with Crab Apple, especially when the White Chestnut type is focused on cleanliness and/or order. The Crab Apple/White Chestnut patient will enter a room and tell you, in his first sentence, what is wrong with it or wrong with you. This patient inevitably fixates upon what needs fixing or changing in every situation and with every person. The White Chestnut/Crab Apple type may also become obsessed with personal hygiene and may become germ-phobic, or, like Lady Macbeth, spend a good deal of time scrubbing his hands.

Perhaps the most negative quality of the White Chestnut type is his sheer relentlessness. Once he has fixated upon a subject, he cannot let it go until or unless he exhausts it or himself, whichever comes first. This is all well and good if he fixates upon an academic or scientific subject. In these cases, White Chestnut types are as happy as can be, and can actually accomplish much for the good of all. But if the White Chestnut type fixates upon something within the home, or some project on which he can use as an axe, then he can be as highly destructive as he can, when well focused, be creative. (White Chestnut types have an uncanny ability to turn almost anything that they fixate upon into a weapon they can use to wound others.) White Chestnut types will see their marriages fail simply because they have exhausted their partner. They will see their business shrink in the same way, because others simply become too exhausted to deal with the process the White Chestnut uses to exhaust himself enough to sleep.

## Positive Qualities of the Type

As the White Chestnut type evolves from his old obsessive patterns of thought to a more positive posture, the important change is that the White Chestnut type at long last gains some control over himself, his thoughts, and his behaviors. He will not lose his innate intelligence, or even his energetic drive. But where he once was the victim of his own thoughts and a slave to his addictions, he now stands in a state of emotional and mental balance and is able to pick and choose his thoughts and actions.

After the White Chestnut has worked to release his obsessive thoughts, he can stand back and watch these thoughts rush at him and by him, without ever wanting to cling to any of them. Or better, the White Chestnut may just experience a calm end to these thoughts and peaceful nights of sleep in their place.

The White Chestnut type is still capable of great focus and still has great powers of concentration. But this ability has been brought into balance with the other aspects of the White Chestnut type's character, making him even more capable of accomplishing great things and certainly more capable of working and living in harmony with others.

## The White Chestnut Child

The White Chestnut child worries through many restless nights. These children worry about schoolwork, about a visit to the dentist, and about punishments they might receive. They are children who often seem older than they are, in terms of their chronic and very adult state of worry. Parents of White Chestnut children need to help them be children, to live in the moment, not replaying the past or worrying about the future.

It is my belief that we are now finding White Chestnut children to be very common, where once there were very few of this type. This has a great deal to do both with the nature of our world today—and certainly with the technology available to everyone—as well as with our expectations of our children. We are creating an ever-growing number of anxious and driven children who actually believe that they must work very, very hard, almost from birth, to achieve all they can and earn satisfaction from their parents.

## The White Chestnut Adult

While I have to this point mainly described the White Chestnut type from the perspective of the workplace or to study, I want to stress that these areas are not always their focus. Certainly, the White Chestnut type may obsess over any thoughts. For instance, they may be elderly patients who fixate over memories of family events that happened a half century ago (combine White Chestnut with Honeysuckle in these cases). The

White Chestnut mania may appear in adults of all ages, all classes, and both genders. The important trait is that the mind intrudes upon the patient's ability to live his life in a balanced manner, with comfort and clarity, rather than focusing on the subject of the chatter. When it comes to obsessive thoughts, any chatter is possible.

This is the patient who suffers from mental agitation. As if a part of the mind is restless, like a leg jiggling and jiggling. Their mind seems never free to float and to imagine. Instead, their thoughts are trapped by compulsive and obsessive behaviors. Their life energy is literally being drained away by minute details and petty hurts and fears that are blown out of all proportion.

No matter the age of the patient, from early youth to old age, when the mind begins to close in, when the patient feels that he no longer, even for the briefest time, controls his thoughts, but that they control him, use White Chestnut.

### The White Chestnut Animal

By all means, give this remedy to terriers. Give it to them often. It will help.

Use this remedy for any animal that is obsessive, especially if the animal obsessively bites or scratches himself.

### White Chestnut and the Homeopathic Pharmacy

Our homeopathic type that seems most similar to White Chestnut is Argentum Nitricum, a remedy made from silver. These people are sweet and likable on the surface, but under the surface they are beset with obsessive thoughts that upset them night and day.

### Issues that Suggest White Chestnut

Aging; allergies; carpal tunnel syndrome; colds; drug abuse; exhaustion; headache; hypertension; infections; insomnia; jaw pain; laryngitis; mouth pain; neck pain; nightmares; rheumatic pains, especially those that are affected by the weather; shoulder pain.

### In Conclusion

The White Chestnut type can fool you. They are often highly verbal, well spoken, and very opinionated. They may jump from topic to topic, especially if those topics are related, at least in the mind of the White Chestnut. Because of this you may think at first that their minds are rather fluid, that they do not fixate. This is how they will fool you. White Chestnut types are often intelligent enough, and they are certainly willful enough, that they can keep moving forward for quite a long period of time. They can seem very successful while still covering their inner tension and exhaustion and the fact that they are, in truth, running on fumes.

Once the need for White Chestnut is uncovered and the remedy is given, I have repeatedly found that is has nearly instantaneous results. The White Chestnut relaxes almost the moment the drop is placed upon his tongue. And the White Chestnut is very happy as a result of this relaxation.

Unlike many other types, you never have to worry whether or not the White Chestnut is taking his remedy. Once he learns that he will sleep if he takes it at bedtime, he is more than happy to take it. In fact, this is one of the types who may, if you are not careful, take his remedy too often.[17] When you give the remedy to a White Chestnut you must remember that he is somewhat compulsive and that he has a highly addictive nature. Therefore, he must be fully instructed as to how and how often he should take his remedy. Once he has been "programmed" with the appropriate use of the remedy, you need not fear. His own obsessive nature will do the rest.

But where the remedy White Chestnut will do a great deal of good for the patient, it may not do the whole job. By this I do not mean that you will likely have to combine the remedy with others, although this is certainly the case. What I mean is that you may have to help the White Chestnut find adjunct therapies that will help him bring balance into his life.

In addition to using Bach's White Chestnut remedy, patients of this type often also need to turn to yoga, tai chi, or some other form of movement and breathing to help support their emotional balance and well-being. Gentle forms of exercise such as these will not only help exhaust the White Chestnut enough to help them relax, but they will also help them breathe correctly. In their tense state, most White Chestnut types forget to breathe and take rapid, shallow breaths that only tend to increase their inner tension (and raise their blood pressure). Yoga and tai chi—or any other form of gentle motion and deep breathing—used in conjunction with White Chestnut and other appropriate remedies, can help White Chestnut types turn their lives around.

## CHESTNUT BUD · THE REMEDY FOR THOSE WHO HAVE OBSESSIVE BEHAVIOR

Bach says that his Chestnut Bud remedy holds great promise "for those who do not take full advantage of observation and experience, and who take a longer time than others to learn the lesson of daily life. Whereas one experience would be enough for some, such people find it necessary to have more, sometimes several, before the lesson is

---

17. Remember, because Bach remedies are, in some sense, homeopathic remedies, you can do more harm by taking them too often than you can by taking too little. It should only be taken once or twice a day in constitutional cases. If the remedy is taken too often, it will actually have less impact than it could if it was taken more appropriately. The true strength of these remedies comes into play when they are taken for a longer period of time, with more time between doses, than if they are taken too often in multiple doses.

learnt. Therefore, to their regret, they find themselves having to make the same error on different occasions when once would have been enough, or observation of others could have spared them even that one fault."

- **Chestnut Bud is both an acute and a constitutional remedy.**

## Botanical Information

The remedy Chestnut Bud is made from the horse chestnut (*Aesculus Hippocastanum*) tree, the same plant that produces the remedy White Chestnut. But where White Chestnut is made from the tree's white flowers, Chestnut Bud is made from the tree's buds.

## Chestnut Bud in General

As far as I am concerned, everyone needs Chestnut Bud, and, if I have anything to do with it, everybody gets Chestnut Bud. I say put it in the public water supply instead of fluoride—it will do more good. I strongly feel that is the most underused remedy in Bach's pharmacy.

> As far as I am concerned, everyone needs Chestnut Bud, and, if I have anything to do with it, everybody gets Chestnut Bud. I say put it in the public water supply instead of fluoride— it will do more good.

It is the Homer Simpson of remedies: overweight, out of shape, caught in a trap of his own stupid thoughts and beliefs, wanting to change but never able to, always with a new plan, a new diet, a new relationship, all of which fail. Each time the Chestnut Bud catches himself doing the same stupid thing once again, all he can say is "D'oh!" And then he does it all over again.

If there's a reason why we all love Homer Simpson, it's because we are all just like him. Or like Ralph Cramden, or like any other of the dozens of fictional characters who dream of getting rich quick, of better lives and jobs, more beautiful mates, but who lack the ability to change themselves in any way that could bring about a better tomorrow. Chestnut Bud is the remedy for those who are mired in their actions, their considerations and opinions, in their lives. It is the remedy for those who have bad habits—who still smoke even though they know it will likely kill them. For those who cannot learn a lesson the first time, who have to repeat the same mistake again and again before they can, through pain and humiliation, finally get it into their heads not to do it again.

We have all heard insanity defined as the same action repeated with the hope of a new and different result. If that is insanity, then I fear we are all insane. We all have, in our lives, made the same foolish mistake again and again, touched the hot stove more than once, not learned our lesson when the lesson that needed learning was obvious to everyone, even ourselves. And, therefore, we all need Chestnut Bud.

We all, inside ourselves, understand and relate to the universality of the Chestnut Bud state. If there is anything that describes the Chestnut Bud state, it is that old Dusty Springfield song, "Windmills of Your Mind." "Like a circle in a circle," the song goes, "Like a wheel within a wheel."

That's what's inside the Chestnut Bud's feverish little mind, and the cyclical nature of his life. Like White Chestnut, a remedy that has a great deal in common with the Chestnut Bud (after all, they are made from the same plant) the Chestnut Bud type is both fixated and obsessive. But where the White Chestnut is obsessive in his thoughts (and these obsessive thoughts sometimes lead him into obsessive behavior), the Chestnut Bud is instead trapped in obsessive patterns of behavior, anything ranging from bad habits to compulsive ritual behavior. Either way, the Chestnut Bud's life tends to be something of a minefield, with any number of things that can set him off. Some are prisoners of luck, dependent upon numbers, colors, or horses names to guide them. Others are prisoners of their own behavior, and have to drive to work by certain roads, or get a specific table in a restaurant. Still others are prisoners of bad habits they cling to as if they were not destructive, but instead were their greatest source of creative strength.

It is easy to write about this remedy with tongue in cheek, just as it is easy for us to feel superior to the stupid little Chestnut Bud, making the same mistakes over and over again. That is, until we remember how many times we ourselves have drunk alcohol to excess, or eaten something we know will upset our stomachs, or allowed ourselves to be trapped in the same upsetting reassessment of our relationships with loved ones. Almost all of us need Chestnut Bud at some time or another to set ourselves free from wrongheaded patterns. You and I, therefore, have nothing to feel superior to when dealing with Chestnut Bud. We have only to face our own negative patterns, however large or small, by which we cripple our lives.

However much I must resist the temptation to shorten the name of the remedy and simply call it "Bud," it is important to remember that while the Chestnut Bud type can be benign and even cheerful, bringing more harm to himself than others, the Chestnut Bud state is still destructive. By becoming obsessive in his patterns of habit and behavior, the Chestnut Bud type limits his ability to function freely and damages his ability to accomplish his goals. He will undermine himself, often actually defeat himself, at every turn. The Chestnut Bud type is the one who, when success is all but assured, will manage at the last moment to snatch defeat from the jaws of victory. And in doing so, he will leave those around him stunned at his accomplishment once again.

Interestingly, one aspect of the Chestnut Bud's negative state lies in direct opposition to White Chestnut's. Where the White Chestnut type tends to be a victim, both emotionally and physically, of his own tendency to overfocus, Chestnut Bud has issues with lack of focus. Where White Chestnut hones in on a topic of interest or study and focuses on it until either the topic itself or the White Chestnut type himself is exhausted, the Chestnut Bud has trouble keeping his attention or his focus riveted long enough to gather or retain information. The Chestnut Bud has trouble with details, with keeping his interest fixed long enough to organize them, and with his physical ability to recognize and utilize them. Between the eyes and the brain of the Chestnut Bud type is a sort of disconnect that can make it difficult for him to learn, especially to learn by reading. Many of those who constitutionally need this remedy have learning disabilities, many of which are associated with attention deficit disorders and with actual physical issues of vision relating to eye motion and yoking. While Bach's statement that Chestnut Bud types are those who "take a longer time than others to learn the lesson of daily life" is most certainly true metaphorically, it is very often literally true as well. Not only are Chestnut Buds given to missing the point that life itself seems to be trying to teach them, requiring them to make the same mistakes over and over in their lives, but they often have difficulties in learning in the classroom as well. Chestnut Bud types, who are slow to learn and unwilling or unable to concentrate on the task at hand, ironically require a great deal of focus on the part of teachers, parents, and employers who try to instruct and motivate them.

Chestnut Bud types are another of our remedy types who seem to lack an inner sense of motivation. They tend to always choose the short-term pleasure over the long-term goal. Those around them, who worry about them and their physical and financial health, will assume that it is a matter of education—that if the Chestnut Bud can only see the folly of his ways, he will surely try some new tactics for success. They slowly come to realize that the Chestnut Bud type is very often quite aware that what he is doing is not in his own best interest, that some of his actions can be self-destructive. In fact, he is often more aware of his own mistakes than are those who try to instruct and correct him. The problem is not that the Chestnut Bud does not know that what he is doing is not working in his own best interest. The problem is that he doesn't know a way out.

In some ways, therefore, the Chestnut Bud resembles the Walnut type, who is always standing at the crossroad, looking ahead to a new day and a new way of traveling through life, but who requires a kick in the pants to get him on his way. With the Chestnut Bud, the situation is more serious, however. It will take more than a single kick to move him in a new direction. The Chestnut Bud type is mired in his own obsessive behaviors. He clings to his habits as if his life depended upon them. (This is something of an irony, since many of his habits are life-shortening or life-ending, not life-sustaining.) The Walnut state tends to be transitory, something we visit while moving through the particular milestones of life, but the Chestnut Bud state, like the other Chestnut states, is a hammerlock. It contains the patient and imprisons him.

In some ways, the Chestnut Bud state also resembles the Wild Oat state. The two can look alike and patients needing the two remedies may even be drawn together, finding each other to be kindred souls. Often the two remedies will be needed concurrently in the treatment of a single patient. But Wild Oat types are motivated—if that is the word for it—by a sense of meaninglessness and futility. They perceive life as chaotic at best and the universe as a random place. This undercurrent of perceived futility undermines their attempts to establish themselves in life. They drift, moving from experience to experience, always searching for the thing that will cut through their sense of meaninglessness and ignite a true flame of passion within them. When they do find something they can feel passionate about, they cling to it, in a way that can seem obsessive, until the passion is gone. And then they move on.

While the Chestnut Bud type may display some behaviors that are similar to the Wild Oat type, his motivations are different. The Chestnut Bud type moves through life with a sense of confusion rather than a sense of futility. He is like a traveler to another land who only understands a few words of the language. He is slow to learn, slow to understand. He is also very accepting of his own foibles, and often finds humor in his own mistakes. He is self-deprecating and always willing to forgive himself when he repeats his mistakes again and again. And he is also stubborn and fixed in his habits and in his intellect. Where the Wild Oat is among our most fluid of types, the Chestnut Bud type, along with the other Chestnut remedies, is among our most fixed. He is a creature of habits, a buyer of specific brands, who cannot bear when his favorite beer is out of stock. He is confused and angered by the sort of change the Wild Oat relishes.

This is not to say that the two remedies Wild Oat and Chestnut Bud are never used concurrently. They are a very powerful combination. The patient who needs them in tandem is one who is careless in the extreme. Who moves through life without focus, without path, and without care, clumsily crashing into everything around him. This patient tends to project himself as being much younger than his years. He will, as an adult, dress like a child and show interest in things of childhood—games, comics and the like—long past the years in which these interests are appropriate.

In everyday life, remember to use Chestnut Bud when any habit has gotten out of hand. It can help patients stop smoking, change their diets, finally make changes in their lives that they have been unable to make for many years.

It is also very helpful to those who are careless and/or clumsy, especially when these are linked to a lack of focus or lack of interest. Since the Chestnut Bud type tends to be highly egocentric and interested in himself and his wants and needs above all else, this remedy can help us open ourselves up to the people around us and create a sense of compassion to counterbalance a focus on selfish things, even when it is used acutely.

Chestnut Bud's lack of focus very often results in a state of absent-mindedness or very selective memory. Those needing the remedy will forget things they want to forget, as well as things they do not consider interesting or important (like birthdays and anniversaries), no matter how important others may consider them to be. Even in acute treatments, Chestnut Bud can work wonders for absentmindedness and can restore a working sense of memory.

### Negative Qualities of the Type

The Chestnut Bud type is in a negative state in which they can never learn from experience: either their own or another's. Therefore, they are as incapable of learning from books as they are from their own experiences. They can, for instance, be told that the ice is too thin, or they can have actually have already fallen through that ice on two past occasions, but they will still stubbornly start walking out across the lake. As a result, they can, at best, seem naive and childlike and much younger than their years, and, at worst, they can seem backward in terms of their mental development.

Chestnut Bud types can be those for whom each day is truly a new beginning, as if their memory had been cut away during the night, leaving them to learn again every basic lesson of life. Or they can be those who have very clear memory, but do not let their own inner wisdom guide them when that guidance would require them to *not* do in a given moment the thing that they very much want to do. They cannot, for instance, resist the lure of the ice cream sundae, even if they are fifty pounds overweight. Nor can they use the fact that they are failing in school as enough reason to stay at home and study.

Left to their own devices, Chestnut Bud types end up living a life that is very messy. And they have no desire to clean up the messes themselves. In fact, they are quite willing to live, often literally, in the messes. If they are to be cleaned, others will have to do it. And given that their life has many such messes, financial, emotional, educational, and literal messes of piles with stains among them, cleaning up after a Chestnut Bud takes a great deal of time and effort, more than most of us are willing to give for long.

### Positive Qualities of the Type

Chestnut Buds are magnificent students of life. They move through the schoolhouse of life and take notes, learning from every experience and teaching all this information in a way that is both interesting and helpful. Further, they do not waste their time, but use each day to gain all the experience and information that they can.

### The Chestnut Bud Child

This is a natural type for a child. They are, after all, in the business of learning the lessons of life and cannot be faulted for needing to repeat a lesson more than once. So this is very often an acute remedy for children, to be used when a child seems stuck by a particular issue and needs help learning it before he or she can move on.

Some children can need Chestnut Bud constitutionally, however. Often these children reveal themselves in the school setting by their learning difficulties. Very often they will be identified as "special needs" students or students with attention deficit disorders.

Let's be clear on this. Chestnut Bud students' issues with learning very often have more to do with their own egocentric nature than with their actual ability to read or learn. Let's face it: Chestnut Bud types are motivated by their short-term desire for fun and excitement more than they are by anything else, so they often have trouble learning things they are not interested in. They don't care, for instance, about spelling or about dates in history books, so they put no effort in learning them. And, as they are obsessive types, they tend to be very stubborn. They will be all but impossible to budge once they have decided they are bored or have no use for a particular subject. The teacher who demands that the student work hard and learn something is the teacher that the Chestnut Bud student will decide is "out to get him."

This is not to say that some Chestnut Bud types don't have more serious learning issues. As noted above, reading comprehension can be a serious problem for Chestnut Bud types. They are also given to vision issues—often their eyes fail to work well together as a team, making it hard for the Chestnut Bud to replicate or use the information he has just read. Remember this is an absent-minded type. He will have problems trying to recall things, even things he read only minutes ago.

Many young people pass through a Chestnut Bud phase in late childhood and early adulthood. It is difficult for the best of them to concentrate as their bodies change and their hormones rage. This is also a time when children are beginning to experience a little personal freedom as their parents and their culture give them greater latitude. Therefore, young people at this age are beginning to explore, and experience things, both good and bad, that can be locked on and turned into life-long habits.

It is very important that parents of those moving through a Chestnut Bud stage recognize it for what it is, and realize that the habits—both emotional and physical—formed at this time can be clung to for many years to come.

### The Chestnut Bud Adult

Along with two other Chestnut remedies, Red and White Chestnut,[18] Chestnut Bud is an obsessive-compulsive remedy type. Chestnut Bud types are trapped in repetitive and habitual patterns that retard their personal growth in mind and in spirit. They are also

---

18. It is perhaps important to note again that the remedy Sweet Chestnut is a chestnut in name only. It is taken from a plant that is unrelated to the horse chestnut from which the other chestnut remedies are taken and, therefore, does not share any of the attributes common to the others.

prisoners of their own bad habits, which is why this remedy is often very helpful for those trapped in addictions such as alcohol, tobacco, food, and drugs.

The need for Chestnut Bud is not linked with any specific stage of adulthood. It can occur at any time. It is, however, a long-lasting pattern that is very hard to overcome once established. Those needing Chestnut Bud as their constitutional remedy most often need to take it for an extended period of time. This remedy can be slow to work, so don't be discouraged if there are no instantaneous results.

As noted above, adults who need Chestnut Bud often seem younger than their actual age. This may not be a good thing; they can seem a little foolish, because they act in a manner that is not in accord with their true stage in life. In the same way, they can look a little garish and even silly because they wear the hairstyles and clothing of much younger people. Sometimes they can appear a little out of phase with reality, especially when they continue to dress and wear their hair and makeup in a style that suited them thirty years ago, as if those years had not passed.

Finally, Chestnut Bud adults are also supremely self-centered. They may never realize the myriad ways they offend and bore others as they continue on, always amusing themselves.

### The Chestnut Bud Animal

Happily, I have never come upon an animal that I felt needed Chestnut Bud constitutionally. It is, however, helpful in working with animals and breaking them of bad habits. Use it, for instance, when you are trying to get your new dog to stop chewing on the furniture or when your cat claws the couch. It can also be a helpful tool in housebreaking animals.

And Chestnut Bud is excellent for animals that seemingly cannot be trained. Animals that make the same mistakes over and over again and animals that seemingly cannot be housebroken all respond to Chestnut Bud.

### Chestnut Bud and the Homeopathic Pharmacy

Among the thousands of remedies in the homeopathic pharmacy, none deal so clearly with issues of habitual behavior than those that are carbon based. All of our mineral remedies are slow to work and deep in action, and the compound remedies, formed by mixing carbon with some other mineral substance, certainly deal with a certain sluggishness of nature and slowness to learn. But the chronic Chestnut Bud state involves an ongoing wrongheadedness, a pattern of wrong thinking and bad decision making that controls the patient's life. The homeopathic remedy most similar, therefore, is Calcarea Carbonica, a remedy famous for its inability to make the correct decision in almost any instance in life, and for its tendency to stay stuck in one place physically as well, like the clam from whose shell the remedy is made.

## Issues that Suggest Chestnut Bud

Addiction; allergies; breathing problems; candidiasis; cellulite; cystic fibrosis; digestive disorders, especially acid reflux; eating disorders; functional conditions of all sorts; gas pains; headache; indigestion; immune dysfunction; overweight; skin conditions; snoring; ulcers.

## In Conclusion

Certainly, it can be gleaned from the material above that the Chestnut Bud type seems to be rather young (certainly in the energy he brings into any situation), and rather egocentric. I have, to some extent, dealt with the fact that a Chestnut Bud of middle age or older can seem somewhat grotesque—acting, speaking, and dressing as if they were a generation younger than they are, and also with the fact that many Chestnut Bud types would do well to pay attention to what is happening beyond the tip of their own noses. I have not, as yet, mentioned the shallowness of the type, however.

And it is important.

Part of what makes the Chestnut Bud state so destructive is the fact that it robs the patient of his or her ability to understand the intricacies of life. The Chestnut Bud type is not only slow to learn and unwilling or unable to change, he is also quite fixed upon only exploring the depths of life that will get him what he needs right now. It is a simplified view of life, what life requires, and the rewards it can offer. It has the emotional depth of a baby who wants the breast, wants to be rocked, wants to be changed, and very little else. In my opinion, the Chestnut Bud type who does not receive treatment remains frozen in time at the point in his life when he entered into the Chestnut Bud state of being. A patient who developed the Chestnut Bud's needs and wants and life patterns at an early age will literally never grow up. In a very real sense, he never learns from life's lessons because he is not equipped to learn from them. He lacks the emotional depth and the intellectual range to parse the subtleties of life.

Because Chestnut Bud types are clumsy creatures, and creatures of habit most often related to personal comfort, they lack motivation to push forward and to push deeper to a richer understanding of what life is and what it can offer. Because of this, they defeat themselves and cheat themselves out of experiencing all they could. They never share themselves fully with others, or grow toward wisdom through experience and the manipulation of details.

Is this something we all do, to some degree or another? Yes. At the end of a hard day we all choose the movie on television and turn off the news channel, just as we want to have a glass of wine at the end of that day. We all often choose our short-term pleasure over our long-term goal. And the degree we do this is the degree to which we need to look at our behavior, our habits, and our relationships with an honest eye and wonder, "Should I be taking Chestnut Bud?"

# 10

# Considering the Seventh Mood: The Faces of Loneliness

Perhaps if we are truly secure and happy with our true self, we can never be lonely. But the fact that Bach has gathered together the three remedies in this small group for the sake of those who are lonely suggests that Bach himself felt that loneliness is universal, like despair and fear, and that none of us are truly secure within ourselves. The remedies gathered here are those that will allow us to soothe our complaints relating to the void within ourselves that we call loneliness, and allow us to be brought into a state of emotional balance in which we can be fully at peace with self.

Each of the three remedies in this group feels the hollow core of loneliness, and each displays a different pattern of emotion, thought, and behavior as a result.

Two of the remedies, Water Violet and Heather, stand in direct opposition to each other in terms of behavior. Water Violet, in her loneliness, retreats from the world, while Heather uses his sense of loneliness as a force that drives him into the world and, indeed, all too often into the lives of those who unwillingly become the targets of his interest, however briefly his intrusion is allowed. Water Violet and Heather, are, therefore, forms of archetypes for the concept of loneliness. The Heather is that intrusive person who is rather pathetic in his need for attention and physical and emotional contact. The Water Violet, on the other hand, is the hermit who has shaped his world into a table for one.

> The remedies gathered here are those that will allow us to soothe our complaints relating to the void within ourselves that we call loneliness, and allow us to be brought into a state of emotional balance in which we can be fully at peace with self.

With the Impatiens type, we have something different, and something of a chicken-or-the-egg situation. An argument could be made that the Impatiens behavioral pattern is based in loneliness, while another, perhaps more compelling argument could be made that the Impatiens type's behavior is not a result of his loneliness, but that his loneliness is a result of his innate restless nature. The Impatiens type often finds himself cut off from those around him simply by the way his mind works—his indistinct sense of time and his tendency to emotional and mental restlessness—not as a result of some circumstance or trauma. Where the Water Violet often withdraws after the death of a loved one and the Heather loses contact with the world through a change of locale or other shift in circumstances, the Impatiens seems to be born to his part, and is set apart from others in an almost physical way. Only another who shares his inner clock and lack of focus can understand his motivations.

## Loneliness and the Homeopathic Pharmacy

There is a void in the homeopathic repertory where concepts relating to loneliness should be. It is surprising that our homeopathic forefathers did so little research on an emotional state that touches each of us, either acutely or chronically, at many points in our lives.

Still, there are some remedy types known for their tendency to feel alone. Chief among these are Lachesis, who is often set apart by his keen intellect and who, like the Impatiens type, will often use a barrage of words in place of human contact. He will take the stance that he has no need for that contact but is quite content with his thoughts and labors. In the same way, a Sulphur will often substitute philosophy for human contact and, as a result, will be quite lonely, while presenting a mask of smug contentment.

More obvious in their loneliness are Phosphorus and Arsenicum, both of whom dread being alone. But where the Phosphorus type will make this an emotional issue, with many a Phosphorus types crying through the night to get their parents to come into their room and give them company, the Arsenicum will actually experience a worsening of their physical symptoms when they are left alone.

The Lycopodium displays his loneliness in a different way. He will not want to be totally alone, but will not want to have to put up with other people either. Therefore, the Lycopodium will want to have others in the house, and will take comfort from hearing voices or the television in other rooms, but he will not want to actually have to be with them. The Ignatia Amara type will also, in her grief, want to have others in the house, but will not be able to deal with them directly. If she is forced to come into contact with others, it often becomes explosive, as she will use a wrong word or gesture as reason enough to run from the room.

And then there is the Rhus Tox type, who will become servile rather than be left alone. The Rhus will stand for almost any humiliation or bad behavior if the other will simply not leave her alone. And, finally, there is Pulsatilla, who so loves company and any sort of stimulation—physical, mental, or emotional—that she withdraws into a deep depression if left alone for too long.

The idea of loneliness is rather simple, really. For Bach, it came down to just three patterns of behavior. You could yield to the loneliness and withdraw, which is a very "yin" response. Or you could fight your loneliness and push outward, demanding that "attention must be paid," which is a very "yang" response. Or you could simply ignore your loneliness and, instead, rage within yourself, filling yourself with so much chatter and motion that you don't have to notice or deal with how lonely you are.

For Bach these are the patterns by which human beings deal with loneliness. And these are the faces we present to the world when we are trapped within this emotional state.

All the remedies in this chapter are fairly balanced in their uses, which is to say that they all are as effective as acute remedies as they are constitutionally. For many, loneliness is a fleeting thing, something that time and life will clear away rather effortlessly. For some of us, however, the pattern of loneliness can become a long-time heavy burden once it is set in place.

> Unlike some of the other groups of remedies, the remedies in this group do not fall into a common pattern of behavior. Some groups, like those who are Controlling or in Despair, are, as a group, aggressive in their behavior. Other groups, like those who are Indifferent, are rather passive in theirs. The remedy types gathered here, however, display a full range of behaviors, from emotionally aggressive to very passive.

Unlike some of the other groups of remedies, the remedies in this group do not fall into a common pattern of behavior. Some groups, like those who are Controlling or in Despair, are, as a group, aggressive in their behavior. Other groups, like those who are Indifferent, are rather passive in theirs. The remedy types gathered here, however, display a full range of behaviors, from emotionally aggressive to very passive. They are linked together by their sense of aloneness, their lack of emotional support (or, perhaps, their "perceived" lack is more correct, since in many cases, the patient who is lonely is surrounded by others who wish to help and support them, but whose love and attention go unnoticed or unwanted; this is common to the Water Violet, who fixates on a lost love) and the fact that they move through a world of couples on their own.

## REMEDIES FOR THOSE WHO ARE LONELY

- **Water Violet**—for those who are aloof

- **Heather**—for those who are needy

- **Impatiens**—for those who are impatient

## WATER VIOLET · THE REMEDY FOR THOSE WHO ARE ALOOF

Water Violet, writes Bach, is the remedy "for those who in health or illness like to be alone. Very quiet people, who move about without noise, speak little, and then gently. Very independent, capable, and self-reliant. Almost free of opinions of others. They are aloof, leave people alone and go their own way. Often clever and talented. Their peace and calmness is a blessing to those around them."

• While Water Violet may be used from time to time as an acute remedy, it is, more often than not, a constitutional remedy.

• Water Violet is one of Bach's original remedies, the Twelve Healers.

### Botanical Information

The water violet (*Hottonia Palustris*), also known as "water wysteria," is a pond plant. It requires a good deal of sun to grow well, but is not fussy about soil content or temperature. It is a bushy plant often found planted in dense clumps in water gardens. It is also an indoor plant that can be found in tanks and aquariums.

Water violet is native to Europe and especially common in Ireland.

The water violet flowers in May and June. The plant self-pollinates and is hermaphroditic.

### Water Violet in General

While Bach groups Water Violet among his remedies for those who are lonely, there is no better remedy for those who are trapped in a state of grief. This is not a remedy for those who have experienced a loss—whether it is the death of a loved one or the end of a relationship—very recently, but for those for whom grief has become a way of life.

Water Violet is an excellent acute or constitutional remedy for the patient who has become cut off from human contact due to grief. She has pulled in emotionally until she stands quite alone in the world, in her viewpoint.

The negative emotional state of loneliness typified by the remedy Water Violet is not limited to grief, however. The aloof loneliness of the Water Violet type, which can range from simply introverted to arrogant to a hermitlike existence—need not be caused by grief, although that is common. Anything that separates the patient emotionally from others can be the root cause of this state. And the patient feels emotionally isolated even if he or she is living among millions of other people in a large city. The Water Violet type adapts to her state of loneliness by becoming aloof, by seeking to be as completely independent as possible. Water Violet types, above all else, do not wish to be a burden upon others in any way—physically, financially, or emotionally, so they erect a sort of wall around themselves. This wall can be made of many different materials, from slippery, invisible glass to barbed wire or solid stone.

Water Violet types, therefore, are eager to keep any contact they must make with others as brief and shallow as possible. This lets them create and maintain a façade that makes them appear stronger, happier, and more capable than they are. They never share their own problems with others, no matter how long or how well they know them, although they may be quite willing to listen as others tell them their troubles. A Water Violet type may be willing to issue advice—but this advice somehow often seems to issue from on high, with a trace of arrogance that informs the troubled party that the Water Violet can only advise them theoretically, because he or she (the Water Violet) would never be caught up in such an ugly mess.

Mess is another thing, along with sloppy human contact, the Water Violet type tends to avoid. They insist that their homes be meticulously clean and that their meals be simple and well balanced. They cannot tolerate excess in any form, whether emotional or sensual. They do not like strong stimuli, from loud noises to bright lights. When Blanche Dubois puts a paper lantern over the naked hanging light bulb in A *Streetcar Named Desire*, she shows her Water Violet sensibility. In fact Blanche typifies the emotional disconnect of the Water Violet type with her inability to understand or cope with the attitudes and behaviors of those around her, and her own aloof and somewhat judgmental attitudes. And she is an excellent example of the Water Violet blend of arrogance and emotional fragility.

> When Blanche Dubois puts a paper lantern over the naked hanging light bulb in A *Streetcar Named Desire*, she shows her Water Violet sensibility. And she is an excellent example of the Water Violet blend of arrogance and emotional fragility.

The Water Violet type begins a process of disconnecting from the emotional reality she once knew when the betrayal or loss of the original emotional injury first occurs. Sometimes the process is very abrupt; the Water Violet suddenly moves and starts a new life. Most often, however, it is a slow thing, and the Water Violet begins to shutter the windows one by one. Her friends notice slowly, one by one, that they have not heard from her for weeks or months. When they attempt to contact her, she at first gives vague excuses and finally stops returning their calls.

With the emotional injury that they have sustained, Water Violet types make a decision on a deep emotional level that they will have to make a go of it alone. It is important to note that they do not think this is their own choice. In their perception of the world this hollow new life is thrust upon them. Either they have lost the one person who truly understood them, or their love and trust have been so betrayed that the wound, festering as it still is, will not allow them to ever trust again. And so, they sol-dier on, alone.

They often develop a refined sense of existence in their solitude, showing deep interest in what they consider to be the best things in life, cultural and philosophical things. They will study the great philosophers or the world religions, turn their atten-tion to fine art, to classical music and to opera. Often they will find an emotional solace in great art, and will feel a connection with it—with paintings, dance, or music, prima-rily—that they do not feel with other humans. Their love of culture and of the arts, therefore, becomes the way they stay connected with the human race. The passion the artist puts into his work affects Water Violet types deeply, as this is the only passion that they will allow themselves.

In that the Water Violet type is the most emotionally unavailable of all of Bach's types, this remedy stands in direct opposition with those that are open and available emotionally, like Cerato and Centaury, although Water Violet may be just as emotion-ally vulnerable. The Water Violet type has to expend a great deal of emotional energy to keep up her façade. When she feels her strength is waning or her façade is cracking she will respond by withdrawing even more.

Water Violet types tend to be very concerned with their homes. Their homes will be far more to them than the walls that protect and surround them, although that is an important aspect of the home because Water Violets are very interested in protection and in walls. But their homes *in toto* will represent them, their independence, and their artistic sensibilities. Therefore, the appearance of their home, and the possessions it houses, are very important to the Water Violet. Even more important is that the home has the appropriate blend of public and private spaces. Now, make no mistake, the Water Violet's whole home is a private space. The Water Violet type is very careful about who gets invited inside. But even those who come inside are never invited past the public spaces. You might think of the Water Violet's home as a series of apartments, some available to others and some only for the Water Violet himself. Or you might think of it as a maze, with the Water Violet's own bedroom in the center.

When a Water Violet feels emotionally exhausted or threatened, he will retreat into his bedroom and will not move from it until his emotional balance is restored. Often, the move to the bed will have apparently physical causes. Headaches and back pain are common reasons for bed rest.

But the Water Violet's whole lifestyle is based upon, as the Greek's put it in their dramas, *strophe* and *antistophe*, which were the terms for the movement of the Greek chorus on the stage. Loosely put, the Water Violet's life is one of advance and retreat, based upon the state of his or her emotional independence on a given day, and colored by the physical symptoms that are closely linked to that emotional state.

Another aspect to the Water Violet negative emotional state is rigidity. Along with her almost staged movements of advance and withdrawal, the Water Violet has both physical and emotional rigidity. The Water Violet type, with her strong sense of what is and is not appropriate in terms of behavior (proper manners are very, very important to her), totally lacks spontaneity. There are behaviors that are allowed and others that are not, and there are behaviors that are not only allowed but are required in nearly every one of life's events and situations. Water Violet knows them all, and expects you to know them too. With her strong sense of what is and is not appropriate, the Water Violet not only does not behave in a spontaneous manner, but will not tolerate such high jinks in others either. This emotional rigidity may well manifest itself physically as well, and the Water Violet type is given to chronic joint stiffness and pain. Even Water Violet types who do not have physical stiffness will tend to carry themselves almost as if they do. They tend to walk with head up and with a stiff and heavy gait.

Finally, there is the sense of pride that is part of this remedy's emotional core. The Water Violet is typically very proud of his achievements. He feels that he should be very proud because he has made himself independent and capable (at least in his own mind) and is now his own best product. Water Violet types invariably fall into this trap of pride to some degree or other. Some are merely arrogant, while others allow themselves to climb up onto the papal throne of infallibility.

Pride can be a big issue for the Water Violet type and especially for those who come into contact with him. After all, in their minds all Water Violet types, male or female, see themselves as Queen Elizabeth II, wearing a hat, waving gently to those who have come to look at them, and never carrying cash.

Others often perceive the Water Violet type to be haughty, aloof, and uninvolved. They also can seem emotionally cold and lacking in any sort of liveliness or humor. But remember, when dealing with the Water Violet type you are again dealing with a masked personality. Beneath this patient's thick veneer of superiority and entitlement is a very vulnerable, very lonely being.

As a remedy type that most often stems from a sense of grief, loss, or betrayal, Water Violet has similarities with other emotionally unavailable types. Perhaps chief among these is Willow. While the Willow type seems to be more negative and more destructive in his attitude and behavior pattern than the Water Violet, the two types do have much in common. Each shares feelings of anger that are the underpinnings of their behavior.

But where the Water Violet is haughty and emotionally aloof, the Willow type is vindictive. Willows tend to feel they have axes to grind and scores to settle, which connect them to the world and other people in ways that the Water Violets are not. After all, both love and hate create long-lasting chains of interplay between people. The Willow forges these chains of bitterness with their bare hands, but Water Violet withdraws and leaves others to their fate instead. While these two remedies may, upon first glance, appear similar—each is rigid, stoic to one degree or another, and somewhat haughty—their motivations could not be further apart.

Another of our remedies for those who are grieving is Chicory, but like Willow, the Chicory type works from a very different set of motivations than the Water Violet. The Chicory type not only desires emotional contact with others, she insists upon it. The Chicory type is clingy at best and domineering and smothering most of the time. The Water Violet type would be shocked and alarmed at the ways Chicory is willing to manipulate the people she wishes to control through her pretense of love.

Note that Chicory is most often helpful for patients in the first stages of grief. Combined with Sweet Chestnut it can be very helpful to those who have a loss of emotional control as a result of their loss, and are still feeling the first shocks of grief. (Star of Bethlehem can also be added to help with a state of shock, especially in cases of sudden death.)

Honeysuckle is the other remedy often given to those who grieve. Like Water Violet, it is given to those who have passed through the first stage of shock following a loss, and have moved into a quieter, longer-lasting grief that colors and controls their entire lives. Where the Honeysuckle will close herself in her home—a home that has become a shrine to the life she once had and to those she loved. She will enter into a golden haze of memory in which all that was is better than all that is, aching for a past that has slipped out of her fingers. The Water Violet, on the other hand, will not fill her life with memories in her retreat. She will, instead, avoid those memories, especially if they are at all painful, and will fill her life with activity, with cleaning and organizing, with the arts, which give her passion she cannot otherwise feel, and, all too often, with doctors to treat her myriad ills.

Honeysuckle and Water Violet can be used in conjunction for the patient who is experiencing a withdrawal from life that blends Water Violet's aloofness with Honeysuckle's deep sense of nostalgia.

Water Violet is often combined with Star of Bethlehem. It is an excellent combination that is very helpful in allowing the Water Violet to deal with the original trauma that caused her emotional withdrawal, no matter how long-lasting it has been.

Two remedies can help those Water Violet types who tend to be rather aggressive in their haughtiness and in the few contacts with others they allow. The first is Willow, which is mentioned above. The patient needing both Willow and Water Violet will feel deep feelings of betrayal that are the source of this joint emotional state. Both types can commonly feel betrayed, even if the person who "betrayed" them did so by dying, something that certainly was not their choice of action. So these two remedies work very well together with patients for whom a sense of betrayal is a strong theme.

The other remedy that works well with aggressive Water Violet types is Holly.

Patients who need these two remedies together deepen the Water Violet's innate sense of aloofness and superiority into something deeper and more destructive. They are misanthropes who find that they can barely tolerate the presence of others. Often they will demand more of anyone they consider to be their "inferiors"—lawn men, cleaning ladies, and cashiers at the drug store—than is commonly considered tolerable. These Water Violet/Holly types, therefore, have a great deal of trouble in finding anyone who will tolerate their attitude for long. (If a strong streak of perfectionism enters into the picture, if the Water Violet shows a strong need for cleanliness and order, add Crab Apple to the mix.)

Many of our Bach types have other types that stand in direct opposition with them. In the case of Water Violet, the opposite remedy is Heather, another remedy grouped by Bach for the treatment of those who are lonely. (Heather follows Water Violet in this chapter.)

Both are remedies for lonely people. But the life strategy each adopts to cope with their loneliness is in direct opposition with one another. Where the Water Violet retreats and fixates upon presenting herself as somewhat superior and independent in all things, the Heather type intrudes into every conversation and everyone else's personal space. No doubt the typical Heather would, upon meeting a Water Violet, consider her to be a snob, and the Water Violet, after fleeing from the Heather, would say that she is a coarse bore.

Like Oak, with which it combines quite well, Water Violet types can seem stoic and, more important, older than their actual age or as if they themselves belonged to another age. They seem rooted in the way things used to be, almost stubbornly ignoring the way things are. The remedy type Honeysuckle also presents itself this way. Any or all of these types may wear hairstyles and clothing from a generation ago—a time before their travails began.

As an acute remedy, Water Violet is used to treat feelings of shyness or any momentary feeling that cuts off our sense of contact with others. The whole issue for the Water Violet is human contact. When we feel a disconnect, especially one in which we feel we are "tainted" by emotional or physical contact, we should start running for the Water Violet dropper bottle.

### Negative Qualities of the Type

Many Water Violet types not only give off an air of superiority; they also can actually believe themselves to be superior. They can be overly proud, and can look at others with a withering stare. They do not want to give or take advice. They do not want to deal with humans on a purely human level, but seek always to pull things to their highest level. While this makes for a nifty philosophy, it also lets Water Violet types set the rules in determining just what makes for the "highest level." In this way Water Violets can be very domineering and controlling. Having lost their ability to emotionally reach out to others or to have others reach out to them, Water Violet types can be cruel and dismissive in their way, leading those who do look upon them with true affection to feel that they are just not good enough in the Water Violet type's eyes.

### Positive Qualities of the Type

The Water Violet type truly cares about the impact of thought, of philosophy in our lives in both the negative and positive aspects of the emotional state. He will take the time and the energy to explore all that he feels needs to be explored. He does not concern himself with popularity or surface issues. As such, both positive and negative Water Violet types are given to deep study and can accomplish much in the way of research or education. But Water Violet types must have the emotional strength of their most positive emotional state before they can develop the compassion and the ability to communicate and put all they have learned into action.

At his most positive, the Water Violet type is the most compassionate of people, allowing each to find his own path, offering wise advice only when asked. He will help transform both individuals and communities for the better, usually while quietly working in the background. Positive Water Violet types make excellent teachers, especially on the college level. They share all they have studied with a sense of passion and have a unique ability to connect both intellectually and emotionally with their students.

### The Water Violet Child

If there is another child more likely to answer in monosyllables, I don't know him. The Water Violet child, who most often combines shyness and an odd sense of superiority, will project a persona that is both older and more sophisticated than the child's actual age would suggest.

The keynote terms for the Water Violet child are "self-assured," and "self-contained." The Water Violet type is often a "little professor"; a child who seems like a miniature adult, who speaks with and feels more comfortable with adults than with other children. This is a child who plays it very close to the vest, emotionally speaking; who speaks or acts out very little according to their feelings. They need to learn that they can and should reach out on a human level and give their emotions equal force to their intellect.

### The Water Violet Adult

Adults who find themselves in a Water Violet state are in a very real state of confusion. Somewhere and somehow, they have lost their ability to communicate with others. They have lost the emotional connection they once felt for and with other humans.

Instead, their attempts at human relationships become clumsy. Because of this, Water Violet types withdraw. This withdrawal can take many forms, from withdrawing into polite chatter or to actually withdrawing physically from the world. Often, their physical state—riddled as it is with chronic if vague conditions—will be the excuse that allows Water Violets to retreat.

The perception of haughtiness that is commonly applied to the Water Violet may or may not have basis in reality. Certainly, many Water Violet types will, over time, come to think of themselves as more refined and somewhat superior to others. But many mask their clumsiness in human contact with an emotional aloofness that is interpreted by others as haughty and superior, although the Water Violet does not mean it to be taken that way.

The Water Violet state, while it projects a sense of age and gravitas upon the patient, is not linked to a physical age or stage of life. Water Violet types may be found at all ages and in both genders. Although it is often considered to be a somewhat feminine state because of its sense of refinement and quest for appropriate behavior, it can be found in both men and women.

### The Water Violet Animal

I have never found Water Violet to be a particularly good remedy for animals, although I have used it with success for animals who withdraw when ill.

### Water Violet and the Homeopathic Pharmacy

There is much that relates the Natrums—sodium-based remedies including Natrum Muriaticum, which is made from table salt—as a group with Bach's remedy Water Violet. They especially share a tendency toward emotional withdrawal and a strong need to be alone when they feel exhausted or sick. Also, both will tend to consider their home to be their castle and will not want to have this castle disrupted in any way.

But the remedy Ferrum Phosphoricum also has much to relate it to Water Violet. Like Natrum Mur, Ferrum Phos is often used in cases for which we have a distinct lack of symptoms. The Ferrum Phos fever is just a general fever, without Aconite's or Belladonna's keynote symptoms to lead you to a remedy. So we use Ferrum Phos when the patient is busy not telling us about themselves, just as is the case with Water Violet. The Water Violet patient will talk about their thoughts, their philosophy, but not about their heart or about their true issues.

### Issues that Suggest Water Violet

Asthma and breathing problems; gall stones; guilt; hay fever; headaches; itching; joint stiffness and pain; kidney problems; lung problems; overweight; sexual dysfunction; sexual guilt; skin conditions, especially eczema.

*In Conclusion*

While extravagant is a word that you might not, at first, think of as describing the Water Violet type, there is a sort of extravagance that is common. The Water Violet, because he is cut off emotionally from others, neither giving or receiving human contact, tends to want to "reward" himself in several ways.

First, the Water Violet type may be something of a gourmand or may be a fancier of fine wines. He can, like television's effete radio talk show host Frasier Crane, or, even more so, his brother Niles, set himself up as being an expert on the topic and will thrill to a dinner in a very fine restaurant or will actually go out of his way to attend the meeting of a wine-lover's club.[1]

In the same way, Water Violets will commune happily with others who share their specific passions, as long as the conversation stays on the subject of their joint interest or only includes other topics like antique collecting or home décor, things the Water Violet feels are appropriate topics for conversation.

Water Violet types are also often passionately interested in scientific and pseudo-scientific topics of study and, especially, in religion. They will most typically withdraw from the world and from community action when they become passionately involved in their church. They are especially drawn to churches that offer a good deal of mystery in their faith, such as the Catholic and Episcopal churches, or to those that claim to have secret knowledge, such as Christian Science. Water Violets are loyal people. Once they have decided that a topic is worthy of study, they delve into it as deeply as possible. In the same way, they are devout worshipers, although they are not very likely to attend the morning coffee after the worship service.

## HEATHER · THE REMEDY FOR THOSE WHO ARE NEEDY

Heather types, according to Bach, are "those who are always seeking the companionship of anyone who may be available, as they find it necessary to discuss their own affairs with others, no matter whom it may be. They are very unhappy if they have to be alone for any length of time."

---

1. Note that the Water Violet type, while always aloof from those he considers common, will actually go out of his way to speak to or spend time with those he considers his equal. What human contact he does form is invariably formed with those who share his quite specific interests in the arts, religion, or fine dining. Conversation with these people is always confined to their joint interests, but it can be highly pleasurable for the Water Violet, who loves the interplay of ideas. If the person who was so delightful at the concert the night before makes the mistake of intruding into the Water Violet's life with a phone call that suggests that there could be more to their relationship than just the single topic of conversation, they will be quickly rebuffed by the Water Violet, who will add them to his list of bores.

- **Heather is both an acute and a constitutional remedy.**

## Botanical Information

This particular heather (*Calluna Vulgaris*) plant is an evergreen groundcover that is native to much of Europe. Its flowers are very small, but form in clusters of pink to mauve to purple blooms that erupt in late summer and autumn.

Heather prefers to grow in full sun. It does not like the wind, although it can grow in desolate locales and in barren landscapes.

Note that there are more than 1,000 types of this particular species of heather plants. Many have been cultivated into gardens across the globe. Most often, it is used as a foreground plant, often planted in the front of a perennial border.

## Heather in General

The negative emotional state of the Heather type is connected to the need for recognition, acceptance, and attention that is within us all. Heather types crowd others, emotionally and physically, and force themselves upon those who do not approach them first. The Heather type who is not given attention will demand it. And that same patient will be almost totally incapable of being alone. He will prefer anyone's company, no matter how much or how little he actually likes the other person, rather than being left on his own. In the same way, the Heather patient will announce his personal business to anyone who he can make listen. And he will tend to ask others for their advice and opinions, again, whether or not he really values the other person's advice.[2] The Heather type, along with the patient who needs Chicory (a remedy that blends very well with Heather), is perhaps the most emotionally demanding and emotionally needy of all the remedy types. It is most certainly a toss-up between these two types as to which is the most self-centered.

Heather types are most certainly motivated by their own needs, and only by their own needs. In their particular blend of brazen intrusiveness and emotionally vulnerability, they can tend to forget that others have emotional needs of their own. This is perhaps because the Heather state itself suggests a rather infantile emotional viewpoint. Despite their chronological age, Heather types are frozen in the childish state we

2. In this behavior, the Heather type can resemble the Cerato patient, who will also ask advice from nearly anyone. But where the Heather asks advice solely as an attention-getting ploy, and seeks to "seduce" others with the flattery of admiring their intelligence or wisdom, the Cerato type asks for help because he is so insecure of his own ability to judge a given situation that he believes even a stranger on the street will have a better take on reality than he does. The Heather type is very emotionally needy and wants reassurance of being liked and wanted, but he does not share the Cerato type's lack of intuition and weak sense of self. Quite the opposite in fact, the Heather type is dynamically self-centered.

all pass through, but which most of us soon grow beyond: the state in which we all need our mother's full and loving attention. The state in which we must always have total approval of all that we think, say, and do. On the deepest level, Heather types feel that they cannot trust life to bring them the love and attention they actually need, so they seek it on a continual basis and seek to control both its quality and source. In their willful and egocentric need for attention and approval, the Heather type seeks not just to be in the photograph, but to be dead center.

> In their willful and egocentric need for attention and approval, the Heather type seeks not just to be in the photograph, but to be dead center.

Since Heather types want to control the source of the attention they receive, they will quite often fixate upon one person and will focus a good deal of time and effort in trying to seduce that person into paying them heed. Along the way, of course, the Heather type will take up with any or all others who pass her way, as she will choose any alternative to being alone. But she can spend a good deal of time mooning over one person, only to suddenly conclude that that person will never return her attention (often she will say that the other person is not worthy of her time) and move on to another target. Because of their overriding need for attention and their underlying sense of deep loneliness (remember, this is a remedy for those who are lonely), patients who need the remedy Heather on a constitutional basis are likely to have a history of unhappy and unfulfilling relationships. And since the dynamic of a loving relationship is the chief desire of a Heather type, many of these types will be deeply alarmed and confused by their apparent inability to maintain a satisfactory and stable relationship in their lives. (And "loving" here can take on many different shades of meaning. Many Heather types truly yearn for a loving and stable parent-child relationship, but, instead become involved in a string of relationships that confuse the nurturing of a parental relationship with the passion of a sexual encounter.) Just as any number of the other Bach types seem incapable of realizing that their destructive patterns of behavior deny them the goal they desire, the Heather type often do not understand that their aggressive and clumsy demand for love makes the chances of actually finding it all the more remote.

Often, in their loneliness and confusion, the Heather type will seek a tool they can use to help them to be "brave" enough to continue to approach others after they have experienced a few emotional failures. Like the Agrimony type, Heather types may turn to alcohol to help fuel their drive for attention and to free them of inhibitions, so they can give themselves permission to take full advantage of whatever attention they receive. This combination of the Heather type's neediness and lowered inhibitions will often lead him into downright dangerous relationships, especially sexual relationships. Heather types, who, again, are never amongst the most discerning of folks, will most of the time choose the companionship of strangers over sleeping alone—especially through the long, dark hours after the bars have closed. They will often have one-night stands and brief sexual encounters and take part in sexual experimentation. Especially in their younger years, Heather types often confuse sexual attraction with approval or emotional attachment. This can lead to emotional outbursts (especially when the Heather feels that they are being deserted by the partner who wanted nothing more than sex)[3], to roller-coaster mood swings, and even manic-depressive behavior. It can also lead to other disastrous results, disease and pregnancy chief among them.

While the Heather type is usually childlike, and may even speak in a somewhat childish voice, they can also begin to seem a bit desperate and, in a strange way, older than they really are while they are still very young chronologically. They can seem world-weary, as if they have already written the unhappy ending for each new relationship in their own minds, even when it has just begun. In earlier days, that same Heather type would have entered each relationship believing that this could be "the one," and that all would be made right in the world once he or she connected with their new potential partner. But with time and disappointment, this early naïve emotional state is replaced by a more cynical outlook. Thus, the Heather state is, like all the other Bach states, a continuum. Some Heather types may be very open emotionally and very upbeat. Others can seem permanently wounded and, while still open to possibility and quite needy, very negative in their expectations.

The key to understanding Heather types is that they are deeply, deeply lonely. Heather types are like the twins who were separated at birth that we see on talk shows, who spend years knowing that something is profoundly missing in their lives, but not knowing what, until, one day, they are told about their twin or they find their twin quite my accident. And then it all makes sense—the loneliness, the sense of loss that could not be explained. Heather types share this sense of loss and of loneliness that makes them feel as if something has been ripped away. Perhaps the Heather state is created by the loss of love at an early age. It certainly is one of our states in which the patient seems to have frozen in time at an early age. Perhaps it is caused by a lack of approval from a beloved parent or from a lack of nurturing while young. While the cause may be unclear, the fact that the patient feels unloved and unappreciated and has decided to do something about it is quite clear. Where the Water Violet type shares the Heather type's deep loneliness but adapts a strategy of independence and emotional aloofness as a means of coping, the Heather takes quite the opposite strategy. He

---

3. The fear of desertion runs deep in Heather types. This can hardly be surprising since they are motivated by a desire to never be alone. Heather types will attempt charm, threats, and even suicide to keep from being left alone once they have connected, however briefly or shallowly, with another person.

becomes extremely aggressive in his search for his missing half and for his solution to his sense of loneliness and loss.

Is it surprising then, that Heather types can be quite unrelenting in their need for attention? They can be downright annoying when you are trying to have a serious conversation with someone else or trying to enjoy a quiet dinner with a friend. If you are intruded upon by an aggressive Heather type—who will do anything short of setting his hair on fire to get your attention—you just have to remember that his behavior is yet another negative emotional state common to us all. It is something that you yourself have been guilty of, to a lesser or greater degree. In other words, try to be compassionate when confronted (and that is the word) with a Heather type.

Perhaps in combination, Heather works best with Chicory. Indeed, the line between these two distinct emotional states can be blurry at times. The Heather state often evolves into a Chicory state over time. Once the patient who demands attention and wants never to be alone manages to form anything that could be called a family, he or she will often rule that family with an emotional iron fist. The patient who, in her Heather state, feels that she is the child who was not loved enough by her mother, can, in the Chicory state, become the mother whose love must be both earned and obeyed. And the moment that the Heather finds that her love object is pulling away, or suspects that desertion is imminent, is the moment when the self-centered Heather type can take on the pattern of emotional control consistent with the self-obsessed Chicory. Thus, these two remedies work well together and are often needed, either concurrently or one following the other (usually, use Heather first) in order to balance the patient's emotional state. Sometimes you will also have to include the remedy Sweet Chestnut, for the patient who is high strung and who loses control when faced with what she perceives as desertion.

In cases where the patient is less emotionally destructive, if no less annoying, vanity is often the chief emotional attribute of the Heather type. If the patient is almost outrageously vain, if they behave as the coquette, the combination of Heather and Honeysuckle can help. This blend helps those who are wildly emotional and nostalgic, almost sickly sweet in their appreciation of a flower or a box of chocolates. For the patient who seems to be obsessed with self, with his appearance and ability to charm others, especially those of the opposite sex, combine Heather with White Chestnut to give the patient a chance to think about something other than himself for a change.

If the patient is very aggressive in his emotional demands or unrelenting in his behavior to the point that you find yourself wanting to shoot him with a tranquilizer dart, consider adding Vervain to the Heather. Add Cerato to the mix if you don't think one dart would be enough to slow him down. All three of these remedy types can be extremely extroverted. All these, and Centaury and Agrimony, can seem to be "on" and will make bids for attention. All five of these remedies mix well, just as all can work well singly, but I usually would not use more than three at a time to avoid clouding the issue with too many different remedies on the same theme. Note that Heather and Agrimony are often used in combination for those who are using alcohol or drugs to fuel their sense of goodwill and their extraverted behavior.

In the acute context, we all could use a jolt of Heather on a regular basis. Think of this remedy any time your ego is wounded, any time you think you are not getting the attention or recognition you deserve. Any time you find yourself "acting like a big baby." Take Heather when you are feeling left out of a situation and find yourself pushing your way in. When you are just plain talking too much, take Heather. And when you are feeling lonely, and out of sync with others, especially if you find yourself the odd man out at a party, or when you are in a crowd of strangers at a business convention, politely excuse yourself, go to the bathroom and take Heather. Then don't come out until you feel that you won't do or say anything you will regret later.

## Negative Qualities of the Type

The Heather type is selfish, period. He lives in a state of wounded ego and is, therefore, constantly needy. Because of the wounds to his ego, he overcompensates with feelings of vanity, whether they are earned or not. He feels out of touch with others and quite lonely, so he overcompensates with aggressive and intrusive behavior. The Heather type who does not receive enough attention, or who does not receive it quickly enough, or for a long enough time, or from the source that he desired, will continue to up the ante to get the full attention of another person. He crowds people, overwhelms others with his energy output as he seeks attention. He cannot bear to be alone. These are individuals with wounded egos, who need constant support to feel loved and appreciated.

Because of this, because his focus in life is in satisfying his need to be loved and wanted (especially wanted), and because his own behavior makes this less likely to happen, the Heather type leads a life that is limited by his own motivations and behaviors. Because he places so much effort in one area of his life, he tends not to achieve the success that he could in any other area. Certainly, like the rest of us, the Heather type wants both balance and success in all aspects of life. But that balance eludes him just as his search for emotional connection often yields unsatisfying results.

Heather types who are mired in a state of destructive thought and behavior seem very negative people. They are quite often those who others simply avoid, especially those who have already experienced their emotional blackmail. For this reason, they often go underrated, as workers, students, and emotional partners. Sadly, this is because the Heather type often fails to show others just how much he does have to offer. Instead he projects himself to be both needy and childishly naïve and demanding.

## Positive Qualities of the Type

The patient who has moved into a positive Heather emotional state has dealt with the wounds his ego has received over the years, and with his need for attention, his feelings of vanity or low self-esteem, and his deep sense of loneliness. In short, the positive Heather is a fully matured adult. Finally, in his state of emotional balance, he is aware of his own needs and the needs of others, and he has learned to give, as well as take. He can freely give his full attention and his love and life energy to others, should it be needed. Positive Heather types are vibrant, strong individuals who are good listeners and have a wonderful gift for drawing other people out of their shells and making them feel good about themselves.

## The Heather Child

This is perhaps our most common negative emotional state for children. In fact, it may even be considered a normal state and not a negative emotional pattern for children of a very young age. Very young children, who must depend upon their parents for everything in life, naturally will demand attention when they need it or want it. But as a child grows beyond this early stage, he most often will develop beyond this early, grasping need for attention.

The child who continues with the early pattern of demanding attention well beyond the age for which it is appropriate is a Heather child. This is a whiny child. A child who clings to his mother's skirt and demands full parental attention anywhere and any time. They demand attention while their mother attempts to shop at the grocery store. They cannot bear for mother to talk on the telephone, or father to watch a football game on television.

The Heather child will become obsessed with his body and with what is wrong with it if he has been injured or has become ill. He will spend a good deal of time telling others exactly what his symptoms are. Like Heather adults, Heather children talk too much, and talk only about themselves. Like Heather adults, they can be very vain, and will certainly demand that they are the center of everyone's attention, whether it is appropriate or not.

The Heather child can be disruptive in school. Here, too, he will need to be the center of attention and will be nearly inexhaustible in his demands that he be stroked and petted. The Heather child soon decides that negative attention is better than no attention at all, and will continually up his ante of attention-getting behaviors, good or bad. Often he will become the class clown to get and keep the focus of the classroom.

## The Heather Adult

No one talks as much as Heather types of any age. They are endlessly fascinated with their own lives, with their own troubles, heartaches, and illnesses. It never quite occurs to them that others have experienced similar things, or that others may also want to speak. Heathers feel that they will almost cease to exist, at least as far as other people are concerned, if they sit quietly.

Heather types love attention, love to be physically touched and patted. They love to be reminded of just how good they look, how great they are, and they are not above putting the words into other people's mouths, if that is the only way they can get them to say them.

As I have noted above, the Heather state is naturally a state of youth. It contains many of the emotional highs and lows and follies of youth. Heather becomes an increasingly desperate and cynical state when it lingers into adulthood and middle age. Adult Heather types are often given to having both sides of a conversation at once, either in their own heads or out loud. The presence of the other person becomes, over time, a necessary evil. But the Heather already knows how the relationship will end, and what the other person is thinking. This, of course, is a matter of perception for the Heather. He may or may not have a real knowledge of the other person. But, again, it really matters very little whether the Heather type is on target or not, since he doesn't really care what the other person is thinking. Only what he perceives them to be thinking is important.

As I have noted above, the Heather state is one that I believe, over time, develops into other states, often the Chicory state of controlling false love or the bitter Willow state. Heather types can also drift into a Wild Oat state, usually fuelled by alcohol or drugs, in which they perceive life and all its aspects to be meaningless and their hope for love to be futile, like everything else.

The Heather state does sometimes re-appear in elderly patients, who can achieve both an almost incredible state of vanity and an uncontrollable willingness to intrude upon others and demand attention at any given moment. These Heather types will have even less ability to rein themselves in emotionally than other, younger Heather types. They will place their desire for company above all else, and will do almost anything to get it.

### The Heather Animal

This remedy can be extremely helpful to owners of demanding animals. Animals of any sort that simply demand attention, or who, by their behavior, place themselves at the center of the household, making everyone in it constantly aware of their needs and wants.

### Heather and the Homeopathic Pharmacy

Is there a homeopathic type that is more emotionally demanding than a Pulsatilla? Or one that is more capable of moods that roll upward and downward like a roller-coaster?

Pulsatilla is a remedy that is taken from the "wind flower," and the Pulsatilla type is buffeted by her own emotions like a little flower buffeted by the wind. Often those who are near the Pulsatilla don't know what they said or did to make the Pulsatilla cry, or laugh, or suddenly jump into their lap. Like Heather types, Pulsatilla types want attention and love physical contact.

### Issues that Suggest Heather

Aging; alcoholism; allergies; drug addiction; hay fever; deafness; immune dysfunction; skin conditions; psychosomatic ailments.

### In Conclusion

One final note: Be aware that people of all ages who are just going into therapy, or are becoming a part of any psychological, spiritual, or therapeutic group that requires that they face themselves and their patterns of thought and behavior can often lock themselves into a Heather pattern of behavior for a time. It can also be common for those who are in recovery for substance abuse or are facing aspects of addictive behavior in their lives.

After all, one of our most valuable therapeutic tools is talk. If we encourage patients to talk about their thoughts and feelings to work through old patterns and establish new ones, can we then blame them if they have trouble knowing when to stop talking?

We often become very self-obsessed in our excitement when we are first discovering ourselves or are first discovering a valuable new pathway to self-understanding and forgiveness. And in this state of obsession, we often talk too much about ourselves and just plain talk too much. This is something that everyone, therapists, patients and family and friends alike, must be aware of and willing and able to endure for a time so the patient can work through all the stages of their emotional or spiritual healing and move into a healthier state of being.

All healing, after all, is a process, and a rather sloppy process at that. The Heather state of behavior is very common and is perhaps necessary for those who pass through it on their way to recovery.

## IMPATIENS · THE REMEDY FOR THOSE WHO ARE IMPATIENT

Bach notes that Impatiens "wishes all things to be done without hesitation or delay. When ill they are anxious for a hasty recovery. They find it very difficult to be patient with people who are slow, as they consider it wrong and a waste of time, and they will endeavor to make such people quicker in all ways. They often prefer to work and think alone, so that they can do everything at their own speed."

• While Impatiens is more often needed constitutionally, it does have acute applications as well.

• Impatiens is a component in Rescue Remedy.

• Impatiens is one of Bach's original remedies, the Twelve Healers.

### Botanical Information

Also known as "ornamental jewelweed" and "policeman's helmet," impatiens (*Impatiens Glandulifera*) is an annual flower that is grown for its color and for its ease of care.

It is grown throughout the British Isles (its nickname of "policeman's helmet" came about because the shape of its flowers resembles the British policeman's helmet of the 1950s) and is particularly prized in Ireland, where it grows in profusion. Impatiens is actually native to the Himalayas and is also known as "Himalayan Balsam." In a natural setting it can be found growing along riverbeds throughout Europe.

Today, it can also be found in gardens throughout the world. It grows in thick clumps and each plant can quickly sprout many branches. It needs to be held in check in the garden, as it can be highly invasive. In some parts of the world, it has escaped cultivation and become an invasive weed. For this reason, it is often planted in container gardens and on porches and walkways.

Impatiens prefers to grow in sun to part shade. It flowers throughout the summer. Its flowers appear in a number of different colors from white to pink to purple.

### Impatiens in General

It would literally kill any constitutional Impatiens type to know that this remedy is listed last of the thirty-eight remedies described in these pages, especially if the Impatiens was expected to read the other thirty-seven first. Impatiens types flip through the pages of books to find out who "done" it. They read with their eyes jumping from line to line, thought to thought, and not word by word and, in the process, they often miss key pieces of information. They spend most of their time, in their minds at least, waiting. Impatiens types feel as if the rest of the world and time itself is moving too slowly, crawling along while they race ahead. They are natural scouts, racing in front of the mass of humanity to see what is beyond the horizon. Because Impatiens types have a distorted sense of time,[4] they tend to be restless, often bored, and, worst of all from the viewpoint of others, quite irritable.

---

4. Here's a very simple test to illustrate the Impatiens type's sense of time. Sit them down and hold a watch in your hand. Ask them to tell you, without checking their own watch, when three minutes have passed. Most Impatiens types won't get past a minute and a half before they are quite sure that three have passed. Watch the Impatiens type's face while the test is underway. The look of total concentration and, quite likely, agony on his face is a dead giveaway.

Impatiens types have a personal sense of time that is out of whack with reality. Impatiens types are forever living just a few seconds ahead of the rest of us. And while this can be an excellent skill if you are appearing on *Jeopardy,* it can be a distinct handicap anywhere else. Impatiens types see things quickly and target the details within the landscape faster than most. They assess situations quickly and make swift judgments as to any action required. Their minds race ahead of the moment in which they are living. They are quick to solve problems, and quick to finish tasks. Most often they have a good deal of anger around this particular issue, and feel that others should pick up their speed to match their own. They feel they are most often required to do more work than others simply because they capable of working faster without sacrificing quality. In fact, most Impatiens types prefer to work swiftly and would feel punished if they were forced to slow down. So they feel strongly that others need to speed up and they should neither be forced to slow down or do more work than others. For this reason, Impatiens is best working alone. At times Impatiens are overly critical, especially when it comes to how swiftly others can learn and make use of what they have learned. They tend to judge others in this context and to believe that others are lazy or unwilling if they can't keep up. They also find it hard to believe that others couldn't move more quickly if they would only try. At times they are downright rude if other people don't get the point or finish the task quickly enough to suit the Impatiens.

In his irritated state, the Impatiens type can talk down to others, letting them know quite clearly that he feels they are just not that bright. In the same way, the Impatiens type will be given to overexplaining his ideas, and will tend to make sure that he has repeated his major points at least twice, so that the slower listeners will be able to keep up. The Impatiens type will very often fail to understand that his behavior is somewhat demeaning to the listener and that he has insulted others with both his method of speaking and with his general demeanor.

Because of this, the Impatiens type can be difficult to deal with when he is in any position of authority. He will tend to tell everyone exactly what to do and how to do it, and, more often than not, will end up doing it himself, because that is what he really wanted to do to begin with. Remember, a key to understanding the Impatiens type is that he wants to work alone and, in truth, he does work better alone. He is suited to tasks in which he can put his inner passion to work without being observed or restricted in any way. Where it is the quality of the finished product that is important. By his very nature, the Impatiens type neither wants to be in charge of others or have others in charge of him. Unlike the Vine type, who is deeply attracted by the notion of being in charge, the Impatiens type values personal freedom above all else, in both work and personal relationships. If this can be understood and respected, then all is well. If a boss or a partner of any sort fails to understand this basic tenet of life, then it is only a matter of time before the Impatiens type will move on, often very disruptively.

Often, just as Impatiens types want to work alone, they will want to live alone as well. They can feel crowded very easily. And they cannot bear the feeling that they are impeded in any way. Therefore, they are slow to marry, although they may be perfectly happy with the relationship. The restrictions implied in the actual act of marriage may be more than they can bear. In the same way, they may demand separate bedrooms throughout their lives, no matter how happily they are married. Given that the Impatiens type often has chronic issues with sleep (more on this later), and are highly sensitive on the subject of sleep, they may not be able to sleep in the same room with anyone else. Even as children, Impatiens types may have tremendous difficulty working or playing with others ("Does not play well with others" will be a common comment on their report cards) and an even harder time sharing his personal space.

It is safe to say, therefore, that Impatiens types are somewhat misunderstood by those with whom they come into contact. They are often considered to be more difficult than they truly are, especially if those in partnership with or authority over them do not understand that, above all else, Impatiens types pretty much would prefer to be left alone. This is not to say that they never want human contact—they can most certainly be charming hosts and loving members of the family—but that they want it on their own terms. And those who care for them must understand that Impatiens types, unlike many others, tend to see themselves as individuals first, as "solo creatures" within their societal groups.

What others may fail to understand is that the Impatiens, like the other types in this group, is a prisoner in his own state of loneliness. As with the Water Violet and the Heather types, the Impatiens type feels cut off from others and his natural sense of community is both conflicted and tenuous at best. In the case of either the Water Violet or the Heather, the patient needing the remedy has experienced a severing of his ties to others. Often, the Water Violet has experienced a literal loss, through the death of a loved one or the rupturing of a deep relationship. And the Heather type has commonly experienced a lack of nurturing in childhood and has stayed emotionally frozen at the stage of life in which he experienced his loss of nurturing love. Either way, the patient knows full well that they are lonelier than others, and adapts a behavior—independent aloofness for the Water Violet, invasive demands for attention for the Heather—by which they might cope with their feelings of loneliness. In other words, these patients are actually motivated by their loneliness.

With the Impatiens type, something very different is happening.

The loneliness experienced by the Impatiens type has a very different quality from that of the other two types associated with this mood. It is the result of the Impatiens type's own way of thinking, instead of being the result of a specific trauma or a link to any stage of childhood development. Of all of Bach's types, the Impatiens type seems perhaps the most constitutional. It can have acute applications, for those times in all our lives when we are feeling just plain impatient with those around us or with our present set of circumstances, when we yearn for change that does not occur as quickly as we think it should, and, as a result, become difficult to deal with or just plain angry. More commonly, however, if you need Impatiens, you need it constitutionally, and have for some time and will for some time ahead.

The loneliness of the Impatiens type seems linked to the Impatiens type himself and the way his brain is wired. This is a quick intellect and, therefore, a restless one. The Impatiens type thinks well on his feet, and is very quick verbally as well. This can manifest itself in wit, or in sarcasm, or in criticism. They are very quick to see the flaws in plans and to criticize those flaws. They will quickly assess, judge, and dismiss the thoughts of others, and then will turn to all assembled with an expression on their face that says, "Next?"

> The Impatiens type thinks well on his feet, and is very quick verbally as well. This can manifest itself in wit, or in sarcasm, or in criticism. They are very quick to see the flaws in plans and to criticize those flaws.

There is no single trauma that results in the Impatiens state. Indeed, it differs from the other Bach types in that it is not the result of any negative emotional state at all. The emotional state that presents itself in irritation and, commonly, a somewhat overbearing and know-it-all attitude is instead the result of a mental state. The Impatiens patient's mind, for whatever reason, runs faster and sometimes better (although the Impatiens type's speed manages to trip him up in foolish mistakes that others, thinking more slowly, would very easily catch) than do others, and his inability and disinterest in slowing down is a great source of frustration. If anything, the emotion the Impatiens type most commonly displays is intense frustration, which is the source of their irritation and cynicism.

The Impatiens type is forever frustrated. Frustrated with himself, and highly self-critical (as he tends to demand more of himself than he does of others) whenever he makes any sort of mistake or performs under the level of his capability. Frustrated with everyone else, especially when he feels they are moving or thinking too slowly. And frustrated with inanimate objects. When the Impatiens type gets frustrated, he tends to throw inanimate objects, or to become very sure that they are "out to get him." Because his mind races ahead, missing details, and skipping steps, he often misplaces things and blames others for moving or taken them, only to find them months later. Because his mental focus often does not match its speed, his memory can be surprisingly poor and scatter-shot.

Often the Impatiens will come across looking more intelligent than he actually is. Others are often intimidated by what they perceive to be a razor sharp intellect because he thinks and answers back so quickly, only to be disappointed by him again and again as he makes (and repeats) foolish mistakes. (Chestnut Bud can often be a remedy to help Impatiens types focus in more and learn from their mistakes.)

His scattershot speed can affect his physical body as well, undermining his health as it does his emotional balance and intellectual accomplishments.

For instance, along with White Chestnut, Impatiens is our best remedy for insomnia. The White Chestnut type will not be able to sleep because his mind is fixated on specific and often tormenting thoughts while his body is very tired, where the Impatiens type is wired. It is as if he has had several cups of strong coffee. The Impatiens type may, therefore, have trouble quieting both his mind and his body so he can sleep. He will often walk the floors at night, or give up and go down to the kitchen for some food. Often, Impatiens types will get into a pattern of behavior in which they must eat to adjust their blood sugar before they go to bed.

Or, like children who do not want to sleep, Impatiens types will become involved in books and read long into the night, or will prowl the Internet or watch old movies on television. The White Chestnut, the other type known for insomnia, suffers more from his insomnia because he is trapped in a cycle of thoughts and regrets that torment him. The Impatiens type tends to accept his insomnia more cheerfully. He will tend to think of it as just another way he is different from everyone else. He may also just decide, over time, that he will only sleep four or five hours a night and will spend the rest of the time working.

Just as the Impatiens type is given to insomnia, he tends to suffer from hypertension and can develop serious heart conditions as well. Like the White Chestnut, the Aspen, and the Vervain types, the Impatiens type seems to live life a little harder and drives himself into serious illnesses at an earlier age than most. Where the Oak type will wear himself out slowly and steadily, the Vervain, the Aspen, and the Impatiens types especially will wear themselves down sooner. They seem to live their lives at a faster pitch, as if they were vibrating faster than anyone else. Whatever the core cause, Aspen's anxiety, Vervain's intensity, and Impatiens' sheer speed and irritability are not without consequences.

The Impatiens type tends to suffer from chronic pains of all sorts. In fact, the remedy is so helpful for those who feel pain that this is the reason that Bach included it in his Rescue Remedy mix. Impatiens is a remedy to consider in any case that involves pain, whether acute, like toothache (combine it with Vervain for the patient who is frantic from tooth pain) or chronic. Impatiens types are given to all sorts of muscle aches and pains, and to chronic tightness of their muscles. They tend to respond well to massage and to acupuncture treatments, both of which help them relax.

Obviously, Impatiens types will find a great deal of benefit from any sort of therapy that leads to relaxation. They do very well with yoga and dance, or any other sort of physical therapy that stresses breathing as a form of relaxation. Just listening to calm music can have a profound effect on any Impatiens types. They are also highly sensitive to colors (again, as are Vervain types) and should be, whenever possible, surrounded by calming things.

White Chestnut[5] and Vervain are perhaps the most common among the remedies that are most often used in conjunction with Impatiens. But Impatiens and Scleranthus are also an excellent blend. Think of this combination for patients who are high-strung and unstable. For patients with highly unpredictable behaviors who are capable of very high highs and very low lows.

In acute circumstances, think of Impatiens first and foremost as our most valuable pain remedy. For any sort of situation in which there is sudden pain, such as injury or toothache. Also think of it for those times when you are very nervous and therefore not thinking clearly, such as the moments before public speaking or taking an important test. Think of this remedy as one that can help you to meet any deadline with a minimum of stress or fuss, especially those deadlines of any sort that can get you so worked up that you can't find your car keys. Or situations in which you are so frustrated that you want to throw those car keys. Impatiens will help.

## Negative Qualities of the Type

The negative Impatiens type is isolated by the fact that they live their lives slightly in the future, while others are living in the present. They are isolated by their own speed of thought and speech. Others may respect or even be intimidated by them, but they do not particularly like them, especially if they are forced to work with them. The negative Impatiens type is an iconic slave driver for whom no one can work quickly enough or effectively enough. They are harsh critics. Because they are driven by a sense of frustration with nearly everything in their environment, they can be irritable nearly all the time, often without apparent reason. This leads those around them to wonder "What are they angry about now?"

The negative Impatiens is also given to bouts of exhaustion and sudden hunger because they are burning energy with the same speed that they are thinking and working. In the same way, they can be given to sudden emotional or mental breakdowns or to physical complaints that suddenly appear with great severity.

## Positive Qualities of the Type

The irony of the negative Impatiens emotional state is that the Impatiens type, who is fixated on achievement and independence and very proud of his speedy intellect, quite

---

5. Personally, I find White Chestnut and Impatiens combined to be perhaps the best mixture of Bach remedies available. I use them together so often that they have become one remedy in my mind. I think of them as my personal "rescue remedy."

often does not understand that the speed that he so prizes causes him to be erratic and actually limits his abilities. Because the Impatiens prizes speed over skill, he can be clumsy, both physically and mentally, and destructive emotionally. He may fail to see the destruction he leaves in his wake or to fully understand why those who agreed to work with him once will refuse to do so again.

If the Impatiens type can make the transformation from negative to positive, he does, indeed, have to learn to slow down a bit. Just a bit. But, in doing so, his keen intellect has the chance to move with a bit more care and to see the details that once were so easily missed. Thus, the Impatiens type who finds a positive emotional pattern and learns to slow down a bit and balance his emotional energy is capable of accomplishing much more, and of greater quality, than he could before.

While positive Impatiens types tend to remain strongly independent, they are also patient people. While they still maintain their speedy intellect, they are able to finally understand that this is a gift that they own and other people do not. Therefore, they are able to happily wait for others to catch up, while still enjoying their own abilities to the fullest. They become gentle, where once they had been irritable and rude.

Perhaps most important, positive Impatiens types learn to live "in the moment," and, in doing so, fully integrate themselves into their lives. They become aware of their bodies in a manner that lets them know when to work and when to rest. They become aware of the world around them and of the other beings in it, giving them increased compassion for those they love. They become fully capable of interacting with others, and, finally, of being able to look another person directly in the eye and stay completely connected with them, without projecting their mind to other places, other times. As such, they are finally capable of actually living their lives instead of rushing through them.

### The Impatiens Child

I am not sure just when in childhood the Impatiens state first shows itself, just as I am not sure if there is any emotional trauma or wound that is the basis for Impatiens behavior patterns. But I do know that there is such a thing as an Impatiens child and that he or she will exhibit a predictable set of behavior patterns.

The Impatiens child becomes bored faster with any school lesson, toy, or movie than any other child. They will add anger to their boredom if the source of their mood is not removed and some new interest brought forth. They tend to also become bored with people, especially with their friends, moving on to new friendships very quickly. They are excitable and restless children who need to find their calm center and learn the regular pace of life that is both healthful and workable for the average person.

It is important to note that, even as children, Impatiens types tend to drain themselves of their vital force, especially when frustrated or irritated. In other words, they do not spend interest in reaction to stress, but instead spend principal. They will drain themselves of life energy and will not stop to rest until their reserves are exhausted. This means that parents are likely to find their Impatiens child running from room to room. Later, when they suddenly realize they haven't seen them in a while and go looking for them, they find them asleep under a table or on the couch, having exhausted themselves so much they don't make it to their bed before collapsing. Impatiens children (and adults) who are not taught the lesson of balancing their energy and resting when they need to will often exhaust themselves into illness.

In the same vein, let me also note that Impatiens children will not want to be sent to bed. They see bed and sleep as a sort of punishment. They want to be where the fun is, where the excitement is. They will fight sleep until they are so exhausted that they can fight it no more.

Impatiens blends well with the remedy Vervain for the child who is high-strung and hyperactive. It can also be used in conjunction with Vine for the child who is aggressive with other children. Often Impatiens and Aspen are very successful in the treatment of children who are both high-strung and highly sensitive. Impatiens/Aspen children will have nightmares. They will motivate their hyperactivity from a place of anxiety and will overreact to any negative emotions or insecurities in the household.

Acutely, use Impatiens for the child who is throwing one of those embarrassing fits or temper tantrums in a public place. It will quiet the child quite quickly and allow him to behave more reasonably.

### The Impatiens Adult

There is no specific stage of life that is more common to the Impatiens type than any other, but it often links a bit more to youth and young adulthood than to middle age and beyond. In the same way, while I cannot say that it is a man's remedy, it is perhaps found a bit more often in men than in women. What is important in understanding the remedy type is the fact that once the Impatiens state is set in place, it is a long-term pattern. Just as there is no specific trauma or stressor that can be identified as the "cause" of the pattern of impatience and frustration, there is no set method for its removal. It is, therefore, one of our true constitutional Bach remedies.

Time is the great enemy of the Impatiens adult. Time is perceived by the Impatiens adult as a hindrance at best and a choking harness at worst, not just in the ongoing war between time and self in the daily struggle for getting things done, but also on a spiritual and emotional level. The Impatiens adult needs *gentling*. He needs to stop and listen to his or her own heartbeat, to learn the pace at which we are meant to live our lives. In the same way, he needs to learn to be more gentle with others. The Impatiens type's frustration is the enemy of all that is calm and gentle. Therefore, the Impatiens type must learn to calm down if he is ever going to achieve all he wishes to in life. He must face the fact that he will have to slow down if he is to blend in with the rest of society. He needs to realize that slowing down is, in reality, a new gift—a new ability—not just a sacrifice of his old methods and what he sees as his greatest gift: his speed.

## The Impatiens Animal

This is a great remedy for animals that are just plain uncooperative, especially when they are irritable as well. It combines well with Vervain for high-strung animals with unpredictable behavior. Consider Impatiens for animals that are hard to train, that have a great deal of energy to spare and that tend to dominate other animals and any humans they do not respect.

## Impatiens and the Homeopathic Pharmacy

While the remedy Lycopodium, with its need to succeed, comes to mind when considering a homeopathic parallel to Impatiens, the remedy Lachesis, perhaps the most intelligent homeopathic type, comes closer to matching the Impatiens type's sheer speed of thought, action, and speech. Like Impatiens, Lachesis can seem arrogant and can become very unpopular through their natural gifts for speed. Also like Impatiens, Lachesis speaks quickly and at great length.

## Issues that Suggest Impatiens

Abuse; anger; cramps; eating disorders; fatigue; irritable bowel syndrome; headaches; hypertension; infections; insomnia; itching; low blood sugar; migraines; muscle aches and pains; muscular dystrophy; rashes (especially those that itch) and other chronic skin conditions; twitches and tics.

## In Conclusion

I have not yet mentioned the physical clumsiness of the Impatiens type. Because they tend to rush ahead, often without thinking (making this one of our remedies for impulsive types), Impatiens types often have the tendency to trip over their own two feet. Once again, this is because they tend not to be fully present in their own lives. Because they rush ahead in their minds to what will be happening in a few seconds, because they are restless to the point of never being content to live life now, they often miss things—details, like the flight of steps right in front of them.

For this reason Impatiens types are prone to injury. They will often injure themselves because they are not paying full attention to what they are doing. Or they get very frustrated with an object and throw it, smash it, or hit it, and, in doing so, injure themselves.

This carries over into other aspects of life. It should come as no surprise that Impatiens types have a strong connection with physical speed. This can be embodied in two ways. Some Impatiens types—fewer in number than the other group—are actually afraid of speed. Because they are speeding so much internally, they greatly respect phys-ical speed. Therefore, they will become terrified if they are being driven at a high speed, and will actually be rather slow and cautious drivers when behind the wheel.

These Impatiens types will often comment that they feel as if they are flying up or out of control when they move swiftly. They will say that they feel as if the car will leave the ground and crash when they are in a speeding car.

More common are the Impatiens types who love both speed and thrills. They will drive fast, and, given their level of concentration, will be prone to accidents. Because of their fast reaction time, they will tend to feel rather invulnerable behind the wheel and will count on the speed of their reactions to keep them safe. Then they will be caught not paying enough attention to the task at hand and will have an accident.

This sort of Impatiens type will love the fast rides at the amusement park. He will love high speeds in anything, and may be addicted to video games that involve fast reactions.

This sort of Impatiens type will also be prone to road rage, and will take his full frustration out on anyone who is unwilling or unable to travel at a speed that is fast enough for him. Other drivers will want to stay out of his way and hope that he passes them by before he gets angry or careless.

Others may find themselves getting out of the way of the Impatiens type in other situations as well. The fact that the Impatiens type has not learned how to be gentle robs him of the ability to be at peace with others (either physically with inanimate objects or small pets, or emotionally with anyone other than another Impatiens, with whom he can share his restless viewpoint). Those who know his explosive frustra-tion—road rage or otherwise—are wary of him and avoid him.

I cannot emphasize enough that the price the Impatiens type pays for the way he lives his life is loneliness. And while the Impatiens type may happily accept this as a trade-off for his restless exploration of life, the core loneliness of the Impatiens type is caused by the fact that he is either unwilling or unable to have his own mind and body live fully in the moment in which he is alive. He robs himself of being able to fully understand anything other than himself by not making real contact with the world around him. Therefore, the loneliness of the Impatiens type is deeper than that of the other remedies.

# PART THREE

# Using the Bach Flower Remedies

*"The patient of tomorrow must understand that he, and he alone can bring himself relief from suffering, though he may obtain advice and help from an elder brother who will assist him in his effort.*

*"In the future there will be no pride in being ill: on the contrary, people will be as ashamed of sickness as they should be of crime."*

—EDWARD BACH

# 11

## Taking Cases

If I were writing strictly about homeopathy in these pages, I would just state the "three laws of cure" as Samuel Hahnemann developed them and, in doing so, give you a solid basis for the use of the remedies. All homeopathic treatments follow the same pattern: remedies are given singly, in the lowest possible effective potency, and with the fewest number of effective doses. And the remedy selected for use is chosen by virtue of the fact that it, in its full range of actions, most closely mirrors the physical, emotional, and mental symptoms that the patient is experiencing because of his disease.

In the same way, homeopathic philosophy teaches us that the goal of our treatment should be concurrent with the patient's needs. Which is to say that a simple acute treatment carries with it the goal of restoring the patient to the same level of health that he enjoyed before the onset of his condition. Thus, the patient who is given a remedy because he is suffering from that cluster of symptoms we call as common cold will, at the end of the treatment, be left in the same condition that he was in before the cold. Any other more chronic conditions, such as sciatica, will be left untouched by the treatment.

The practitioner who is working more deeply, who is giving the patient a constitutional treatment, is working toward another goal. Constitutional treatments always carry with them the goal of substantially changing the patient's health for the better, on a more or less permanent basis. Constitutional treatments (and constitutional remedies) are those that touch on every aspect of the patient's life and being, and affect, quite literally, every cell in his body. Just as acute treatments are selected on the basis of a range of symptoms, body, mind, and spirit, objective and subjective, constitutional treatments take into account all of the patient's symptoms, positive, negative, or benign. But here the net is cast wider. The practitioner who is giving an acute remedy often has to work swiftly. Therefore he will not need a full medical history before treating the patient who has cut his knee on the playground. The practitioner who is considering a constitutional treatment must be much more thorough by virtue of the changes that treatment may potentially cause. A full medical history will be taken. And the case taking itself—the gathering of the symptoms and the selecting of an appropriate remedy—will be a complex thing.

Many homeopaths will dedicate two or more hours to a complete case taking. Some will also require some of the same medical tests that allopaths will, to identify the patient's disease state. In addition to this, the homeopath will have to spend several hours refining the symptoms, identifying which are most important to resolving the case, and selecting one remedy, from the more than five thousand available to him, that is the single best choice for the patient. In homeopathic practice, this remedy is called the "Simillimum." It is what every homeopath searches for in the service of his patient—the exact right remedy in the exact right potency and the exact right number of doses.[1]

Part of Edward Bach's conscious rebellion from what he saw as the overly complex practice of homeopathic medicine involved a complete simplification of the process of case taking. In the same way, he both streamlined and simplified the goals of treatment. For Bach, the goal is always the same: the healing of the patient.

This runs parallel to Hahnemann's goal of treatment: the curing of the patient. And I think it is important that we take a moment to consider the difference.

## Bach Vs. Hahnemann

On the very first page of his great work on the subject of medicine and homeopathy called *The Organon of Medicine*, Samuel Hahnemann writes that "The physician's highest and *only* calling is to make the sick healthy, to cure, as it is called." In this simple statement, he establishes a format for the practice of medicine that is quite in opposition with the one that Bach developed in his lifetime of work.

The difference between the goals of homeopathic and Bach treatments is the difference between the viewpoints of the two men who developed them. Hahnemann, for all his creative foresight and revolutionary zeal, still held with the allopathic notion that the doctor could somehow cure his patient, while Bach moved a step to the side and offered the same patient the possibility of curing himself instead.

This difference is widened by the way in which each system of medicine viewed the patient himself and his very nature. And, especially by the way each doctor would define illness itself.

1. Homeopathic treatments may also move even deeper than the constitutional. Miasmic treatments, which help the patient overcome his or her predisposition to a particular disease or diseases, can be truly transformational and can offer the patient a life free from chronic illness. The word "miasm" means taint. The goal of miasmic treatment is to remove the taint of illness from the patient in total: in body, mind, and spirit. Therefore, miasmic treatments are the most complex and require a homeopath of some skill to be resolved completely.

To begin with the radical concept of cure, we need to go all the way back to the beginning of medicine as we know it, to the ancient cultures of Western civilization.[2]

> The difference between the goals of homeopathic and Bach treatments is the difference between the viewpoints of the two men who developed them. Hahnemann still held with the allopathic notion that the doctor could somehow cure his patient, while Bach offered the same patient the possibility of curing himself instead.

The idea of medicine, after all, is not innate to mankind. At some point in prehistoric times, some individual had to come to the conclusion that a dynamic intervention between the suffering of the patient and his hoped-for recovery could take place using the tools at hand—a blend of herbs, teas, or poultices of some sort most likely. Until that time, life, death, suffering, and recovery were left in the hands of fate or of God, depending upon the viewpoint of the patient. Since that time, we have not only had to take the responsibility for discovering and refining those products we call "medicinal," because of their ability to interfere with the disease process, and for the development of systems of practice by which those medicines can be used to their best advantage. Part of this process has to do with making drugs both safe and effective. On this aspect of medical treatment, I believe that Hahnemann and Bach are in total agreement. Both believed that medicine must always be benign. For this reason, each sought methods by which the drugs in their pharmacy were completely safe, offering the patient a pathway back to health that could never complicate his case or cause him harm.[3]

Bach and Hahnemann, however, would differ on another aspect of medical practice—the way in which the patient himself is considered as a being. Allopathy, homeopathy, and Bach treatments each have a single definition, if that is the word, for the patient's own state of being, and how the patient should be considered as a being in terms of treatment.

Before the development of what we now call allopathic medicine in ancient

2. Please don't think for a moment that I believe that Western civilization is solely responsible for medicine by this. By ignoring the concepts of curing and healing the sick in the rest of human civilization, I seek only to zero in on how we, as people living in the Western world today, developed our ideas. Certainly other cultures throughout the world developed powerful healing tools, some similar to our own and some not. But that is a study for another book and another time.

3. This is certainly never the case in allopathic medicine. Allopathic drugs so commonly cause dangerous side effects and disease states of their own that allopathic practitioners have a name for the classification of diseases that are actually caused by allopathic treatments. The fact that this classification actually exists and that allopathic doctors seem all too willing to continue to practice their toxic medicine in spite of this is, to me, one of the great arguments against allopathic medicine.

Rome, during the first and second century A.D., the patient was seen as a solid and whole being. For Hippocrates and the ancient Greeks, the interior of the patient's body was largely unknown, unmapped, and unimportant to treatment. Medical treatments given by Greek doctors were similar in some ways to those given today by Naturopathic physicians. They tended to be rooted in nutrition and exercise and in the emotional well-being of the patient. In fact, a patient treated by Hippocrates himself on the island of Cos (off the coast of Greece) was as likely to be prescribed watching two comedies in an amphitheater as he was to be given a prescription for medicine.

Note that the concept of the patient as a whole being had a different context then than it does today. Today we are quite aware of the idea of body, mind, and spirit being taken as a whole. Our religions, if not our medical practice, stresses our wholeness.

But the wholeness assumed by the ancient Greeks was more literal. It was the belief of a people whose technology had not allowed them to take x-rays or remove and weigh various organs. Therefore, to the ancient Greeks, the wholeness of the patient's being was a mysterious and wonderful thing. Some, no doubt, assumed that the patient's body was a solid whole—that it was not made up of specific organs, but consisted of fluid or energy or a mass of solid flesh.[4] This gave the ancient practitioner a viewpoint of the patient as a mysterious thing, and, in doing so, a wonderful freedom of treatment that we have lost today. Because the patient was largely an unknown, it was far more difficult to make assumptions about him or his treatment. Instead, each new patient had to be seen as a new mystery to be solved, as a being whose functions were unknown and whose diseases had to be studied, considered individually, and treated on a totally individual basis as well.

Ancient Western medicine was, therefore, very different from the Western medicine of today. This has always made me wonder why modern allopaths chose Hippocrates to be the father of their medical system, when he practiced and thought about his patient and the very definition of medicine so differently. (If, for instance, there is a general practitioner who understands nutrition and individual nutritional needs, I have never met him. Even those who consider themselves versed in nutrition, tend, in my experience, to know less than the average clerk in a health food store.)

The modern practitioner of Western medicine has a firm grasp, both on what they consider to be the nature of the patient and his disease, and on the way that patient should be treated medically. For the allopath, the patient is a mechanical thing, a being

4. I am, of course, speaking in terms of medical treatment and not of physical appearance. While the Greeks, of course, saw dead and living humans cut open, physicians did not think in terms of treating the patient's heart or lungs. They would have surely put a bandage on a wound, but they treated the whole patient in order to heal the lungs or heart. It was the Romans, the fathers of allopathic medicine, who became fixated with the parts to the point of ignoring the whole, just as we unfortunately do today.

made up of a number of parts. These parts have been mapped and their functions explored for many centuries now. In fact, it was the ancient Romans, under the influence of a doctor named Galen,[5] who actually "invented" the allopathic viewpoint. The Romans were the first to cut open the corpses of the dead to systematically explore what was contained inside. In doing so, they developed the concept of the patient as being the sum of his parts. Today, we even see these parts as interchangeable. The kidney you are born with is not necessarily the one you will be using when you die.

When Samuel Hahnemann codified the system of treatment that he would name homeopathy, he insisted upon a return to the philosophy of medicine practiced by Hippocrates and the consideration of a patient as a whole being. He demanded that all aspects of the patient, visible and invisible, be taken into consideration in treating the patient. He worked with symptoms on all levels of being—body, mind, and spirit—in selecting the remedy that could most appropriately be used to treat that patient. He also worked with both objective and subjective symptoms—those that could be witnessed and measured by the doctor and those experienced only by the patient—in selecting his remedies. Therefore, in all proper homeopathic treatments, even the most simple and basic acute treatments, all aspects of the patient's being and of the case itself must be taken into account before the patient can be safely and effectively treated.

We have to remember that Bach passed through the study and practice of allopathic medicine, and learned enough about homeopathic medicine to develop a number of important remedies that are still in use today, on his way to developing a system of medicine that was truly his own. So he had an understanding of Hippocrates and of Galen, and a thorough schooling in Hahnemann and his theories and practice before he made a conscious decision to put all he had learned aside, to walk through the fields and begin an ancient process anew.

In picking plants and testing them, in considering the healing virtues of the plants that grew around him, Edward Bach was doing the same thing that the unknown ancients had done. The man or woman who first made the discovery that we could, as rational, spiritual beings, intercede on behalf of those who were ill, who suffered, and help them to recover. Just as ancient man had sought to identify just what plants, what soil, and what sap could possibly bring comfort to those who suffered with illness and free them from its grasp, Bach walked the fields in the last years of his life. He put aside all the medical knowledge he had accumulated in a lifetime of study in the finest schools and hospitals and, instead, trusted his ability to identify for himself—with no

5. Galen had a tremendous impact upon the doctors of his time. Indeed, he should be rightfully considered the "father of allopathic medicine," as he is historically known to be the first who stated "*contraria contrariis curantur*," or "opposites cure." Not only did he give today's allopaths the rationale by which they practice, he also gave them the viewpoint regarding the nature of both the patient himself and of medicine as a practice that still colors allopathic treatments today.

helpful technologies at his side—the substances Nature had to offer to restore the sick to health.

Of course, Bach took with him his lifetime of knowledge and experience when he went back to the beginning, to the process of identifying the plants that could bring healing and then figuring out the method through which they could be made less toxic and safely used. This is what informed him and allowed him to make the great leaps in logic that he made. He could not have accomplished all that he did if he had no understanding of medicine as it had been practiced over the centuries. But, at the same time, he instinctively put aside all he knew and picked the flowers fresh, held them, tasted them—he did all the things that ancient man must have done in his original search for what we would one day call medicine. Bach used all that he had—his mind, his spirit, and his instincts—in developing his new system of medicine. One that called, among other things, for a new way of seeing patients and considering their illnesses.

To Hahnemann, who was, in many ways, Bach's mentor, the patient was a whole being. Hahnemann never for one moment allowed himself, or any who would call himself a homeopath, to think of the patient as a mechanical thing, just as he would never allow anyone to homeopathically treat a "disease." The patient, not the disease, must receive the treatment. If a homeopath treated the disease itself, like allopaths do, then that homeopath made a fundamental error. He mistakenly believed that a disease could, through some sort of magic, be separated from the patient who had the disease. For Hahnemann, Bach, and homeopaths, the patient is the disease and the disease is fundamentally a part of the patient.

This allows homeopaths to avoid one of the greatest errors in medicine, one that allopaths make every day. When you believe that a disease can be treated, then the diagnosis of the disease itself will tend to give you a map to follow to treat that disease. Cancer one becomes cancer two, which becomes cancer three. Each case the same, even though the patient is different. The patient in his wholeness is never fully taken into account, and the disease—which, let's face it, actually differs greatly from patient to patient in terms of severity as well as experience and actual symptoms—once diagnosed, is given the doctor's full attention. If we treat the disease only, then we tend to treat all those with the same disease diagnosis with the same drugs. And this is a terrible mistake.

In homeopathic medicine, three different patients suffering from the same disease will likely be given three different medicines, in three different potencies, and with three different numbers of doses. Because, when we treat the patient and not his disease, we must treat each case individually and can never think that the remedy needed by one will be needed by all.

Yet, Hahnemann tended to hold with the allopaths when it came to the nature of disease. While he felt that all illness was, in the most basic sense, the result of a blockage in what he called the "vital force," the fundamental life energy, he also remained mired in the idea that the flesh must be treated as well as the spirit. For example, most homeopathic practitioners today will request the same medical tests as allopaths. This is because they feel that the "meaty" part of the case is still important, even if it is not the be-all and end-all.

Bach put this concept aside as well when he put aside all he had practiced and learned. Just as he set out to discover the nature of medicine, starting over again in a cycle of discovery that had been explored thousands of years before, he also set out to discover what constituted the true nature of illness and recovery, and the true nature of the patient himself.

Bach had seen first hand, over years of practice, both the suffering of those who were sick and their response to various forms of treatment. Therefore, his own search for a new method of healing was informed by what he already knew was *not* true.

He knew that the patient was not a mechanical thing. That he was much more than the sum of his parts. He knew that all the aspects of the patient's being were certainly present—body, mind, and spirit—and that no real "cure" could take place if the practitioner fixated on the patient's physical being and ignored the most fundamental aspect of the patient, his spirit.

Where Bach differs from Hahnemann is in the importance he gives to a patient's "invisible" nature. Where, for Hahnemann, the patient's mind and spirit were aspects to be explored, for Bach the invisible nature was vastly more important that the visible, completely dominating the flesh. For him, all illness began and was ultimately "cured" within the parts of the patient's being that were intangible and subjective.[6]

Bach took this yet a step further when he came to the conclusion that since the patient is a spiritual being, his path to illness and his path to healing must both be spiritual as well.

In *Free Thyself*, he writes, "We have so long blamed the germ, the weather, the food we eat as the causes of disease; but many of us are immune in an influenza epidemic; many love the exhilaration of a cold wind, and many can eat cheese and drink black coffee late at night with no ill effects. Nothing in nature can hurt us when we are happy and in harmony, on the contrary, all nature is there for our use and our enjoyment. It is only when we allow doubt and depression, indecision or fear to creep in that we are sensitive to outside influences.

---

6. This idea of illness being totally subjective is an important contribution of Bach's. If, as he reasons, we totally throw out the idea that any two patients having a similar experience in illness as being anything more than coincidental, then we remove the idea that anyone is more equipped than the individual himself is to treat himself. The whole idea of professional medical practice, after all, is based on the perhaps foolhardy notion that the practitioners know something about us that we don't know ourselves. By making the experience of illness and of healing totally subjective, Bach puts the responsibility for and the process of healing solely in the hands of the patients.

"It is, therefore, the real cause behind the disease, which is of the utmost importance; the mental state of the patient himself, not the condition of his body."

Bach takes control of our health out of the hands of the medical practitioner even further when he concludes, again in *Free Thyself,* "Health is our heritage, our right. It is the complete and full union between soul, mind and body; and this is no difficult faraway ideal to attain, but one so easy and natural that many of us have overlooked it."

Therefore, when Bach walked through the fields, he was not looking for something new; instead he was looking for something that had been overlooked. That had been trampled underfoot or cut and put into vases. And given all that he had learned about the nature of medicine, health, and healing, he took what was overlooked and used it in a new way. Instead of applying his tonics to the body, as ancient man would have done, he applied them to the mind and spirit. He focused solely on the invisible aspects of the patient's being, with the belief that harmony created in the mind and emotions would lead to harmony in the body as well. He believed that, as the patient is indeed a whole and indivisible being (in other words, what impacts one part impacts the whole—imagine what happens to your happy mood when you slam your hand in a car door and you'll see what I mean) the patient could be moved toward health by bringing any aspect of his being into a state of balance and freedom. So, when the patient's mind and spirit are brought into a state of true harmony, the patient's body will come into a harmonious balance of function as well, because, in Bach's mind, the flesh is a lesser thing than the spirit. So what brings health to the spirit brings health to the whole being.

Finally, but no less important, Bach also sought to simplify what we think of as medicine. Health is, in Bach's view, not something that can be attained only if we only have the right doctor and a large enough amount of money. It is something that each of us can call our birthright, and bring about in our own lives and in the lives of those we love.

## Healing Versus Curing

Think about it for a minute. There is a fundamental difference between the process that we call curing and the one that we call healing.

"Curing" is an external thing. The word itself implies that some outside force acts upon the weakened patient to restore him to strength and health. Now, in our culture, that outside force is most often a doctor.[7] The process of cure is largely one of trial and

---

7. Now, this has not always been the case. For instance, in many world cultures, the members of the family were more likely to call for the elders to come and pray than they were to call a doctor. This sort of thing has been discouraged in recent years, since we have decided culturally that we have more to gain from technology than we do from faith. I cannot help but wonder if we have made a wise choice.

error. A medicine of a sort—and by this I mean allopathic, homeopathic, or herbal—is given, based upon the philosophy of treatment the doctor follows and upon the known history of the medicine and its successful uses. Then the patient and doctor wait to see the results. In allopathic medicine the medicine is often given to mask the patient's symptoms, or to suppress them, while both the patient and the doctor wait for the patient's own vital force (immune system) to fight back and overcome the ailment. Often in homeopathic medicine, which never seeks to suppress the patient's symptoms but to bring them forth and rid the patient of them, both the doctor and the patient still have to wait and sometimes must try several doses and potencies or more than one remedy before satisfactory results are found.

The philosophy of treatment is very different, but the process of the cure remains the same. The patient comes to the doctor and pays him for his education and expertise. The patient, in essence, buys some of the doctor's time, knowledge, and compassion with the hope that the doctor knows something the patient does not. That he knows a medicine that will help, or some change in lifestyle that can modify the situation. When the patient comes to the doctor, he comes with the implied agreement that, because the doctor knows more about medicine than he does, he will do as he is told, take what medicine he is given and put his trust in the doctor. He may not even know the doctor's name, but he quite literally trusts him with his life.

In the process of curing, something external reaches in—into the patient's life and body. And that external thing, in doing so, robs that patient of some aspect of himself and of his personal power. However well-meaning the doctor may be, he robs his patient by placing his efforts in the arena of curing, by taking on the authority role. Even if the patient becomes well, he also becomes dependent. He is dependent upon that outside force for his medicine (especially since more and more allopathic medicines are formulated to manage illness and not end it, making medicine ever more lucrative as more and more patients sign on to take multiple medicines every day for the rest of their lives). He is also dependent upon the outside force for knowledge, since what little information he is actually given about his own condition (let me repeat: *his own condition*) is encoded in medical jargon, and of little use to the patient or his loved ones for understanding the nature of his illness or the implied plan for cure.

Whether that doctor is an allopath or a homeopath, the same paternalistic role-play is inherent in all processes of cure. Certainly the homeopath, in her earth-toned, plant-filled office in her home, is still playing the role of wise expert to the patient's needy child. The roles are the same any time we agree to work to cure, even that wonderful cure that Hahnemann promises in the first aphorism of the *Organon,* and the process of yielding our internal selves to external forces remains the same.

Now, healing is something else again. It is, and must always be, an internal process.

It is the movement toward health that occurs whether or not the process of curing is taking place. Certainly experience has taught us that healing may not take place even if all the doctors agree that the patient has been cured and slap each other on the back. The patient who feels isolated or weak or fearful or, indeed, controlled by outside forces cannot ever be said to have been healed.

Again, the healing process is internal. It is subjective as well. No other man can measure our degree of healing, just as no other being can define just what healing means in each of our lives.

And certainly it is impossible for one man to heal another. We can pray for healing, we can even do things to encourage healing—create a beautiful and peaceful atmosphere or cook nutritious foods, for example—but we can't cause healing to take place or control it.

Yet, I believe that we each can innately sense when it is happening. Just as a member of the Supreme Court once famously defined pornography by saying, "I know it when I see it," we may not really be able to give a working definition of healing, especially since we don't know where it comes from—is it a gift from the God within, an action of the immune system, or an act of will? We know it when we see it happening in others, however, and can sense it when it is happening in ourselves. And we know that the more we try to control the process—to force it to take place on our timetable or within our own definition of terms—the more it seems to elude us.

A Greek homeopath named George Vithoulkas once defined health simply as "freedom." And that is, I think, the best definition that I have ever heard. The process of healing is, therefore, for me, the process of becoming free. Free to live our lives unimpeded, so we can manifest all we can imagine. Free to live our lives without pain or restriction. And, most important, free to live without falling into the negative emotional traps to which we are all vulnerable. The human being who lives without an ongoing pattern of fear or anger or bitterness shaping his thoughts and actions is a human being who is in a state of health. And the human being who has undergone a process of personal transformation that leads to such emotional balance and freedom is also in a process of physical healing. Just as negative emotions lead to weakness and illness, truly positive emotions can only lead us toward health.

And I do not mean this in a strictly spiritual sense. I think that the healing process leads to rather concrete results in terms of changes in a patient's appearance or physical state of health. It certainly has very down-to-earth applications. For instance, the woman who has released her long-term sense of depression surrounding a lost love is far less likely to reach for the ice cream at night and is therefore more likely to lose weight and feel better. And the man who has finally released his long held feelings of inadequacy is far less likely to feel the old anger that once motivated him and allowed him to feel powerful, if only for a moment, and, as a result, has blood pressure that is as balanced as his mood. Certainly spiritual transformation is the ultimate goal of the healing process, but don't underestimate the physical changes that happen along the way. Indeed, these physical changes, which Bach tells us are the least important changes associated with healing, are often the very things most desired by the patient and the reason he began the healing process.

The healing process, being an internal, subjective thing, is therefore something quite opposite from the curing process, which is external and objective (by which I mean that its success or failure must be measured in visible, tangible ways). And Bach is one of the few medical professionals I have ever known to place his emphasis in the process of healing instead of being concerned with curing his patients. This then is the great divide—the concept of curing versus the concept of healing—that separates Bach and Hahnemann once and for all.

Another important aspect of the concept of healing is, of course, the idea that when you are working on healing, the responsibility for the results must remain with the patient and not be handed off to the doctor. If there is a doctor or other medical professional who works with the patient in the healing process, he does so not as the expert who makes the decisions, but as an adjunct who is employed by the patient to answer his questions and work with him in the manner that he, the patient, wishes to be treated and toward the result that he desires.

Certainly this paradigm of treatment can exist, just as the healing process and the curing process can most certainly happen concurrently. But it is not an easy thing to find. Perhaps it is the training of our allopathic and homeopathic doctors that is most to blame. Both are taught that they are, as President George W. Bush once said, the "deciders."

Because our doctors insist upon working solely toward a cure and demand the authority for making the decisions, they rob themselves of their true calling, which is bringing their patient into a full and balanced state of health. That takes a process of healing. It may or may not be accompanied by a process of curing, but it cannot be ignored.

Because of the way in which our medicine is practiced, we abandon the patient to struggle along as best he can in finding his path to healing. Because our doctors have abandoned their responsibility when it comes to healing, and tend to ignore the process entirely as they map out their allopathic or homeopathic strategies toward a cure, the practice of medicine has become a rather hollow thing. The goals of medicine are rather shallow, as they often do not even attempt to heal the wounds deep within. Instead, our doctors applaud themselves when they bandage our surface cuts. And when our doctors leave the room, we patients are left alone to heal as best we can—and often to deal with the ramifications of the cure, which have left us all the weaker as we face our real and deeper challenges.

When Edward Bach placed the responsibility for healing on his patients, he was, in my opinion, only facing reality. Like it or not, we must each take full responsibility for our own health. When we try to shove that responsibility off onto a doctor in exchange for some money, we do a disservice to the doctor and to ourselves. It is a fool's bargain all around—one that neither party should enter into.

Bach's own work with the process of healing was different. While he insisted that we must work toward healing and ignore the process of curing altogether, and placed the responsibility for healing on the patient, he never walked away from that patient or abandoned him to wrestle with his healing as others do. Instead, he used every tool he had at hand—his own knowledge, his experience, and his pharmacy of remedies—to support the patient, even to guide and advise him as needed. The fact that the patient runs the show when it comes to healing does not mean that he does not need or listen to his physician; quite the opposite really. The physician takes on an even more dynamic role in the doctor-patient rela-

> When Edward Bach placed the responsibility for healing on his patients, he was, in my opinion, only facing reality. Like it or not, we must each take full responsibility for our own health.

tionship, because it is based in truth and not in paternalism. The doctor who joins his patient so they can work together to solve the puzzle of the patient's healing must have more knowledge about the nature of disease, of healing, and even of human nature than the doctor who does nothing more than dispense pills. He must be willing to work "in the trenches" with his patient, to know him and feel true compassion for him. That is never a thing that can be rented.

This is the process of treatment with Bach remedies. The remedies themselves do little more than offer the patient a doorway through which they can walk if they choose. They offer a new way of thinking and a path toward freedom.

The person who gives these remedies to another must do so with the willingness of staying with the patient through the whole process. Even if they do not take responsibility for the patient in the allopathic sense, they do take responsibility for becoming a partner in the patient's healing. The person who is unwilling to take on this role—what I call the "role of the physician"—should not take the case, and should never give a remedy. Instead, he might give the patient a book or suggest that he learn more about Edward Bach. That in itself would still be an act of kindness.

Now that we have dealt with healing and curing, with allopathy and homeopathy and with Hahnemann and Bach, we have to actually consider the remedies and how we can best use them.

Before we can touch them, however, it is best if we consider how remedies are selected.

## Case Taking and Determining Bach Treatments

The first rule for case taking is the same as it is for the fight club in the movie of the same name. Just as you never talk about fight club, you should never talk about case taking, at least not in the strict Hahnemannian sense. In my opinion a case taken in preparation for treatment with Bach remedies should never be a clinical thing.[8]

After all, when Bach removed physical symptoms from his healing equation, he eliminated the need for the clinic, the white coat, and the paternalism common to "traditional" medicine. This makes the process of case taking for the purposes of Bach treatments very different.

The first thing the person taking on the role of the physician in giving or suggesting specific Bach remedies must determine is the nature of the patient and the reason why he is asking for assistance. It is also very important for the physician (this is what I will call him, although I do not imply any special educational requirements or specific training, only the role being undertaken) to understand as soon as possible what the patient desires to change and what, if anything, he wishes to avoid changing.

In other words, I strongly believe that no patient should ever be required to change any pattern, any behavior or, indeed, any ache or pain, that he is not yet ready to surrender.

I am always opposed to any physician of any sort taking it upon himself to treat any conscious patient in any manner other than that which the patient himself requests or, at the very least, consents to. And I have found again and again that it is the well-meaning friend or family member who, taking on the physician's role, will overstep the boundaries of appropriate treatment. He or she will either give the patient remedies that he is not yet ready to take, or will fail to educate the patient as he deserves, and

---

8. I know that we have seen the rise of what are called "Bach consultants" or some such in recent years. These are quasi-medical professionals who set up shop to guide individual patients in the selection of appropriate Bach remedies that may be taken singly or in combination. Often they have nice offices into which they invite their patients. They start off with an official case taking which would rival that of any homeopath or allopath. In doing this they do two things. First, they "dazzle" their patients with their supposed "professional" status, having graduated from some course or other on the Bach remedies. Second, they fly in the face of everything that Bach intended in creating his system of medicine, which is largely based upon the concept of self-treatment. In my opinion they denigrate everything that Bach stood for, by taking what, for Bach, was primarily a spiritual process and putting it back into an office (from which Bach himself fled in order to do this work) and by charging patients more money than Bach (who seldom charged any patient anything) would have ever felt decent or appropriate. While teacher and mentors are very valuable to us all as we struggle to learn new things, and while Bach would have applauded anyone willing to share his ideas, we must hold firm to the truth that Bach, as a revolutionary himself, never trained anyone to be a "Bach doctor." Those that he did train were trained to help him work with patients as his own health failed and to carry his message forward from the time of his death. He trained no one to be a highly paid "Bach consultant." I say that if you are not willing to learn about this handful of remedies yourself, then perhaps they are not for you.

ends up giving him a mixture of remedies without telling him what they are or why they are being given.

I cannot stress this enough: before any remedy is given, it is the job of the physician to instruct the patient about what is being done to him and what he is likely to experience as a result, and to receive permission to proceed from the patient. It is never, in my opinion, correct to give a remedy or remedies without this permission. Having received it, it is then only correct to proceed as long as the treatment is limited to those things that follow the patient's wishes.

My experience has taught me that we can only heal at the rate at which we heal and in the manner in which it is possible for us to heal. And that rate and manner is unique to each of us. Therefore, it is impossible for even the most highly trained medical professional to know just how quickly or in what manner healing might take place, much less be able to predict the outcome of the process.

If, as Bach tells us, we become ill by falling out of emotional balance and falling into chronic patterns of negative thought and behavior, we must tread very carefully in untangling the mass of negative patterns. It always amazes me that students of Edward Bach accept his concepts of illness and health very quickly, but then, when the time comes to actually give the remedies, suddenly seem to feel that they cannot cause any sort of issue because they are available over-the-counter, and since they only impact upon the patient's mind and emotions.

Well, physically, that is certainly true. They are benign. They can be used and combined in ways that other medicines cannot, because they are subtle and gentle in their actions.

But think about it carefully for a moment. Since Bach tells us again and again in his writings and teachings that the mind and emotions—the experiential aspects of our spirit—are dominant over the flesh, and that the diseases of the flesh are of a lower level than the diseases of the spirit (Hahnemann would agree with this), then it must follow that remedies that touch upon the mind and emotions are more potent than are those that only touch upon the body. If we follow this logic, then we must be more careful with the Bach remedies than we are with the aspirin and the other drugs we have in our medicine chests. If we don't start out by respecting the remedies and what they can do, and give them out like candy in our first flush of excitement, then we are liable to do a great deal of harm.

How can we do harm with the Bach remedies?

Very simply, by giving them in a manner that more or less forces the patient to deal with issues he is not yet ready to look at, or even to admit.

Each of us has patterns of conduct and thought that drag us into illness. In fact, Bach suggests that we all have patterns that reflect each of his thirty-eight different remedies at some time or other in our lives. In other words, we all have within us the possibility of the full range of negative thoughts and destructive patterns of behavior. None of us is emotionally or spiritually pure, as can be witnessed by the fact that none of us is in a state of perfect health in mind, body, and spirit.

Some of our patterns represent aspects of our personality with which we are very familiar. Some patterns, on the other hand, can be buried deep. And some can reflect parts of ourselves that we cannot yet bear to face.

Before giving Bach remedies to any patient, it is important to first understand where that patient is in his or her life. It may be very simple for you, as the practitioner, to immediately understand the ways a given patient is flawed. You may see these patterns of negative behavior with your own two eyes.

But there is a great difference between your ability to judge the patient's life and his ability to move from negativity to a more positive state—to heal, as it were. Remember, the practitioner has no right to impose any sort of structure or deadline on the patient's process of healing. If anything, such a set of rules would likely impede the patient's healing process and defeat the purpose of your work.

Therefore, above all else, the practitioner must respect the patient and his own decision-making ability. The patient, not the practitioner, must decide what patterns he is ready to examine and perhaps change or discard. In the same way, only the patient can ultimately decide whether or not the treatment has been a success.

The practitioner of Bach treatments who lets his own ego intrude into the process, who chooses to decide when the patient is ready to "heal" from his anger or fear, is a physician who is courting disaster.

In my experience, there is nothing harder than breaking old habits, even those habits that we know are destructive. There is nothing harder than looking ourselves full in the face and admitting that we are wrong in what we are doing or thinking or saying. The willingness to change can only come over time—sometimes when we hit rock bottom, sometimes as a gift from God who gives us insight into our own hearts.

So, each case taking associated with a Bach treatment (or, for that matter, with a homeopathic treatment) should begin in the same way. Ask a simple question: "How may I help you?" and then really listen to the answer. The place where the patient wants to begin, whether it is a fear of dogs or feelings of shyness, is the place where you should begin.

It is my belief that the only thing you really have to do is listen when you are taking another person's case. Just listen. The patient will tell you everything you need to hear. And what they don't tell you they will show you. Your only job, in a very real way, is to witness what they say and how they say it and to help the patient define the course of treatment.

Now, another skill is needed in cases of self-treatment. And that skill is honesty. While none of us is totally honest with ourselves, and none of our diaries tell the whole truth, we all have the ability to admit some truths to ourselves. And, in doing so, we give ourselves a place to begin.

If you sit thinking about which remedy to take and cannot find any flaw in yourself, ask yourself why you wanted to take the remedies in the first place. Ask yourself what things you feel you need to change and ask yourself why you have not changed them yet.

Remember, if healing is a process, then all you are going to do in taking the first remedy or combination of remedies is begin that process. With the patient, you only have to identify a single change that the patient wants to make. If you yourself are the patient, you only have to admit to one little flaw you might want to improve upon. With this restricted permission, you have the ability to begin the healing process by giving (or taking) the remedy or remedies that will help balance that which the patient is capable of balancing or changing.

This system of case taking may not yield the dramatic results you might get by simply giving the patient the remedies you think he needs or that he should, if he were honest with himself, want to take. It will not force the patient to confront himself in ways he is not yet ready. Instead, it allows for the unfolding of the case, and it supports the patient as he makes the changes and adjustments in his life he is capable of making right now.

Further, this system of treatment will allow the patient to have a positive experience of Bach remedies, where the system of giving the remedies you want him to take may result in his refusing to take anything at all in the future. As I have again and again, if you are willing to let go of your ego and let the patient define the treatment, the patient will actually move forward very quickly, and he himself will tell you when he is ready to move forward in his healing process.

Whether your patient is another person or yourself, you must, in case taking, first define what the treatment is and receive permission to continue. Then you must define what the patient wants in the way of change, and you must respect his decision whether you agree with it or not. Then you must listen to the patient and witness his thoughts and words, his demeanor. Then you must consider—usually after the patient has finished and gone on his way, leaving you to your books—what remedy or remedies seem to be the best match for the patient. Like homeopathic remedies, Bach remedies are selected on the basis of the similarity of the remedy's action with the pattern of thought and behavior the patient is experiencing. As each remedy has some sort of continuum of behavior and thought, from acute to constitutional and from positive to benign to highly destructive, you need only identify first the overriding mood of the patient and second, which remedy contained in that mood—which variation of the mood—best defines the patient's state of being.

Then you are ready to treat.

# 12

## Combining Remedies

When we begin working with Bach's remedies, it is best to remember that Bach felt that all of us need all thirty-eight remedies, some perhaps more generally in our individual lives, and others perhaps more strongly at any given moment. But we all need all of them. Therefore, we truly cannot make a mistake in giving or taking any of the remedies.

Remember, Bach also said that his remedies were benign. They cannot cause harm. The remedies can be mixed with any other form of treatment, from allopathic drugs to acupuncture and chiropractics.[1]

In fact, the only remedies I have found that do not work well when they are used concurrently with the flower remedies are Hahnemann's homeopathic remedies. This is because they are too similar to each other in action, and because there is an issue with potency as well. Because homeopathic remedies are made in a wide range of potencies and the Bach remedies are always given in what is considered a "zero" potency or mother tincture, the potency of the homeopathically prepared remedies will overwhelm the weaker Bach remedies, while the Bach remedies will interfere with the potency of the homeopathics. Together they will disrupt when they should cure. In short, at best, they will cancel each other out, and at worst, they can create an unnecessary healing crisis. Note that, in some instances, Bach's remedies can work well with Hahnemann's, but only if the homeopathic remedies are given in a potency high enough to not cause interference. Therefore, if a person is on a homeopathic constitutional treatment and is given a remedy of 1M (1 part in 1,000 in the homeopathic millesimal scale) or above, one can wait a few days for that remedy to "set in" and then follow up with a Bach remedy or mixture of remedies. These will not interfere with

---

1. The one caveat here is that nothing be done in secret. If you are planning to use Bach remedies with a patient who is taking allopathic drugs, the doctor who prescribed those drugs should be told. I believe that everyone on the healing team needs to be fully informed of everything that is being used as part of the healing process. A great deal of trouble can be caused if different treatments are provided by different doctors, each working without knowledge of the other.

each other and will, in fact, assist each other in their work. But given the potencies involved and the complexity of the treatment, such a combination should always be undertaken under the supervision of an experienced professional.

Now some will disagree with me and say that the two types of remedies work well together, no matter what the potency, and others will disagree and insist that we must follow the Law of Simplex and give only the single homeopathic remedy. And we each have to explore this situation and make our own decision, but I truly do not feel that we break Simplex when we *follow* our constitutional with a Bach mixture, any more than we would if we followed a remedy with a chiropractic treatment. The Bach mixtures are different from Hahnemann's and are used differently, and we must respect Bach's rules for their use just as we do Hahnemann's. But the use of both relegates the Bach remedies into being an adjunct therapy, by virtue of the fact that the potentized homeopathic remedies are more aggressive in their action than the Bach remedies.

As a final note, I do not advocate giving the Bach mixture along with Hahnemann's remedy, but only as a follow up in constitutional situations. In acute emergencies, it is best to choose between Hahnemann's and Bach's remedies and follow through from there.

## Using Bach Flower Remedies

Using Bach's remedies is much simpler than using Hahnemann's. For one thing, we have a pharmacy of only thirty-eight remedies, against the many thousands in today's homeopathic pharmacy. As I have already noted, the case taking can be as simple or as complex as one wishes to make it, since no set pattern has been handed down by Bach, unlike the set formats given by several practicing homeopaths. Also, the case taking can be largely intuitive, and can and should involve the patient on a very active basis.

An important first step in the selection and giving of a remedy to another person is to first try and center *yourself*. Now this may be more difficult than it sounds, particularly if the patient is a loved one who is fearful or in pain. Especially in these cases, you must first calm your own breathing—take a brief break from the other person if you need to—and get yourself under control and in a position to be as objective about the case and the patient's plight as you can before proceeding. You may even need to take Rescue Remedy or another Bach mixture before you can proceed in a clear-minded manner. Then, if you haven't already, take the case. Begin by asking the other person what troubles them. Remember, just as with Hahnemann's case taking, it is more important to listen to the other person than it is to put words in his mouth. Try

> An important first step in the selection and giving of a remedy to another person is to first try and center *yourself*. Now this may be more difficult than it sounds, particularly if the patient is a loved one who is fearful or in pain.

to avoid asking questions that lead the patient to a specific remedy you already have in mind. Instead, let him lead you to the remedy he truly needs.

When the case is taken, take a moment to reflect. Again, in acute circumstances you may need to step away from the patient briefly. If the situation permits, you might want to take a longer time to reflect on the remedies and on the patient. Ask yourself: What mood or moods seem to dominate the patient's demeanor? What remedies come to mind when you think of the patient? What are the circumstances of the patient's present situation in life that might define his mood—is he, for instance, in a crisis? If he is, what is the nature of the crisis?[2]

Then think for a moment about the patient in his present state. Is he conscious? Is he fully aware of what has happened to him? How is he reacting to his situation at this moment? Is he angry? Is he afraid? First try to understand which emotional state dominates, then check again to see if he is feeling more than one emotion. If so, notice them as well.

This pattern of case taking belongs to the acute case. It will help you in those times of true emergency, when you will most likely have to decide upon a remedy through the use of your own senses, by witnessing the patient in his duress, and by noticing the details of the situation at hand.

Never be afraid to give Rescue Remedy as a first remedy, especially in case of an emergency situation. It has been my experience that it is often needed as a remedy even during case taking. Even when you are talking with a patient who is dealing with a chronic situation, having the case taken may so stress the patient that he will need treatment for the *case taking* before he can be treated for his true ailment. But be careful

---

2. This is an important question. If it is a crisis, it is important to first ascertain if it is physical or emotional in nature before you select an appropriate remedy or remedies. If it is physical, is it an illness? If so, was it sudden or slow in coming on, and is it acute or chronic? Or is it a physical trauma, like a car accident or other injury? All these things can help guide you to a remedy. If the crisis is emotional in nature, again you must ascertain the root cause as best you can. For instance, the crisis caused by betrayal in love may lead you to a very different remedy than a crisis caused by a sudden downturn in business. And the emotional crisis caused by concern for an injured loved one will need a different remedy than a crisis caused by an emotional injury to the patient himself. You will be able to simplify your remedy selection in a matter of moments by answering this question.

One last note: in Bach treatments, as with homeopathic medicine, in terms of remedy selection it is not only important to discover the cause of the crisis if you can, but it is also very important to understand how the crisis has affected the patient. After all, a loss of love may leave one patient feeling deserted and lonely, while another patient may be filled with rage and a need for revenge. As I say in my homeopathic classes, it is far less important to find out the license plate of the bus that hit the patient than it is to find out how the patient reacted to being run down. So while it helps to be able to categorize the nature of the crisis itself, it is still more important in terms of treatment to understand the patient's current emotional state. You can safely treat him if you can discover this, even if you do not have full details yet on how the crisis developed.

not to give the Rescue Remedy too soon. Give it after the case has been taken. A patient who is quieted by the Rescue Remedy may fail to give you information you need to hear. So give Kleenex during case taking, and Rescue Remedy after.

And, if the case is difficult or if the patient is emotionally fragile, continue the Rescue Remedy while you are considering what other remedy or remedies might be of help.

## The First Remedy

Once you have centered yourself and are sure that you are thinking clearly and objectively as the patient's witness and partner in healing, and once you have completed the process of case taking that is appropriate to the patient's needs and present situation, you are ready to give the first remedy.

As I noted above, Rescue Remedy is often the first remedy given in cases of physical or emotional emergency. But Rescue Remedy is not usually the best first remedy for the many cases in which you are dealing with a patient who has a long-term emotional pattern, or, as he might put it, a "bad habit" that needs to be confronted. Indeed, using Rescue Remedy is just plain sloppy in cases where no particular emergency is presenting itself. While it may do a bit of good in centering the patient and a bit more than that if one of the remedy mix's component parts is of particular use to the patient, it is of overriding importance that you have a knowledge of the Bach remedies that extends beyond Rescue before you give any remedy to a patient.

In fact, you may not be able to identify the core remedy—the constitutional remedy—that the patient needs at first. It may only show itself at a further point in the healing process. Or it may be painfully clear from the moment you meet him. That cannot be predicted or controlled.

What can be controlled, however, is your own knowledge of the Bach remedies. Study them before giving them. As I have always told my students, if you wait until an emergency or until a needy person asks you for help to open the book and learn about the remedy, then you have waited too long to do the patient any good. Always work at your true level of skill when using Bach remedies or homeopathic medicines. If all you have read about is Rescue Remedy, then that's all you can safely give. So, before you give that first remedy, make sure you know them all.

The first remedy is so important. You must ask yourself what you want to accomplish with it. Certainly, in acute emergencies, that is a fairly easy question to answer. You want to calm the patient and help him recover, as much as possible. In very serious situations, you may be working to keep him alive until the paramedics can arrive. In less serious situations, you may only want to help a child get back to sleep after a nightmare, or to soothe a child through the night in spite of teething pain or earache until you can get medical help in the morning.

In constitutional cases, the question becomes more complex.

You must ask yourself how strongly you want to affect this patient's being. You must ask yourself how much you feel the patient can deal with in the present moment in terms of self-discovery and self-acknowledgement.

The answer may lead you right back to Rescue Remedy. If it does, and if, after thinking the case through, it seems the best course of action, then give it. And then watch and wait to see how to proceed. The patient will always tell you or show you how to proceed if you only watch and wait.

More often, by working through these questions, you will have an idea of a single remedy. After you have thought the case through, the thing that dominates may be that the patient is riddled with rather concrete fears that limit his life, such as fears of crossing bridges or taking elevators. If so, begin with Mimulus. And then wait and watch. Witness the changes that take place, sometimes almost instantly, sometimes over days or weeks. Again, let the patient react as it is natural for him to react, in his own time and his own way.

I believe that, in constitutional cases the best way to begin is with a single remedy. (Acute emergencies need to be dealt with as they need to be dealt with—if several remedies are needed at once, then give them—and don't forget to treat any others who are close to the patient, as their fears and distress can affect the case as well.) Maybe it is my homeopathic training getting in the way, but my experience has shown me again and again that you can only know the true effect of a remedy and, indeed, the effect that the Bach remedies as a therapeutic system will have upon that particular patient by giving a single remedy to begin with.[3]

So I recommend that you begin, whenever possible, with a single remedy. And, for the purposes of this argument, I consider Rescue Remedy to be a single remedy, because the workings of this mixture have been noted for decades. Other remedies, as we shall see, can be added as needed, but I believe that the cleanest way to begin, the way that will most often lead to the simplest and swiftest positive outcome, is with a single remedy.

## Combining Remedies

Since Edward Bach had practiced allopathic medicine, he was familiar with a school of medical treatment that saw no issue in giving a patient more than one medicine at a

---

3. I know that I have already addressed the concept of polypharmacy (simultaneous use of more than one medicine) in these pages as well as in the pages of my companion book, *The Healing Enigma*, but let me just say that if too many remedies are given in a case, especially at the beginning of a constitutional case, it can get very difficult to tell what remedy did what, and which emotional symptoms are the result of the remedies and which are native to the patient. So starting slowly is the best way. After all, when Bach said that we all need all thirty-eight of his remedies, he didn't mean that we should take all thirty-eight at once.

time. Indeed, in modern allopathic medicine, the profit margin of the industry seems to be dependent upon getting a patient on as many medicines as possible and keeping him on them for as long as possible.

While Bach certainly would have a problem with that whole idea now, he did come from a background of treatment that permitted multiple medicines. The fact that he had studied homeopathy so deeply means that he also had read and understood Samuel Hahnemann's viewpoint against polypharmacy.

In developing his own system of treatment, freeform as it is, Bach sided with the allopaths and not only blesses the concept of polypharmacy in Bach treatments, but actually practiced it himself by all accounts.

Perhaps I am biased on this point. Perhaps because of my own training in homeopathy, I do not see the fact that Bach used more than one remedy at a time as license for those using the remedies today to combine them every which way and to overprescribe the remedies in doing so. Bach remedies are as much homeopathic medicines as they are allopathic in the nature of their creation, so it seems to me that they come into their best usage when they are administered homeopathically. By this I mean they should be used with some caution, and careful consideration must be given when they are combined with other remedies or when they are given in multiple doses.

I have, for instance, found that the Bach remedies work powerfully when two are used at a time. And, I must admit, my own experience has shown me that some of the remedies, like White Chestnut and Impatiens, work so well together—creating a kind of synergy that improves the patient so dramatically—that I have to conclude that the two together work better than either does alone, polypharmacy or not. As you work with the Bach remedies, I am quite sure you will find combinations that, used together, sing a sort of duet that is more beautiful than either singing solo. I encourage you to learn these combinations. Lock them away as your "secret recipes," as I have. Once you know that Chicory and Sweet Chestnut have a particular power to help the patient who is in the first terrible stages of grief over the loss of a loved one, you will know to use that combination again and again.

So although I usually start, when possible, with a single remedy,[4] I often quickly add another. In many cases, this duet of remedies can be helpful in the long term; for example, the driven and mentally overactive patient who needs that combination of

4. Let me say as a little side note: when you are in doubt about how to begin, and no single remedy suggests itself to you, try Wild Oat. Remember, Wild Oat is one of Bach's two "primary" remedies, along with Holly. But where Holly can cause disruptions and aggravations, Wild Oat is an easily tolerated remedy that can help clarify confusing cases. Because it is useful for patients who can't identify their path in life or who are out of balance with the world around them, it can be useful for most, if not all of us, all the time. When in doubt for a place to begin, give Wild Oat instead of Rescue Remedy, which may be of no help at all if there is no ongoing emergency.

White Chestnut and Impatiens may find that it is all he needs in the long term. Or he may need another remedy added soon. Only time will tell.

When possible, I strongly suggest that all remedies be used and/or added one at a time. And then carefully watch and wait after adding a new remedy, noting all changes in the patient's behavior. If the remedy is not helpful or if it stresses the patient by bringing up things he is not ready to deal with, remove that remedy and go back for a time to what was used before, to give the patient a chance to bring himself back into balance. Then add another remedy if the need for one seems apparent. This is the way I build Bach mixtures.

Note that I will sometimes add a duet of remedies I know to be helpful to specific patients or in specific circumstances. In my mind, some of these duets have become like a single remedy because I know their action in combination. I may increase by two remedies at a time in these specific cases, again waiting and watching for changes afterward.

> When possible, I strongly suggest that all remedies be used and/or added one at a time. And then carefully watch and wait after adding a new remedy, noting all changes in the patient's behavior.

How long should you wait before changing your mixture, adding or subtracting remedies? That depends upon the situation at hand, upon the patient, and upon the remedies used. Emergencies, of course, require swifter responses than do chronic conditions. Some remedies work faster than others. The individual listings for the remedies in these pages can give you some clues as to each remedy's actions and the speed of those actions.

Because I approach Bach treatments through homeopathy, I tend to be very conservative in using the remedies. This means that I am not quick to change remedies or recombine them. In my opinion, those who change remedies often and change a patient's mixture every few days are likely to so muddle the case that it can become impossible to tell what is going on after a while. In these cases, the patient will have to stop taking all Bach remedies for a time, until the case has cleared and his natural patterns of thought and behavior reemerge.

Finally, there is the question of just how many Bach remedies may be used at one time. Those who approach Bach remedies from the herbal tradition tend to be most liberal when it comes to this question. They tend to just ladle them on, as many as they think are needed.

Those who come to Bach treatments from allopathy tend to settle on a set number and say to use that many, whatever *that* is. Some say that Bach remedies work best when no more than five are used at once. Others say that, since there are seven moods, you may use up to seven remedies.

Coming from a homeopathic tradition, I wish I could give you a definitive, simple answer to this question, but I can't. After all, my own education teaches me that they should be used one at a time. So by admitting that I have found that they often do work better in combination, I am already walking out onto thin ice.

I can simply say this: you should give no more remedies than absolutely need to be given. This is a patient, after all, not a guinea pig. You have no right to try out new combinations on him just to see what will happen.

If you can bring the patient into a state of emotional balance with only one remedy, then by all means just give the one remedy. If two are needed, then keep it to two. But don't fall into that error in logic that pervades our culture by thinking that if two are good, then certainly three will be better. When it comes to medicine—any sort of medicine—more is very seldom better. It can be a great deal worse, in fact.

I don't think I would ever give more than four or five Bach remedies at one time, no matter the situation. Let me explain why. I feel that each single remedy is like a radio station, broadcasting directly into the patient's mind. Each is broadcasting a particular message. The patient will be able to hear and understand one message very clearly. Two can also be heard and understood, especially if they are broadcasting messages that enhance one another. But each time you add a remedy, you are adding another broadcast. If you combine too many, you jumble the messages into noise the patient can no longer understand. You create confusion instead of clarity.

The number of remedies a patient can handle at one time differs from patient to patient. If you add them one at a time, it will be simple for you to know when he has reached his limit. If you add them as a group, you will have no way of knowing if you are using too many or using them too often. Again, all you will create is a muddle.

It seems to be a cultural thing with us that we want to get things moving very quickly. A chronic condition that has been in place for twenty years needs to resolve itself in two weeks, or we feel that we have failed. So we throw in more remedies to stir the pot. And, in stirring the pot too hard, we drive the patient away.

Remember that you don't have to use all the remedies that seem to present themselves in a patient's behavior patterns at any one time. If you take the case and see seven remedies that you feel the patient strongly needs, then refine the list. Choose the one that dominates and motivates. Give it, and go from there. Keep the list of seven nearby and add them as needed, singly or in duets. Don't give too many at one time. Rotate in new remedies over a period of time, as the original remedies complete their work and are no longer needed. Keep the original remedies close at hand, however, as they may present themselves again later for continued use.

Keep your eyes on the patient. Let him tell you or show you how he is to be treated and when his mixture of remedies needs to be changed. If you combine the remedies in this way, you will see great results.

# Left-Brained and Right-Brained Constitutional Treatment Approaches

There are two ways to approach treatment when treating patients who have deeply engrained emotional patterns that may involve complex layers of hurt and response to being hurt, and therefore need constitutional care. I think of one as the "left-brained," or systematic approach, and the other as the "right-brained" or intuitive approach. I think it will be of some help to outline each of them here. (I tend to stress the left-brained approach over the right.)

## *The Left-Brained, Systematic Approach to Treatment*

The systematic approach looks first not at the individual remedy types, but at Bach's seven moods of negative emotional patterns. Once the case has been taken, the practitioner first breaks it down by considering the patient's more general state of being as well as what motivates him in his particular pattern of behavior. Is he, perhaps, lonely? Is he fearful? Is he controlling? And so forth. This may not be as easy as it seems on the surface, as some moods are presented subtly, while others may be displayed quite aggressively. Do not make the mistake of thinking that aggressive behavior is always the dominant motivator. Sometimes quiet insecurities or fears are the true wellsprings of behavior.

Look to see which of the seven moods are present in the patient's patterns of emotion, thought, and behavior. Separate these moods out, if you can, into those three categories: emotion, thought, behavior. Those moods that seem present in all three categories are more pervasive than those only present in one. A patient may seem fearful, for instance, but not act upon his fear, which is a real indication as to the remedy needed.

After you have worked to identify what moods are present in the patient's patterns, and have tried to separate out just how each mood is presented, then refine your search further. Take each mood, one by one, and, even if you have studied the remedies time and time again, get out your reference books and read the remedies that pertain to that mood once again. Identify which remedy or remedies define the patient's experience of the aspects of that mood. And try to identify just how—by what behaviors—he is embodying them.

This should give you a list of moods in order of dominance, and the remedies within each of those moods that pertain to the patient at this time in his life. If you have any indications of past moods and remedies that have already been passed through and have been resolved or suppressed, note these as well.

This gives you the list of all the remedies that may be needed by this patient at this time. Add and subtract from that list as you work through treatment, and as some issues come to the surface and other issues are resolved.

This is a systematic approach to the Bach remedies, which will yield as few surprises as possible over the course of treatment.

### The Right-Brained, Intuitive Approach to Treatment

Those who approach the Bach remedies with their right brains dominating will tend to be less systematic, but no less helpful, if they can manage to keep their emotional connection with the patient strong.

This approach to treatment demands that the patient and physician have a strong bond of trust and a relationship that allows the patient to always speak openly and frankly. (For the patient who is involved in self-treatment, it involves a tremendous ability to be honest with oneself, which is why I suggest that those self-treating try to be more systematic in their remedy selection.)

The intuitive approach to Bach treatment is just that: the practitioner and the patient may not even do an actual case taking. There may be no formal question and answer session. Instead, they may talk about anything, especially about politics or religion or anything about which the patient feels passionately. The practitioner will want to see how the patient reacts to life and to those aspects of life that he feels strongly about. As the Bach remedies are used in treatment of our emotional states, the intuitive practitioner will need to get an understanding of how the patient's mind works, of his emotional patterns and responses, so he or she can identify which remedies will be of the greatest help.

The intuitive practitioner will not break the case down into moods and then into patterns within moods. He will still refer to his reference books, however, refreshing his memory about the details of each remedy, just as a homeopath revisits his *Materia Medica* again and again, always searching for the Simillimum. The intuitive practitioner also keeps good notes, of his original feelings about the patient and the case, and how those impressions change as the case unfolds.

Each Bach practitioner will tend to fall more into one camp or the other, and will be either structured or intuitive in their practice. The best practitioners, of course, bring both their right and left brains to the task when they are working. They try to be, at once, structured and intuitive and always open to the needs of the patient.

## Dosing and Bach Remedies—Frequency, Quantity, and Duration

Having resolved the issues of how to begin a course of treatment with Bach remedies and how to combine those remedies during the treatment, all that remain are the questions regarding how often the remedies should be taken and when and how treatment should end.

As to the appropriate method of determining the number of needed doses, I tend to fall back, once more, on my homeopathic training. According to the Three Laws of

Cure, all homeopathic remedies are given one at a time. In using Bach remedies, I try to stay true to the spirit of this principle, while still following Bach's own principles of treatment, as outlined above.

According to the Three Laws, remedies should also be given in the lowest possible effective potency. Bach has solved this issue for us. Where homeopaths have to wrestle with the concept of just what would be the "lowest effective potency" for a particular remedy and a particular patient, Bach made his remedies in only one potency, the so-called "zero" potency of a mother tincture, a medicine that has been diluted in water, but has not been succussed into succeeding levels of potency, as a homeopathic remedy would be.[5]

Therefore all Bach remedies are given in the single potency Bach intended for them. It is this state of being—directly between homeopathic and allopathic drugs—that gives the remedies their unique and subtle gifts.

The final Law of Cure is problematic. In homeopathic medicine we always give our remedies as needed, in the fewest number of effective doses. If a single dose effects a cure, a second dose is never given.

Now, this can be difficult for Americans. We always think that more is better. Even our American homeopaths tend to want to give just one more dose "for the road," and they spoil many cases by doing so.

It is a principle of "classical" homeopathy that more cases are spoiled by giving too many doses than in any other way. The true power of a remedy is never revealed in the first dose, which optimally cures quietly, without complications, but in the repeated doses. It is by the use of repeated doses that remedies are proven, artificially creating new symptoms that bring needless discomfort to the patient.

The same holds true with Bach treatments. Just as too many practitioners ladle on too many different remedies and make a muddle of their cases, too many give doses too often or for too long a time. Just like Hahnemann, Bach never intended that patients take his remedies every day for the rest of their lives. They were developed to be used when needed, and stopped when not needed. It is the allopath's trick to have every patient on multiple medicines for as long as possible. The allopath is a smart business-man, and has figured out that there is a lot more money involved if the patient's illness

5. I am well aware that there is a company out there that has decided to potentize Bach's remedies in order to make them fully homeopathic. Apparently those responsible for these abominations feel that Bach himself lacked the knowledge and skill to potentize his remedies, even though he managed earlier in his career to make seven homeopathic bowel nosodes that were fully potentized and proven as homeopathic remedies. Before trying these remedies, remember that Bach knew exactly what he was doing when he chose his very simple method of preparing very low-potency remedies that balance between the homeopathic and allopathic. The remedies are bastardized into a shape and form that Bach never intended when they are made fully homeopathic and thus taken out of balance.

can be maintained and managed and not cured. The homeopath and the Bach practitioner are supposed to be more foolish: they are expected to help their patients become fundamentally healthier, until they no longer need treatment.

Therefore, the Bach remedies are to be given as needed, and anyone using them should consider them like homeopathic remedies. They work best when given in the fewest number of doses needed. I don't hold with the idea of giving the remedies three or four times a day, unless the patient is too young or infirm to take them any other way. Or unless the patient is a dog, who can't tell you his symptoms.

In most cases, especially constitutional cases, the patient must learn when he needs his remedies. On a stressful day, he may need them four times. On a calm day, he may not need them. If he does not need them, he should not take them at all.

Think in the long term in constitutional cases. Think of using the remedies as cleanly as possible, to create as few muddles and disruptions as possible. If they are well-selected and well-used, the remedies should help the patient clarify his issues and resolve and release them. He should not be turned into a slave to the remedies, anxiously clutching them at all times.

The patient should take the remedies on a limited basis as he undergoes this learning process and becomes familiar with how they make him feel. He may start out taking them once a day until he learns what his triggers are and what things make him want to take them.

If you are combining the remedies, he may take one remedy in the morning and a second remedy or duet of remedies at bedtime. This is especially true if the patient has nightmares or insomnia, or any other condition that makes nighttime hard to bear.

Truthfully, if you are going to use the remedies correctly, you are going to have to find your way with each new patient. Each patient represents a new way of working. Each patient will need his case taken in a different way, appropriate for that patient only. Each will need the blend of remedies special to him. And each will need to take the remedies as many times as his personal schedule demands.

As for the other questions of how long a Bach treatment should last and when should we end them, the answer is really very simple: it is not for the practitioner to say. Because Bach remedies are an engine for healing and not a mode of cure, only the patient himself can decide if a treatment is helpful or if it is complete. Those in the patient's life, his loved ones and coworkers, can tell you whether they see positive changes in the patient's demeanor, and you will be able to see them for yourself, but only the patient can define his own healing. Therefore, the practitioner should look to the patient for these answers.

Some books may tell you that you should see a change in four weeks, or that you should, as a rule of thumb, give a remedy for a month for each year that the problem being treated has persisted. I find these measuring sticks to be ridiculous. They attempt to know what is unknowable. Some patients react very quickly to the remedies. Often age is an indicator; very young patients tend to change quickly and elderly patients may stubbornly cling to the patterns with which they are comfortable. But this is not always the case. In the same way, animals tend to react to the remedies very quickly and make major changes at amazingly fast rates. But some dogs or cats may prove very stubborn and may need long-term treatments for what seemed, at first, to be very simple conditions.

So the answer remains the same as before: the patient will tell you when he is ready to stop treatment. Or, if he is not a verbal type or is not consciously aware that he is finished, he will show you by the changes in his demeanor—the changes in his life.

To get the answers to these very important questions, you only have to pay attention to the patient. Give the remedy. And then wait and watch and pay attention. Put aside your ego and your expectations. You will be surprised and perhaps very pleased with the results.

## Dosing: FAQs

Beginning users often have many questions about how and when to use the remedies. The idea of dosing can seem complex, but, in reality, it is really rather simple once you get the hang of it. It's important to remember that Bach wanted to create a system with very few rules, so using the remedies is really not a difficult thing.

*How long do you wait if there is no change after a remedy is given,*
*since some are slow acting and some are faster acting?*

You ask a question for which there is no simple answer. In acute circumstances, you might wait only minutes before trying another remedy. In constitutional cases, you wait days or even weeks before moving on. Each patient is different and, indeed, each remedy is different, so you can't make simple sweeping statements that would satisfy this question.

The basic rule is that if you feel you need to take a remedy, take it, even if you only took it a moment ago. And if you feel that you don't need it, don't take it, even if you skip a day or two, or a month. Bach felt that the actions of his remedies were cumulative, so when you take your next dose, you begin working emotionally where you left off—in other words, the progress you make is considered to have been permanently made. Because we are dealing with emotional insights into our own lives, the remedies do not work like allopathic medicines do. They don't "wear off." So the use of the remedies is a very simple thing—a matter of desire more than need.

Now, when you are giving the remedy to another person, things work a bit differ-

ently. In acute situations, you have to keep watch to make sure that the remedy is helping the person in hysterics or in whatever crisis they are in, and if there is any sign that
they have not yet absorbed the trauma or dealt with their shock, the remedy should be
repeated as needed. As with homeopathic remedies, more remedies are needed in more
doses for acute emergencies than are needed for constitutional cases. And doses will
likely have to be repeated with less of an interval in between for acute cases than for
constitutional cases.

If you are giving a remedy to another person in a constitutional context, the most
important thing is that you don't, in your desire to help the other person, force them to
take the remedy more often than they want to. Most often, constitutional treatments
are begun twice a day, in the morning and evening. Some do better with once a day
when they come home from work. Others do well taking their remedy mix at bedtime.
It depends both upon the patient and the remedies used when during the day they will
work best. Remedies that help the yang type to be calmer and more centered are best
used after work or at bedtime. Remedies that help the vague or distracted to become
centered and more active are best used first thing in the morning. During a crisis, of
course, even constitutional remedies should be used at any time of day and as often as
they are needed.

The heart of learning to dose with Bach remedies is learning to pay attention—to
ourselves or others, depending upon who is being treated. When I say that they are best
used in any context—acute or constitutional, for ourselves and others—as needed, I
mean just that. Learn to watch for signs that the remedies in the same mix or with a
remedy or remedies added or subtracted. Look for signs of emotional stress, the return of
old patterns, and the uncovering of new patterns, both positive and negative. I wish
that I could give more specific rules to follow, but I promise you that, as you use the
remedies you will increase your knowledge of them and your awareness of their use. In
time, you will know when it's time for the next dose.

### If the remedy makes a patient "more so" in a negative way during its process of cure (let's say it makes him more angry) how does the physician deal with this?

You don't. Any change that impacts upon the mood being treated is considered good.
A "healing crisis" that increases the negative mood should only last a few hours or a
couple of days at most. The Bach remedies do not have the power to create long-term
crises. If the remedy is correct, the patient will improve. If the remedy is incorrect or of
lesser value to the patient, nothing will happen. That is why the short-term negative is
considered a "good" thing. Because when a remedy is simply not right for the patient,
nothing happens at all. Therefore, no change would be considered the worst outcome,
with an immediate change for the positive being the best, and a short-term change for
the worse somewhere in the middle.

*When one combines allopathic and Bach remedies, should they be administered separately, or does it not matter?*

It doesn't matter at all. Bach remedies may be taken while a patient is on allopathic drugs. They may be added to food or drink or taken on an empty stomach. These things don't matter, but it is important that all doctors are aware of all medicines being taken, including Bach remedies. I never believe in secrecy when it comes to medicine.

## Mixing, Using, and Storing Bach Remedies

All Bach remedies come in liquid form. The floral essences are stored in alcohol, which serves to preserve them and retain their potency. The concentrated remedies are available from health food stores nationwide and are sold in dropper bottles.

Remedies may be taken directly from the bottles of concentrate as purchased from the health food store. If a patient is taking a single remedy, he may simply drop the remedy onto his tongue from the bottle of concentrate. This is especially common with Rescue Remedy. Or they may be used singly by adding them to water, as discussed below in terms of combined remedies. When a few drops of the concentrate are added to the water in a fresh dropper bottle, the initial bottle of concentrate will last much longer, lowering the cost of the remedy.

Remedies may also be blended together and taken in liquid form. When remedies are combined, they are usually put into fresh amber glass dropper bottles. To make a mixture of remedies, add two or three drops of the concentrate of each remedy to the empty amber bottle. Then add fresh water to the bottle until it is about two-thirds to three-quarters full. (I use filtered water because I prefer to use water in motion instead of water that has been bottled, especially if it has been bottled in plastic.) The bottle is then topped off with alcohol, most commonly with brandy.

If a particular patient does not want to use the alcohol, by all means leave it out. The only difference is that the potency of the remedy will dissipate, and the combination remedy will likely have to be remixed every few days, instead of lasting indefinitely as it will when alcohol is used as a preservative. If the patient hesitates even to ingest the small amount of alcohol that is present from the concentrate, then the remedy can be used topically instead of being taken by mouth. To use the remedy topically simply have the patient place a couple of drops on the pulse points of both wrists and have them rub it into the skin. It is important to note that no one else should rub the remedies in, because it would dose the practitioner as well as the patient.

All Bach remedies may be taken topically or orally. My experience suggests that remedies have a more potent effect when taken orally, but either method will elicit a response. Remedies may even be taken orally and topically at the same time, or one remedy may be used orally and another topically, as needed.

Bach remedies may also be given in food or drink.[6] This is especially helpful with animals. Simply add the needed remedies to your pet's water dish for best results.

In fact, water is perhaps the very best method for dosing. Just as water serves as the best medium for taking homeopathic remedies, it is also an excellent medium for Bach remedies. Many patients report that they receive best results when they place a few drops of their combination remedy in about a quarter glass of water. The patient then sits quietly for a few minutes, sipping their remedy. Improvement can be almost immediate when Bach remedies are taken in this way.

Remedies should never be stored in the direct sun or in places where conditions will be too hot or too cold, such as glove compartments, as this can impair their potency. In the same way, remedies should never be stored where they will be in a strong electromagnetic field, such as on top of a refrigerator, television, or microwave oven. They should be stored in a somewhat dark, temperate place.

If prepared correctly and stored properly, Bach remedies in their concentrated form will remain potent for many years.

---

6. In another departure from traditional homeopathy, Bach saw no reason why the patient should wait for an hour or so after eating or drinking in order to take his remedy. In fact, Bach felt that the remedy could be given in food or drink with no loss of potency.

# 13

---

# Rescue Remedies
# and Other Blends

In her loving biography, *The Medical Discoveries of Edward Bach, Physician,* author Nora Weeks dispels some of the myths surrounding the development of the Bach Flower Remedies. Among these myths is the story I had always heard about the discovery of Rescue Remedy.

As I understood it, Rescue Remedy was created on the fly, as a result of an emergency in which a group of Bach's neighbors brought him a sailor who was near death from drowning. Bach ran his hand over his remedies and quickly selected five. He blended them and moistened the dying man's lips with the mixture. Within minutes, the story goes, the man opened his eyes, fully conscious. Within days, he was well.

Nora Weeks, a close associate of Bach, tells a different story. According to Weeks Bach did not create his Rescue Remedy in a moment of need. Instead, since his remedies were a balance of herbal and homeopathic medicines, he began researching the use of remedies in combination early on. Over the years, he made a number of combinations, always closely verifying their impact. Among these different mixtures was his early version of Rescue, which only contained three remedies at first: Clematis, for fainting and unconsciousness; Impatiens, for pain; and Rock Rose, for panic. He found this Rescue to be very successful in treating a wide-range of patients in times of crisis. As he continued his research he added two more remedies: Cherry Plum, for hysteria and irrational behavior, and Star of Bethlehem, for emotional trauma. With the five remedies, Bach felt that he had his final, polished formula.

It is said that for the rest of his life, Bach always had a vial of Rescue Remedy in his pocket and that he handed it out freely whenever it was needed.

According to Weeks, however, that sailor did actually exist. As she tells the story, "On one occasion a man who had been strapped to the mast of a wrecked barge for five hours in a terrible gale was brought ashore by the lifeboat. He was delirious, foaming at the mouth, helpless and almost frozen, his life was despaired of.

"As he was being carried up the sands to a nearby house, Bach repeatedly moistened his lips with the Rescue Remedy, and before the man had been stripped of his clothing and wrapped in warm blankets he was sitting up and in his right mind, asking for a cigarette. He was taken to the hospital, but after a few days' rest he had completely recovered from his dreadful experience."

## Rescue Remedy

Bach polished his formula for Rescue Remedy at the end of his research. Soon after, he declared that his work was finished and spent what little remained of his life using his existing remedies either singly or in combination for the treatment of his patients. Bach also took this time to teach his principles of treatment to those who volunteered their time and energy to help him with his work. Chief among these was Nora Weeks herself, so her account of Bach's life and work, biased as it is in favor of Dr. Bach, remains our definitive source for information.

Rescue Remedy is an odd sort of thing, really. While it is to Bach remedies what Arnica or Sulphur are to homeopathy—the first remedy a lay person is likely to come into contact with when they first hear about a particular modality of treatment—it is no more a universal treatment than they are. Just as the homeopath who always gives Arnica in acute crises and Sulphur as the constitutional remedy of first choice will find that he has more patients unhappy with their treatment and with their symptoms unchanged than he has patients who walk away cured, the Bach practitioner who gives Rescue Remedy to all patients in all states of emergency will find that many patients are not helped by the blend.

> You must, when using Rescue Remedy, remember that it is a generic thing. It was created with the idea of doing the greatest amount of good for the largest number of patients. Remember, all really effective Bach treatments, like all really good homoeopathic treatments, are always chosen to be specific to the patient.

Indeed, it has always surprised me just how Rescue Remedy has wormed its way into so many purses and glove compartments (which is not a good idea, since these get too hot in summer and too cold in winter to keep the remedy potent) and why so many people swear by it. Sure it's a nice blend of remedies, but it is nothing more than that. The five remedies contained in Rescue Remedy have no more affinity for each other than any other five remedies. No more, no less. Which is to say that they will, in the combination called Rescue, do some patients a great deal of good, other patients some good, and still other patients no good at all.

It all depends on the patient, and on his reaction to the emergency.

You must, when using Rescue Remedy, remember that it is a generic thing. It was created with the idea of doing the greatest amount of good for the largest number of patients that you can when using a combination that is not uniquely created for each patient. Remember, all really effective Bach treatments, like all really good homoeo-pathic treatments, are always chosen to be specific to the patient. The fact that they might have helped his friend or his mother does not mean that they will do this partic-ular patient any good at all.

So, by all means use Rescue Remedy. Carry it in your purse or pocket, if not in your glove compartment. But when you use it, have only the expectations that are appropri-ate: that it will do no harm, and that it may do some degree of good. Perhaps a great deal of good, perhaps only a little.

To get really good at using the Bach remedies, we have to move beyond generics. This is why I get so upset when I see the myriad of blended remedies now on health food store shelves. Often these remedies (which are not, I might point out, sold by the Bach Foundation, but by private companies) will have clever or sweet names like "Happy Dreams" or "Quiet Times." And they are certainly safe to use. They may work or they may not. They are not and cannot be blended for the use of a specific patient, whether human or animal (and I see them a lot in organic pet stores).

How much better it would be to learn enough about the individual remedies and their actions, and enough about case taking and management to be able to mix the remedies yourself. Certainly the mixing is simple and the mixed remedies will keep for a good long time—certainly long enough to be effective, if not as long as those that come "factory mixed." More important, the remedies put into combination for the use of a specific patient, whose emotional state is known and whose reaction to stress has been noted, can be far, far more effective than the generic blends. (And you can always give them cute names and create little pastel labels for them if desired.)

Now, I realize that I may be perceived as hypocritical in writing this. After all, the individual listings for remedies in this book contain all sorts of information on what remedies, in my experience, bring out the best in each other. But I have tried to walk a fine line. While on the one hand, I want to discourage what I call "quid pro quo" pre-scribing (which is to say that we should never blend remedies based upon a situation—we must always blend based upon the patient's specific emotional needs), I also know that it is important to share my experience in using the remedies. Therefore, through-out the book, I have tried to avoid absolutes in language. I have tried never to say that this remedy or these remedies will *always* work. Instead, I have tried to say that I have known this particular treatment to work well for patients with this sort of an emotional response. Therefore, I have tried to give the reader a head start in combining remedies, without ever trying to undermine the practitioner's need to do his own thinking and his own blending of remedies.

And I believe that one of the things a good practitioner will be able to blend for any given patient, especially after the two have worked together and are familiar with and trust each other, is a "rescue remedy" that is not generic, but is specific for his needs. Something that patient can carry in a pocket or purse for years to come and use as needed.

## Personalized Rescue Remedies

When you create a rescue remedy for a specific patient you must first understand that it is not a constitutional treatment, even though the mixture is blended for the specific needs of that patient.

When you work to discover a patient's own constitutional Bach treatment, you may be looking for a single remedy, or for a blend of two. I have seldom found that more than two remedies will be needed on a constitutional level.[1] More than two remedies— three at the outside—and the mix is no longer constitutional in nature. It may be very effective in treating that patient, but it is not constitutional.

Remember that truly constitutional issues affect many aspects of life. The term refers to the ailments that a given patient is prone to, and has been prone to in a repeated pattern, over a period of years. When applied to emotional health, the idea of constitutionality reveals our patterns of behavior; the patterns by which we live our emotional and mental lives. Like any other pattern, it reveals itself as a continuum, made up of a blend of positive and negative behaviors that reveal themselves based upon the stress level the patient is experiencing at a given moment or in a given period of his life.

Therefore, acute remedies may be very helpful in a moment of true crisis, but the deeper and longer acting constitutional remedies will be helpful for a wider range of behaviors over a longer period of time. Moreover, the acute remedies will be helpful only for moments of crisis, while the deeper constitutional remedies will be helpful for a wider range of circumstances and will help move the patient as a whole to a happier, healthier, and freer way of life.

---

1. For those who have not read this whole book, but are skipping around, let me say that Bach reme- dies will often fall into two general categories of use, just like homeopathic remedies. By their very nature they may be more commonly used either in an acute context or for the treatment of chronic conditions. A handful of Bach's remedies, as noted in the individual listings, are only effective in acute cases and are seldom, if ever, used in long-term treatments. And when I use the word constitu- tional, I am referring to those long-term treatments that are used to help free patients from deeper emotional patterns of thought and behavior that may be of many years' standing. Constitutional treatments, in either homeopathic or Bach practice, can involve many doses of remedy over a long period of time. So the practitioner is identifying the overriding pattern of behavior for a given patient in identifying that patient's constitutional remedy (or remedies, in the case of Bach treat- ments). As the patient is more stressed he will act more and more negatively within this pattern of behavior. So, identifying the patient's "core pattern" of behavior and the remedy known to help bal- ance that behavior is key to using Bach remedies most effectively.

## Creating Core Constitutional Remedies

So it all begins with identifying the constitutional remedy or duet of remedies for the specific patient. My personal combination, as I mentioned before, is White Chestnut and Impatiens. These are the two remedies that are in all of the constitutional treatments I prepare for myself, and in my own personal rescue remedy.

Let's use me as an example. And, using the White Chestnut/Impatiens combination, let's look at how you might go about blending both an individualized constitutional Bach remedy and an individualized rescue remedy.(Remember: this is only an example. Don't use these two remedies in your mix unless they are actually needed by your patient.)

First, consider the difference between these two—the individualized constitutional and acute remedies.

The individualized constitutional remedy starts with the actual constitutional remedy. For me, it is White Chestnut and Impatiens. For another patient it may be Chicory and Willow or Willow and Vine. We start with the single remedy or duet of remedies that most expresses the patient's given pattern of mind and emotion. When you read the individual descriptions of the remedies in this book, consider what remedy or remedy blend, in either its positive or negative characteristics, seems most like the patient. Also consider how negative the patient's behavior is when he is stressed. How far does he go in matching the negative patterns of the remedy?

Answering these questions will help you find what I call the Core Constitutional remedy.

Obviously, to discover this remedy or blend, you first have to find the remedy or remedies that most resemble the patient's own long-term patterns of behavior in their actions.[2]

Once you have discovered this pattern and have identified the remedy or duet of

---

2. Obviously, if you don't know the patient's long-term patterns of thought and behavior, you can't identify this remedy. It often takes a process. If you don't know the patient well or are just beginning treatment, then begin, by all means, with simple acute treatments. Begin with the way the patient is acting right now and give the remedy or blend of remedies that best mirrors this. Sometimes, his present behavior will be an indication of his long-term patterns, and this blend will have huge results. Other times, you will find that this blend does not work on a deep level. Instead, it helps the patient at this moment, and allows you to work on a deeper level at another time. There is certainly nothing wrong with simply working in the moment with a simple acute treatment. However, you will ultimately make a muddle of the case if you keep dosing and continually change the mixture, and never look more deeply at the patient's actions to find the thread of thought and behavior typical to him. So it is best to either use the Bach remedies for acute treatments from time to time or, if you want to use them constitutionally, learn to identify the patient's patterns, and give a blend in which the core remedies remain the same and only a remedy or two changes as needed.

remedies that best mirror the pattern, you have your Core Constitutional and can begin to build from there.

Once you have identified the patient's Core Constitutional, it is wise to begin with that alone, as I have noted before. Then watch and wait. Note the changes that begin to take place before you do anything else.

If the patient undergoes a great healing, then fine. Stop there. Don't try to push for more, but let things unfold.

If the patient experiences some changes, but the two of you agree to work harder, then take the idea of the Core Constitutional and place it within your experience of the patient and his behavior. Aside from what you have already noted that resulted in your selection of the Core Constitutional, what else do you observe when you watch the patient? How does he act when stressed? How does he express his opinions? Is he extroverted or introverted? Does he make strong eye contact or lower his eyes when speaking? Note everything you can about the patient and begin to pick the other remedies that seem to mirror his behaviors.

Add them. Add as few as you can to the Core Constitutional, certainly no more than five in total. And give the patient this mixture. Again, wait and watch, and see what happens.

The fact that the Core Constitutional *is* the core constitutional for this patient means you will seldom, if ever, remove this remedy or blend from any mix the patient needs. What will change, over time, are the other remedies that you have added to this constitutional blend.

And because it is a constitutional blend, it will also change less often than an acute mixture. An acute remedy may be helpful for only a few hours, to bring the patient back into emotional balance during a crisis, but a constitutional blend should be effective in treating the patient and balancing his behavior and emotional patterns for a period of weeks or months. As a rule of thumb, once I have observed positive changes from a constitutional blend, I tend to revisit it on a monthly basis to be sure that it is still having a positive impact. If I find that the patient no longer needs a given remedy, I take it out, but leave the rest of the formula alone. If I find that a new remedy is needed, I add it, but leave the rest of the formula alone.

> I have often found that beginners, when using the remedies, seek to eradicate the personality types they particularly dislike from the face of the earth. This is a big, big mistake.

Therefore, the constitutional formula changes more slowly than an acute formula. I tend to think that it evolves along with the patient, growing with him as he grows.

One important note before we move on: remember that the remedies speak to a continuum of behaviors. The patient or the practitioner who thinks that a bitter and negative Willow type will, with treatment, stop being a Willow is setting himself up for disappointment. The Willow traits will not disappear. Instead, with time and treatment, the negative traits of bitterness and revenge will be replaced with the positive traits of clear-headedness and open-mindedness, and the Willow patient will seek true happiness for himself and others.

I have often found that beginners, when using the remedies, seek to eradicate the personality types they particularly dislike from the face of the earth. They target the aggressive Vines, the bitter Willows, and the impetuous Vervains and try to turn them into quiet Clematis, Cerato, and Centaury types who will do as they are told. This is a big, big mistake. We are who we are. A Willow type may evolve into another type over time. But, with treatment, he will more likely become a positive and emotionally balanced Willow type who has learned to make use of his talents and the positive attributes of his type. This is the purpose and successful outcome of Bach treatments—not to totally reshape patients' psyches according to the practitioner's desires. The last thing we need is a group of Bach practitioners who behave like stern mothers, pointing at our siblings and crying out, "Why can't you be more like him?"

## Creating Individualized Rescue Remedies

Now, getting the formula right for an individualized rescue remedy is tricky; it involves some skill with the remedies, but it is a valuable thing when it can be done.

It blends acute and constitutional treatments. By this I mean you are going to have to know how the patient reacts in his usual pattern under stress as well as what other behaviors are likely to erupt out of him when in crisis to get it right. Will a constitutional Clematis type, passive and dreamy, erupt in aggressive behavior when he feels pushed against the wall? Or will he pull back even more?

If you can track which acute treatments have been successful in the past and which constitutional treatments have repeatedly been used successfully, then you can assemble an individualized rescue remedy.

Now, naturally, this blend will feature some of the acute remedies that are part of Bach's blend: Rock Rose, Cherry Plum, Sweet Chestnut, and Star of Bethlehem are commonly needed. I have found that other remedies are commonly needed as well, especially Aspen, Clematis, Vervain, and Holly. In general, those who need more yang remedies will likely need one or more in this mix. Those who tend to crumble inward and require yin remedies will need some here. Using the Core Constitutional as the base of the remedy, add the other remedies (no more than five total) that best mirror the patient's known behaviors in times of emergency, and you will have an individualized rescue remedy.

Because it uses both acute remedies and constitutionals, the individualized rescue remedy should not be taken on a daily basis. The constitutional blend is for regular treatment as needed, and the individualized rescue remedy is for times of real crisis. It should yield dramatic positive results whenever it is needed, since it is not generic but is blended specific to the needs of the patient.

In conclusion, every time you give a Bach remedy to anyone, including yourself, it is vital that you know why you are giving it and can identify the goal of treatment.

I am not a fan of taking any medicine on a regular basis, no matter how benign it may be. It has been identified as having the power to make changes within a patient's being just by virtue of the fact that it is a medicine. And I don't believe that we should be making any changes without a reason or a plan.

Certainly, Bach remedies can be used acutely as needed. But always keep that phrase "as needed" in the front of your mind. A remedy needed once, to bring things back to balance, should not be repeated. All medicine should be given in the fewest number of doses needed.

That phrase "as needed" means that someone, the physician or the patient or a caregiver, must oversee the dosing. And that phrase "as needed" always implies that, once the dose has been given, someone will be waiting and watching to see if it is ever needed again. The remedies should be repeated or changed only when old patterns return. As long as balance remains, the patient's own vital force should be respected enough to let him move ahead with his life without the interference of medicine.

# 14

# Using Bach
# Flower Remedies

Becoming truly skillful with the Bach remedies involves learning to manage your cases. It may also mean that you yourself may have to learn the lessons your patients internalize as they work with the remedies. And that you may have much to learn from the remedies themselves and from the emotional patterns—good and bad— that they mirror.

## Case Management

Becoming truly skilled with any form of medical treatment, even one as benign as the Bach Flower Remedies, involves more than an understanding of the full pharmacy of medicines at your disposal. It also requires that you have some understanding of the patient who is in need of aid and of the nature of illness itself. Both Bach and Hahnemann wrote extensively about the nature of illness, the methods by which it can be safely treated, and how the patient's natural healing system can be encouraged to return the patient to a state of balance we can equate with "good health."

You must always ask yourself exactly what you are doing when you give any remedy or medicine. Ask yourself if there is a need to treat the patient and if you are skilled enough to treat him. You and the patient must agree on the nature of the treatment. And, finally, you and the patient must have shared expectations as to the outcome of the treatment.

In other words, treatment is a matter of goals. If the patient is in a moment of crisis, then the goal must be to restore balance. There is no reason to do anything else until balance is restored. No point in finding out what their lifelong health has been like, or if they have trouble sleeping; you must work acutely to bring back a sense of self. That can be the only goal of treatment in such a situation.

Remember, in acute treatments we—the patient and the physician together comprising the "we"—are working toward the goal of restoring the patient to the same physical and emotional condition he was in before the present crisis. This goal assumes that the patient was in a state of good health before the crisis, something that may or may not be factual.

That's the problem with acute treatments, and why we must move beyond them at some point if we are to be serious with the Bach remedies. What lies beyond are constitutional treatments; treatments that actually try to help the patient release old negative patterns of thought and action and replace them with healthier modes of behavior.

You can't just work in the moment to do that. You have to go deeper, in your understanding of your patient (even if that patient is yourself) and in your understanding of the remedies and their uses.

You have to learn to be good at taking cases, at recognizing the remedies when you see them played out before you "in the flesh." And making the leap from the words on the page to actual patterns of behavior in a complex and often contradictory human being can be very difficult. It takes study and it takes practice. Those who tell you that you can refer to a chart of Bach remedies and use them effectively without giving it any more thought or time than it takes to read a

> The fact that the remedies are benign makes the task easier, since our chances of causing any real damage are very, very slim. But that does not mean there is no responsibility involved in giving anyone—even ourselves—any form of medicine.

sentence or two are oversimplifying an admittedly simple system of treatment. Just because Bach worked hard for seven years to streamline and simplify homeopathic principles of treatment does not mean that he was intending his treatments to be mindless, or to require no follow-up or study.

It is easier to learn Bach's *Materia Medica* of only thirty-eight remedies than it is to learn even the most basic and commonly used of Hahnemann's over 5,000 remedies, but it still takes some time and effort to get it right. In fact, it can take years and years of practice before you can honestly say that you understand these remedies. Only in recent years, after twenty-five years as a student of Hahnemann and Bach, can I honestly say I have made real leeway into understanding the philosophy and practice of homeopathy and its related therapies.

So study is required. Trial and error is required. The fact that the remedies are benign and we have the capacity within us to respond to them all does make the task easier, since our chances of causing any real damage are very, very slim. But that does not mean there is no responsibility involved in giving anyone—even ourselves—any form of medicine.

I am not saying this to be negative or difficult, but only to stress that you create changes in your patient when you give any sort of medicine. Unless both you and your patient are aware of this possibility, and willing and able to deal with whatever changes occur, it would be better not to give that medicine in the first place. This goes for any form of medicine, from Bach remedies, to herbs and supplements (which are allopathic in nature and can be very damaging to the patient if not used correctly), to over-the-counter medicines. In my opinion, the only safe method of treatment that requires no prior study is prayer.

So start by learning. Learning the process of healing, the remedies and their uses, and case taking. And by learning how you manage a case once you have taken it and given the remedy.

Case management for Bach treatments is a simple thing, at least when compared with allopathic or homeopathic treatments. There is no need for record keeping regarding particular doses or potencies, but it is important to keep notes about the case taking itself, any remedies considered for the case, and those actually used. Make sure to keep simple records of what combinations of remedies were used, during what period of time, and the approximate number of doses per day. Then keep records about any changes that were observed by the patient, his loved ones (if that information is available) and by you, the practitioner.

The actions of Bach remedies are considered to be cumulative. This means that any changes or progress should be permanent. The patient who takes the remedies for a period of time and then stops taking them (whatever the reason) should enjoy their continued benefits. If he begins to take them again, he will likely not have to revisit old patterns, but can begin working from a point of increased health. Therefore, a case should always be revisited before any remedies are taken if a patient decides to begin taking his remedies again after not taking them for a period of time. The same remedies may not be needed any longer.

Case management also demands that you keep records of all the changes you make in a given patient's remedies over a period of time. It also suggests that you keep track of any remedies that may seem called for at some point in treatment but are not being used at present. This list can be very valuable as treatment progresses, because this list of remedies will help you understand your thinking at all stages in the treatment. Often these will be remedies you will incorporate in the combination at some point in the treatment.

Always keep notes that record what the patient thinks of his or her progress. After all, this is fundamentally more important to the healing process than what you are thinking. And keep these notes, as much as possible, in the patient's own words. If the patient says something particularly important or revealing, write it down just as soon as possible in the exact wording the patient used.

When treatment ends for any reason, record its ending, the circumstances, the date, and the remedies that were in use at the time the treatment concluded. In acute cases, treatment ends rather swiftly. The patient is calm once more after a car accident. The treatment ends. The case is simple to record, since the practitioner has given very few remedies for a very short period of time. The patient is restored to a state of emotional balance and has gone about his business. Still, the case merits recording, and its success or failure yields information worthy of study. You can learn what acute remedies were or were not effective for that patient from these cases. You can learn what works best for him and for others who share his emotional "type." Each simple acute case, if well recorded and studied, can give information that will help the practitioner polish his art.

In constitutional cases, treatments usually end when the patient feels the remedies have done all they can. When he feels better for his treatment, or when he concludes that the remedies have not brought him the help he had hoped for. Either way, by studying the increased complexity of the constitutional case, you can learn from your success or your failure. You can learn about the remedies. You can learn about yourself, your skill level, and your own emotional patterns. You can learn about your patient, and you can also learn *from* him.

## Learning from the Patient

In homeopathy, we believe that each new patient is a universe unto himself. That he is totally unique, just as he is totally whole. Each of us is a complete being, in body, mind, and spirit. And each of us functions according to a unique set of "rules." We are all similar beings with similar needs, and we live within a range of functions and beliefs that we call "normal," but the number of factors that allow each of us to be totally unique within that range of normality is nearly infinite. Therefore, we enter into homeopathic case taking with no expectations, only a willingness to feel compassion for and reach an understanding of the totally unique being sitting next to us.

It is the same with Bach treatments. Even though we strip away all that is physical from our thinking and focus on the mind and spirit of the individual instead, that invisible, intangible being is just as complex as the whole person. Nearly anything is possible when we deal with the mind, the emotions, the spirit, and the imagination. And those infinite possibilities must, to some degree, be taken into account.

Since each patient is a new individual, with new viewpoints and new patterns of behavior, we can learn from each new person we encounter.

And since each patient also lives within the range of human thought, human imagination, and physical human life, we also have myriad points of reference—things we have in common through our shared human experience. Although each patient is totally unique, he is also representative of all those who share his basic patterning and adapted to life's stresses with similar conclusions as to how they could best survive or thrive. Therefore, by learning more about the patient, we also learn more about other individuals who follow the same constitutional pattern. And when we learn which remedies combine well for this individual, we learn more about the remedies that combine well for others in his type.

In truth, I don't think it is possible to work with each patient as a complete individual and still be able to function "in the moment." By their very nature many cases, especially acute cases, demand that the case be taken quickly and remedies given immediately. If we cannot learn from patterning, from our own past experiences, and from the recorded experiences of others, we may find that we cannot always treat effectively. If we cannot learn from clinical experience, we will always flail about trying to decide upon a remedy while the patient suffers.

So you have to learn from your patients. Learn what works in the present and place it beside what has worked in the past, to learn what may work in the future. This clinical body of knowledge—your own firsthand knowledge and the recorded experiences of others—will be your single greatest tool when working with the remedies.

But the information will only be usable if it is recorded in a reliable manner. Organization is the key. All serious students of the Bach remedies must learn to write down their findings and organize those records so they are most accessible to themselves and others. While such record keeping may seem silly to those who are only giving Rescue Remedy to their child when he skins his knee, let me point out that if they ever want to do more than that, the pathway to growth as a practitioner demands study, organization, and clinical experience.

## Learning from the Remedies

As far as I am concerned, the greatest teachers in your learning process will be the remedies themselves. The more you study them, the more you use them, the more you will be able to understand about the process of healing and about yourself.

Bach spent seven years of his life working with plants and making his remedies. I believe he began with a plan for just twelve remedies that would be the cure for all of mankind's ills. Once he found his original twelve, he discovered that there were other aspects of human nature—other patterns of negative thought and behavior that were common to us all—that were not contained within the actions of the original twelve. With what I assume was a degree of reluctance at leaving his simple, organized group of a dozen remedies behind, he began to add to them, as he either recognized a particular healing virtue in a given plant or accepted the need to find a remedy for a particular destructive pattern not addressed by the existing remedies.

> As far as I am concerned, the greatest teachers in your learning process will be the remedies themselves. The more you study them, the more you use them, the more you will be able to understand about the process of healing and about yourself.

He added seven new remedies in the next group. Instead of thinking of them as nineteen remedies, he wrote about the original dozen as his primary remedies and the other seven as secondary remedies to be used when the others failed to act.

But he was driven by the need to be able to deal with the full range of human behaviors with his pharmacy of remedies; all the negative and destructive patterns of thought and action. And this is not something that you can fit into easy numbers. Just as the number of remedies that will be needed for a particular patient cannot be predicted as the process of discovery begins.

In the end, Edward Bach discovered thirty-eight remedies. He felt each spoke to a specific pattern of thought and action that could color the life of any human being, for better or worse. More important, he felt that the remedies covered all human patterns of thought and behavior as a group, and that each covered a wide range of positive, benign, or negative motivations as contained within that specific pattern.

Bach, therefore, created a system of treatment that could, quite literally, bring some degree of benefit to every human being. The remedies offer everyone a potential for growth and creative development.

In studying the Bach Flower Remedies, we study ourselves, both as individuals and as members of a race of beings of incredible complexity. The range of behaviors in the continuum of each remedy's pattern of thought and action is a topic for long study. The study of all the remedies and the implications for treatment—metaphorical and actual—that each offers may well take much longer than the seven years Bach dedicated to their discovery. (Remember that seven-year period was preceded by a lifetime of work in the field of medicine.)

Any book on the subject can only give a limited education on this subject, since it only gives the viewpoint of an individual author. So even though books can be a good way of learning the basics, the real education comes from the remedies themselves.

Study them. Take them. Use them. Each remedy speaks to an aspect of human behavior, so open yourself up to the simple fact that each and every remedy represents some pattern of negativity present within yourself—whether you like it or not. Work to find patterns of behavior within yourself that mirror the working of each remedy. That's how you can learn from the remedy, even without taking it.

Work with the idea of possibility. Consider the remedy—like Willow, which has a really bad reputation—and think about it. Instead of immediately thinking, "Well, I'll never need that remedy," think about how you have needed it in the past and how you might need it right now. Think of patterns of behavior—acute or chronic—that you have displayed that show the need for that remedy.

No one wants to admit to really negative behaviors. No one wants to be the Willow or the Holly; everyone wants to be the Star of Bethlehem or the Wild Oat. But, in truth, we all need them all. We all have the full range of potential within us, each remedy type with its most positive aspects and its most negative. By facing this truth—that we all have angels and devils on our shoulders at every moment in our lives—we can learn so much from Bach's research and his remedies.

When you identify a remedy that you thought was totally alien to you at first, but then find the mirror to that remedy within yourself, try taking it. Just put a drop or two on your tongue and go about your business. Later, write about your experience, and the changes, if any, you observed in your own thought and behavior. Even if you never add that remedy to your constitutional mixture, you can still learn about yourself, about the process by which you are healed, and about Bach's pharmacy of therapeutics just by taking a few drops of that remedy.

## In Conclusion

Learn to trust yourself. Trust your instincts as you work with the remedies to heal yourself and heal others, just as Bach trusted his instincts when he wandered like a madman around the countryside, looking for his remedies. There will be many sources of information along the way. There are a number of good books, some excellent Internet sites, and, of course, Edward Bach's own writings, which themselves can fully illuminate your path.[1]

All these sources of information are good. All will help, especially in the early days, when you find yourself flipping through books trying to figure out what to give before just giving up and reaching for the Rescue Remedy.

As I have said before, your best source of information will ultimately be your own experience. The remedies will be old friends to you in time, and their uses will be well mapped in your mind. You will, in time, make your own decision as to how many remedies can be used at once and how well they work in combination as opposed to singly. I think that Bach was very wise in not setting up the rigid system of treatment that Hahnemann did, and in creating a group of remedies whose potencies and actions allowed for and encouraged self-treatment and treatment by lay persons. Because of this, and because of the simple truths that are the foundation of his system of treatment—truths that eluded so many other medical geniuses over the centuries, researchers and practitioners who, unlike Bach, were unwilling to reexamine sources of treatment that had fallen by the wayside—Bach has given us perhaps the most useful, dynamic, and, yes, powerful source of healing available today.

The joke is on those who deride the Bach remedies as a form of quackery. Allopathic drugs may suppress our aches and pains for a time, and homeopathic remedies may actually cure our colds, but only the Bach remedies can change our hearts. Only the Flower Remedies hold a mirror up to each of us, and give us the possibility of true growth, true change, and true healing.

---

1. Turn to the Resources at the back of this book for a short list of the books and other sources of information on the Bach remedies that I have found to be especially helpful.

# Appendices

"The action of these remedies is to . . . flood our natures
with the particular virtue we need, and wash out from
us the fault which is causing us harm. They are able,
like beautiful music . . . to raise our very natures,
and bring us nearer to our Souls' and by that very act,
to bring us peace, and relieve our sufferings.

"They cure, not by attacking disease, but by flooding
our bodies with the beautiful vibrations of our Higher
Nature, in the presence of which disease melts
as snow in the sunshine."

—EDWARD BACH IN
YE SUFFER FROM YOURSELVES

# Resources

Gathered here is a list of the books, organizations and Internet sites that I can recommend to you in your study of the Bach Flower Remedies. I will not list any particular pharmacies or sources for the remedies themselves because they can be purchased in any health food store and also are readily available online.

## BOOKS

Some of the books listed here have been used as resources in the creation of this book, as noted in the text. Others are part of my own library of books on homeopathy and floral essences. All give a unique look at the philosophy of Edward Bach and the use of the Bach Flower Remedies. I have separated the books into two categories: those on Bach and his philosophy and those on the use of his remedies. All are listed in order of how useful I have found them.

### Books about Bach, the Man

*The Collected Writings of Edward Bach,* by Edward Bach, Edited by Julian Barnard. Hereford, England: Bach Educational Programme (1987). If you only own one book on the Bach remedies, this is the one to have. This is the definitive collection of all of Bach's writings and it contains all his major writings, lectures, and even letters. Not only does this book give the reader an understanding of the evolution of the Bach remedies, it also gives insight into Bach himself as a man. It also shows that Bach was that rarest of physicians, a natural communicator as well as a healer.

*The Bach Flower Remedies,* by Edward Bach and F. J. Wheeler. New Canaan, CT: Keats Publishing (1979). This is an odd little book. It is an American publication and presents to the American audience an abbreviated edition of Bach's own writings, including two important booklets, *Heal Thyself* and *The Twelve Healers.* It also includes a repertory of symptoms and the Bach remedies used to treat them by Dr. Francis Wheeler, which, while it is in print individually, can be hard to come by. Wheeler's repertory can be a useful tool in selecting remedies. (As a separate publication, it was published by C.W. Daniel Company, Ltd. of Saffron Walden, Essex, England, 1988.)

*The Medical Discoveries of Edward Bach, Physician,* by Nora Weeks. This is the closest thing we have to a biography of Edward Bach, and, while is it far from complete and very far from objective (Weeks was a close friend and coworker of Bach's), it remains the only picture we have of Bach and the only history we have of his transformation from allopath to homeopath to developer of his own unique system of medical treatment. This book belongs on the shelf of every serious student of the Bach remedies, if only as a sweet and nostalgic look at the man who dedicated his life to their creation. Originally written in the 1930s; multiple reprint editions are available.

## Books about Bach, the Remedies

*Advanced Bach Flower Therapy: A Scientific Approach to Diagnosis and Treatment,* by Gotz Blome, M.D. Rochester, VT: Healing Arts Press (1992). This is an excellent book on the Bach remedies. It not only contains solid, in-depth information on each individual remedy, but also on the combinations that have special importance, in the author's experience. The writing is clear and very well organized. Should be on every bookshelf.

*Bach Flower Therapy: Theory and Practice,* by Mechthild Scheffer. Rochester, VT: Healing Arts Press (1981). This book has become a sort of bible of Bach books in many ways. Since it was published nearly twenty-five years ago, it has forged a special niche among books on this subject. Scheffer was perhaps the first to truly explore the psychological importance of the Bach remedies and to use them in her Naturopathic practice. While the writing (or perhaps the translation) of the text is stilted or oblique at times, this remains an important reference book. Should be on every bookshelf.

*The Encyclopedia of Bach Flower Therapy,* by Mechthild Scheffer. Rochester, VT: Healing Arts Press (2001). As promised by the title, this is an exhaustive look at the remedies and their uses from perhaps the most prominent author in the field. The color plates of the plants from which the remedies are taken are of special interest. While I don't find anything particularly new about this book and consider her earlier work *Bach Flower Therapy* to be a better book, this is still a fine effort. For any bookshelf.

*Mastering Bach: A Guide to Flower Therapies,* by Mechthild Scheffer. Rochester, VT: Healing Arts Press (1996). One of Scheffer's several other follow-ups to *Bach Flower Therapy, Mastering Bach* is an excellent adjunct, as it dedicates a large portion of the book to case studies. The information contained on the treatment of animals and plants with Bach flower therapy is especially valuable. For more advanced students.

*Bach Flower Remedies Form & Function,* by Julian Barnard. Great Barrington, MA: Lindisfarne Books (2003). As the editor of Bach's own collected works, Mr. Barnard is perhaps without peer in his knowledge of the remedies. As such, any book he authors is important and worthy of a position on any bookshelf. And this is, quite simply, an excellent book. It is idiosyncratic, unique, and chock-full of information. I think that this is one of the very best books on the subject and belongs on every bookshelf.

*The Bach Remedies: A Self-Help Guide*, by Leslie J. Kaslof. New Canaan, CT: Keats Publishing (1988). This little booklet is a good, solid bit of information on all things Bach for the beginner. Kaslof, as the President of the Dr. Edward Bach Healing Society of North America, has a solid background in the use of the remedies. Beware of putting too much credence on the questionnaire the booklet contains, however. Good for the beginner.

*Introduction to the Benefits of the Bach Flower Remedies*, by Jane Evans. Essex, England: C. W. Daniel Company Ltd. (1989). This is another good little book(let) for the beginner. It is especially useful for selecting remedies in acute circumstances. Note that this is not a book of thumbnail sketches of the remedies, but, instead, is an overview of the philosophy of treatment with some case studies included. Good for the beginner.

*Bach Flower Essences for the Family*, anonymous. London, England: Wigmore Publication, Ltd. (1993). This is the book most of us start out with, as it is published in conjunction with Original Bach Flower Essences, the company that bottles and sells the essences throughout the United States. This is the thin, green and yellow pamphlet sold next to the remedies in health food stores. And it is good, if the limitations of the text are respected. You will find a thumbnail of each remedy's actions and a line drawing of the flower from which it is made. A solid guide for the beginner.

*The Bach Flower Remedies: Step by Step*, by Judy Howard. Essex, England: C. W. Daniel Company Ltd. (1990). This book is a slim volume, but it is also a fairly well-rounded volume for the beginner. It has a good deal more to offer than the pamphlets listed above, but lacks the depth of Sheffer's and Blome's works. *Step by Step* is just what the title implies, a brief look at each of the thirty-eight remedies, wild praising of Rescue Remedy, and some very short case studies. For the beginner.

*The Illustrated Handbook of the Bach Flower Remedies*, by Philip M. Chancellor. Essex, England: C. W. Daniel Company Ltd. (1989). One of the first books published on the subject of the Bach remedies after the remedies underwent their renaissance in the late 1970s. Chancellor's book has been published in two different editions, one with illustrations, one without (that American edition was published by Keats Publishing of New Canaan, CT). While the information included is certainly complete, I must admit that I have never been taken with Chancellor's style of writing, nor do I tend to agree with his take on the remedies. However, his is a strong viewpoint that may appeal to many readers.

*Flowers to the Rescue, The Healing Vision of Dr. Edward Bach*, by Gregory Vlamis. Rochester, VT: Healing Arts Press (1988). This book gives less of an overview of the Bach remedies than it gives snippets of case studies that illustrate their use on patients from human beings to animals and plants. It is perhaps of greatest interest to those who want to learn more about treating their animals with the Bach remedies.

*Bach Flower Remedies for Men*, by Stefan Ball. Essex, England: C.W. Daniel Company

Ltd. (1996). Maybe I am prejudiced, but I feel that many of the other books on Bach remedies are slanted toward women and the ways women patients specifically feel and express their emotions. Therefore, I find this volume to be excellent, and it gives a unique look at the remedies in that it deals specifically with emotionally stunted males as its topic and the ways in which a male patient feels and expresses his emotions. This is a really good book and it belongs on the bookshelf of every serious student. (Note that the companion volume, *Bach Flower Remedies for Women*, by Judy Howard, a coauthor of Ball's, is not as good. Nor is it, in my opinion, necessary, since most of the books written about the remedies are written by and for women. *Remedies for Women* is published by the same publisher as is *Remedies for Men*.)

*Growing Up with Bach Flower Remedies: A Guide to the Use of the Remedies During Childhood and Adolescence*, by Judy Howard. Essex, England: C.W. Daniel Company Ltd. (1994). I truly recommend this volume to any serious student of the Bach remedies, in that it illustrates how our need for specific remedies and the ways that this need is embodied in our behaviors changes throughout the stages of our lives. This book gives a look at each remedy as seen in the younger patient and of the sorts of complaints, both physical and emotional, that each remedy may be used to treat. This book should be on the bookshelf of every serious student.

*Harmony Is the Healer: The Combined Handbook of Healing Flowers, Colour Therapy, Schussler Tissue-Salts, Emergency Homeopathy and Other Forms of Vibrational Medicine*, by Ingrid S. von Rohr. Rockport, MA: Element (1992). As the title indicates, this book is sort of a catchall for so-called "vibrational medicine." As this book links Bach remedies with homeopathy, I thought that I should list a book that gives more information on the subject. This book, while not perfect (some of the indicated remedies and potencies for homeopathic remedies are downright ridiculous), it has a wide range of topics and gives the readers information on the link between Bach remedies and other offshoots of homeopathy. Not an essential book, by any means, but an interesting one.

*The Twelve Healers of the Zodiac: The Astrology Handbook of the Bach Flower Remedies*, by Peter Damian. York Beach, ME: Samuel Weiser (1986). This is one kooky little book. In it, author Damian takes each of Bach's original twelve remedies and applies them to the signs of the zodiac. Damian incurs my wrath just by associating the remedy Scleranthus with my own sun sign Libra. After all, as a cardinal sign, Libra is anything but indecisive. Damian lets the scale get in his way. One can only guess what Bach might have thought of this. Buy it if you like, but it is certainly not required reading.

*New Bach Flower Therapies: Healing the Emotional and Spiritual Causes of Illness*, by Dietmar Kramer. Rochester VT: Healing Arts Press (1995). This book, and its companion volume listed below, illustrates an idiosyncratic method by which remedies are selected and used. While the book attempts to be modern and even "hip" in its language (patients "freak out," etc.) it is actually a bit stilted (again, it may be the translation). But since Kramer's technique is different, and I tend to champion a fresh viewpoint, I find some value in it. This book is not, however, for the beginner, as it may cause more confusion than enlightenment.

*New Bach Flower Maps: Treatment by Topical Application*, by Dietmar Kramer and Helmut Wild. Rochester, VT: Healing Arts Press (1996). In this follow-up volume, Kramer refines his technique of using Bach remedies. This book offers methods by which remedies can be selected through astrological diagnosis, as well as information on "body mapping," by which the remedies can be used topically on specific parts of the body to direct and strengthen their ability to bring about healing. Like Kramer's other book, this is certainly not for any beginner, but it can offer information that may be of value to more advanced students.

## ORGANIZATIONS AND INTERNET SITES

Organizations dedicated to the Bach Flower Remedies are not as pervasive as are those dedicated to homeopathy. To my knowledge, there is no such thing as a "Bach Flower Study Group," at least not in the United States. Therefore, most of the organizations that do exist have their public face on the Internet. The Internet is also the major source for buying books on the remedies and the remedies themselves, of course. Anyone interested in finding remedies and supplies related to the Bach remedies need look no further than Amazon.com.

The organizations whose workings and websites are familiar to me are listed here. They all have information to offer and I recommend them to you.

**www.edwardbach.org:** This excellent site is sponsored by the Bach Flower Research Programme and edited by educator Glenn Storhaug. This group sponsors an international conference on the Bach remedies, along with other educational events that feature some of the best-known authors in the field. The site is well designed and offers, among other things, a timeline of the workings of the Bach Centre, which has continued the work of Edward Bach since 1950.

**bachcentre.com:** The Centre's own official website, based in Mount Vernon, England, the geographical location where the flower remedies were developed. The site gives information on Bach himself, as well as on the Centre and its foundation. There is also excellent material on the remedies and their uses with humans and animals.

**www.healingherbs.co.uk:** Julian Barnard's own website. Barnard, who is a part of the Bach Centre and a speaker at the Bach Flower Research Programme's conference (I am always impressed with how the various groups dedicated to the Bach remedies work together and never seem to compete or lower themselves with politics or squabbles.) was the editor of Bach's own writings and is one of the leading authors and educators on the subject of Bach remedies. This site has some information on the remedies and is also a source for books and remedies themselves.

**nelsons.net:** This is the only strictly commercial site I will list. Nelson's is a homeopathic pharmacy in London, one of the best, if not the best, homeopathic pharmacy in the world. Therefore, when Nelson's bought the rights to bottle and sell the Bach remedies a few years back from Bach's estate, I thought it was a great idea. They have proven to respect Bach's remedies over these years just as much as they have Hahnemann's over a period of many more years. I invite you to visit this site and learn more about the wonderful company.

**bachflowersusa.com:** This American site is dedicated to flower essences, both Bach's and those of the Flower Essence Society (for more on that group, see the next endnote, "Other Flower Essences"). While the site is less well constructed than the others listed here, and while its creators have decided not to give their names or personal history along with the remedies, the site is still valuable. It also has very good links to other important sites.

**holisticmed.com:** This site is an excellent resource. It has exhaustive links to all the Internet has to offer to anyone interested in any sort of holistic medication, including homeopathy and Bach Flower Remedies. Just visit the home page and follow the links to your area of interest. Under Bach Flower Remedies, you will find links to discussion groups, commercial sites, non-profit sites, and educational sites, as well as information on using the remedies with humans, animals, and plants. Bookmark this site, as you will find yourself using it often.

# Twelve Healers,
# Seven Helpers

In writing about his Twelve Healers in "The Twelve Healers and Seven Helpers," Bach states that "If we treat the mood and not the disease we are treating the real person, and we are giving the patient what is truly required to bring back health." He therefore suggests that the twelve remedies listed below can be just as helpful for those with physical complaints such as headache and digestive upset as they are for emotion upsets, exhaustion, and depression.

Note that, in discussing both his Twelve Healers and the so-called Seven Helpers, Bach considers the patient in a state of illness and specifically how the patient reacts to the fact that he or she is, in fact, physically ill. In that Bach ignored the whole concept of physical illness in most cases, the information listed here may be of particular interest.

Bach writes about the manner in which each of his Twelve Healers experiences pain and/or physical illness in "Twelve Great Remedies." A thumbnail sketch of each remedy type follows.

**Agrimony** (*Agrimonia Eupatoria*): While many other remedy types will try to mask their fear or depression about their illness, no other type will try so hard to mask the very fact that they are ill as the Agrimony. Whatever their illness, the Agrimony type will expend a good deal of energy trying to convince others that they are feeling just fine. And since he will do his very best to make light of his situation, it may take a good deal of objective conjecture to make the remedy selection of Agrimony.

**Centaury** (*Erythraea Centaurium*): The Centaury type may quite literally faint before he will actually ask for help in his illness. He is certainly weak and, often, light-headed because of his illness, but he will most often not want to make a fuss about it, or may simply be too timid to ask for help. The Centaury type, who has a small vital force in the best of times, will become even weaker in illness, and may literally have no energy for any sort of task, no matter how small.

**Cerato** (*Ceratostigma Willmottiana*): You have to watch the Cerato type who is ill very carefully, because he is likely to do just about anything. He will ask you for advice and then choose not to follow it (as is always the case, sick or well). If that advice is as basic as "Go to bed, rest and drink liquids," and he decides not to follow it, he may slide into deeper illness through inaction. Also, the Cerato type who is ill will just plain tend to do stupid things. He will spontaneously decide to eat the wrong thing, or will take too many pills or none at all. Great mischief can result when the basic misguided nature of Cerato is coupled with physical illness, if he is not taken in hand.

**Chicory** (*Cichorium Intybus*): The common tie among all those who need Chicory is that they are fussy patients. No other patients will be so fussy about their covers or the amount of light in the room. This may fool you into thinking that Chicory types are healthier than they actually are. They will still fuss over details while quite ill. They will also demand a great deal of attention and will become even more demanding if they feel they are being ignored.

**Clematis** (*Clematis Vitalba*): The Clematis patient is quite the opposite of the Chicory patient above. The Clematis type, who tends toward daydreams even when well, becomes very sleepy when ill. The Clematis seems to drift in illness, and when sick seems to be very far away. When speaking to him, you will have to draw him back from the place into which he has drifted. The Clematis patient will have little apparent interest in his illness or in getting well.

**Gentian** (*Gentiana Amarella*): The Gentian type wrestles with a tendency toward yielding battles too easily even when well, so they move swiftly into depression when physical illness strikes. The Gentian type will feel there is little reason to struggle against his or her disease, and will not try to regain footing. Instead, he will move deeper and deeper into depression as his physical symptoms increase.

**Impatiens** (*Impatiens Grandulifera*): This is an excellent remedy to consider in any case that involves sharp or deep pain. Especially for cases that involve pains that appear suddenly, and cases in which the patient is suffering greatly from sheer pain. The Impatiens type, when ill, tends to be even more abrupt in their behaviors than he does when well. This is a very difficult patient. He is quick and easy to anger, almost impossible to please. At his best, he could be called "peevish." Like the patient with a sudden toothache, the Impatiens type tends toward lurching about and lashing out.

**Mimulus** (*Mimulus Luteus*): The Mimulus patient will, of course, link fear with his physical illness. As is common to the type, he or she will likely mask this fear with a sense of calm, but, inside, will be deeply afraid. Unlike the Agrimony, the Mimulus type will not try to mask the fact that he is ill, but will mask the fact that he is afraid of what the illness may lead to. He may fear poverty from the cost of treatment, the treatment itself, the pain of his condition or death itself, but he will attempt, to the best of his ability, to seem as if he is coping nicely with the fact that he is ill.

**Rock Rose** (*Helianthemum Nummularium*): Rock Rose is often an important remedy, not only for the patient who needs Rock Rose, but also for all those in the household of the patient. This remedy is often called for in cases of sudden and severe illness. Terror is always in the air when Rock Rose is called for. Either the illness is very serious or it is perceived as being very serious. Often it can be helpful for the infant who suddenly has a fever and seems terrified by his condition. When a patient needs Rock Rose, it is almost always a good idea that the caregivers take it as well so terror can be completely removed from the healing equation.

**Scleranthus** (*Scleranthus Annuus*): Nothing seems quite right for the Scleranthus who is ill. This patient will jump from medicine to medicine and doctor to doctor, with renewed enthusiasm at each leap, only to experience disappointment once more when things don't work out as planned. Scleranthus patients may also exhibit unpredictable behaviors, acting rational and calm one moment, excited and aggressive the next. Those around the Scleranthus will be kept off balance by his ever changing demands and by his erratic behavior.

**Vervain** (*Verbena Oficinalis*): No one else will withstand the amount of pain that Vervain types will. They continue on, trying not only to cope with their illness, but also trying to accomplish their usual life's tasks in spite of tremendous obstacles. This aspect of their personality may leave the rest of us in awe, but the other side of the coin is that no one is so difficult to help during times of illness as Vervain types. They do not want your help or advice. They remain strong-willed and very, very stubborn even in illness unto death. Often they will rise up from their sickbeds to tell the doctors what to do.

**Water Violet** (*Hottonia Palustris*): The Water Violet type will always go into retreat in illness. When well, the Water Violet type will tend to touch upon the rest of the world only lightly, choosing carefully the events and people that bring forth his or her social nature. When sick, the Water Violet type will quite simply want to be alone. Like a sick dog, he may even disappear when ill, as if he were going away to die. He will always want quiet when ill. He will not want company, light, noise, or activity of any sort.

## Bach's "Seven Helpers":

Bach developed the seven following remedies for particular use for patient's who had chronic conditions. As Bach puts it in "The Twelve Healers and Seven Helpers," "When an illness is old, it has become more established and may require help before it responds easily, so that the seven remedies for such cases are called the Seven Helpers."

At the time of their creation, Bach saw these twelve remedies as being the second tier of treatments, that they were most useful in cases of chronic illness in which the best-selected of the Twelve Healers had failed to complete the case.

Bach considered the patient's coloring helpful in selecting among the seven remedies below. Pale patients were grouped toward Gorse, Oak and Olive, while ruddy patients were moved toward Heather, Rock Water, Vine and Wild Oat.

The Seven Helpers are:

**Gorse** (*Ulex Europeus*): For the patient who feels that his case is hopeless, that everything has been tried and that nothing will restore him to health. Look for a complexion with a yellowish tinge, and for dark circles under the eyes.

**Heather** (*Calluna Vulgaris*): The typical Heather type has a very low threshold of pain that he feels that he may endure. Where the Oak or Olive types may struggle on with a great deal of pain, the Heather type insists that he can bear no more while actually dealing with a great deal less. In fact, this remedy type tends toward the ruddy end of the spectrum of human complexions. He may look very healthy, seem to have great vitality, and yet he will insist upon endlessly telling you his symptoms.

**Oak** (*Quercus Pedunculata*): Compare this remedy with Gorse to be sure to make the right selection. The Oak patient, like the Gorse type, may be struggling with a long illness, and yet, even though he feels that there is little hope of a positive outcome, he still has a glimmer of hope. Even if he says that he feels hopeless, he continues to struggle onward to the very best of his ability. This "hard struggle" is keynote to the Oak patient. Look for a pale complexion.

**Olive** (*Olea Europea*): For patients who are depleted. They may have already endured a long illness, or have expended their energy in caring for others. They may have experienced a loss of love or have suffered through conditions that caused them a great deal of stress or worry. But now their strength is gone and they lack the ability to continue to struggle onward. Olive patients may be very needy. Look for pale complexions, which are most common. Look for dry skin that may be prematurely wrinkled.

**Rock Water** (Rock Water): The Rock Water patient will be very strict. Not so much with others, but with themselves. When he becomes ill, he actually increases his strict behavior. He narrows his diet and his lifestyle in order to exclude any supposed cause of illness. As an austere and stoic individual, he will struggle with illness every step of the way, endure any treatment that he is convinced will help him back to health. Perhaps ironically, Rock Water patients tend to have healthy-looking complexions.

**Vine** (*Vitis Vinifera*): Vine patients are taskmasters. In chronic illness they continue to believe that they are quite correct in their opinions and will direct the course of their own treatment. They have been said to be the types who continue to give orders from their graves. They tend toward highly colored complexions, often with very red faces.

**Wild Oat** (*Bromus Ramosus*): This is Bach's all-purpose "Helper." He suggests that this remedy may be given as something of a wild card to any patient who is not responding to another supposedly well-chosen remedy. Bach instructs that this remedy should be given for at least a week before considering a change to another remedy. In that Wild Oat is for those who are unsure of their path, it is logical that, when applied to the idea of treating those who are stuck in illness, it would be helpful for those whose condition remains mysterious even after treatment. If Wild Oat is not helpful itself, it will uncover the true nature of the patient's complaints. While Bach lists Wild Oat under "high colored" remedies, the patient needing Wild Oat may have any sort of complexion, from very pale to very ruddy.

# The Yin and Yang of Bach Remedies

One way to consider the remedies and whether or not a given remedy is indicated for a particular person is to consider the flow of that person's life energy. Some people naturally seem to exude energy, to send it forth into the people around them. These are the people who exert influence upon others, or who may intimidate or attempt to control others. These are the remedies that may be said to be "yang" (referring to the twin concepts of yin and yang, in which "yin" represents the feminine, the principle of yielding, while "yang" represents the masculine, the principle of aggression). The remedies that represent people who take in energy from others more than they yield to others may be said to be "yin."

The following is a list of the remedies associated with each of these principles. Note that not all thirty-eight remedies are listed here. Some belong in neither camp because they are either balanced in their energy or erratic in that they may be receptive at certain times and aggressive at others.

## Constitutional Yang Remedy Types

The remedies in this group are constitutional in type, meaning that those who fall into these patterns of thought and behavior will often follow the same pattern for a long period of time.

**Holly:** The remedy type for pure aggression. The Holly type is motivated into action through rage and jealousy. He can be physically, mentally, and emotionally aggressive, even abusive. Holly is the remedy needed by those who are motivated by any negative aggressive emotion: anger, hate, jealousy, vindictiveness, cruelty, among others. It is also a remedy type that commonly has a strong sex drive and may be motivated by his sexual needs.

**Vine:** The Vine patient typically is both aggressive and domineering. The Vine type seeks power and positions in which he is in authority over others. He can use his power to punish. In a positive emotional state, the Vine type is a natural leader. In a negative emotional state, he is a tyrant. The Vine type is naturally suspicious of others and their motivations. He will be especially suspicious that people are lying to him.

**Impatiens:** Aggressive but not domineering. The Impatiens type seeks independence, not authority. If, however, he is placed in a position of authority, he can be an exacting taskmaster. This remedy type is known for his intensity and his irritability. The Impatiens type will not suffer fools lightly, and will not sit quietly when he feels that his time is being wasted. He can be quite explosive in his anger, which erupts suddenly. Note that Impatiens is also often needed as an acute remedy for cases involving a sudden, sharp pain, like a toothache, that excites and irritates the patient.

**Vervain:** The Vervain type is overly enthusiastic, often to the point of becoming a zealot. He wants to convert others to his way of thinking, and, as such, can be emotionally and mentally domineering. He is not often physically aggressive, however, although he may be very verbally abusive and commanding.

## Acute Yang Remedy Types

The remedies that follow are usually used in acute circumstances, when the situation at hand has so stressed a particular patient that he has been driven to be more aggressive than usual in spite of his normally more balanced behavior patterns.

**Rock Rose:** The Rock Rose acute state involves terror, sweat, the pounding of the heart, and quick, short, gasping breathes. The patient who needs Rock Rose feels as if his life is on the line, like a fugitive running through the night. This is the remedy needed by anyone who has a gun pointed at him. While the Rock Rose type may have low energy reserves, he can use them explosively. Those needing Rock Rose may lash out physically, even if they are not aware of what they are doing.

**Sweet Chestnut:** This state can be similar to that of the Cherry Plum patient, in that both of these types will tend to feel as if they have been backed into a corner and can simply take no more. But the way in which each type responds to this feeling is different. Where the Cherry Plum explodes, the Sweet Chestnut type literally blacks out. The future is blank, a black void, for the Sweet Chestnut type, so they stand in a crisis of faith. And, in this moment of darkness in their soul, they may lash out, at themselves or others. Where the Cherry Plum is very communicative of his emotional state, the Sweet Chestnut will usually attempt to keep it to himself and to stay in control.

**Cherry Plum:** The acute negative emotional state of the Cherry Plum type can be extreme, to put it mildly. The Cherry Plum type will experience sudden thoughts of aggression or violence. They may or may not act upon these fantasies. They are in a state in which they fear that they may simply explode, lose control. Thus, the Cherry Plum type is verbally, emotionally, and physically eruptive. They may threaten or even commit suicide, or may savagely attack others. Something has snapped within the Cherry Plum patient and he will discharge his life's energy in some manner, creative or destructive.

## Constitutional and Acute Yin Remedy Types

In acute situations, when we are seriously ill, it is more common that we, as patients, will take on yin behaviors, including a weakening of will, a slowing of reactions, and a tendency to pull in more energy from others than we give off to them. Therefore, the remedies listed in the yin group can be either acute or constitutional remedies, depending upon the behavior patterns of a given patient.

**Clematis:** The dream state that is common to Clematis types, either acutely or constitutionally, allows them to drift through life or a current stressful situation. It also allows the Clematis type to yield easily to others and surrender to the circumstances at hand, without even seeming to fully notice them. The Clematis type is passive-aggressive. While he never challenges authority or causes a confrontation, he never quite yields either. In a strange way, he takes in more energy than he yields by calmly and quietly forcing others to yield to his behavior.

**Cerato:** Cerato types will willingly yield their personal power to another and will tend to become very clinging, even smothering, in relationships of any sort. They project weak personalities and are cheerful followers, even if, in their hearts, they are quite aware that they are being led astray. In many ways Cerato types are the embodiment of the principle of yin. Cerato types are capable of all but draining the life force from others as they stand, always helpless, always needing your advice.

**Honeysuckle:** Like Clematis, the Honeysuckle type will tend to withdraw from the world around him. But where the Clematis withdraws into fantasy, the Honeysuckle will withdraw into the past, into a glorified memory state in which all that once was is golden. This memory state tranquilizes the Honeysuckle, allowing him to be wistful instead of stressed. The Honeysuckle type is not interested in the present or fully connected with the world around him, making him passive and yielding.

**Centaury:** The Centaury type is the masochist to the Vine or Holly type's sadist. The Centaury type makes a conscious decision to try to please others, to be liked, and, in doing so, yields his personal power to another. They are willing slaves, able to take much abuse from others and unwilling or unable to say the word "no." But Centaury types pull in energy from others as well, in the constant approval they seek and in their strong attachment to those to whom they yield.

## The Yin/Yang Remedy

Finally, there is the remedy that defies categorization, because it embodies the duality of the yin/yang principle:

**Scleranthus:** Scleranthus, the remedy for those who are indecisive, is the remedy type—constitutional or acute—that embodies duality. Because it contains within it the possibility of either or both yin and yang, it most certainly belongs on this list, although it cannot be listed as being just one or the other. Instead, it must be considered erratic. In being erratic, the Scleranthus type exhibits unpredictable behavior and can be aggressive or yielding, or both. Scleranthus types jump from one decision to another, from one topic to another, from one behavior to another. As Joni Mitchell wrote, "Laughing or crying, it's the same release."

# Remedies with Masks

While it may be argued that all negative emotional behaviors are set in place to protect the individual patient from their own feelings of weakness or fear, most of the Bach remedies consider a single behavior or mood in their use. Some remedies, however, acknowledge a dual pattern in which the patient's behavior masks an underlying issue. It can be difficult for the practitioner to witness and understand both aspects of the patient's mood when they select these remedies for another person. The practitioner who accepts the apparent courage of the Mimulus patient may not see the fears hidden behind the air of strength. It is, therefore, important that students of Bach therapy make a special effort to fully understand the remedies listed here.

**Beech:** Masks an inner intolerance with an apparent sense of fairness and a deep concern for justice. In some cases, Beech types will even mask their own judgmental feelings from themselves and will, with sincerity, list (or, more often, their mate will list) their many good works as proof of their saintly nature.

**Centaury:** Masks insecurity and an underdeveloped sense of self with an outwardly cheerful demeanor. This cheerfulness will most often have a manic edge to it and the Centaury will often be seen as "trying too hard." Indeed, the need for Centaury reveals a weak sense of self and a need for both guidance and understanding, both of which the Centaury type will seek from others at cost to themselves. The Centaury type presents himself as being accommodating to a fault to be liked, and he loses his ability to say the word "No" in doing so. He masks his feelings of deep insecurity with a willingness to martyr himself or work relentlessly for the sake of others.

**Agrimony:** Like Centaury, Agrimony covers an inner sense of discord with a surface pattern of joyfulness. Unlike the Centaury, the Agrimony may have a strong sense of self but is unable to cope with his life's circumstances. Agrimony can cover any negative emotional state (including anger, fear, and grief, chief among others) with false carefree behavior. It is important to note that Agrimony will often turn to alcohol and/or drugs to enhance their happy demeanor.

**Cerato:** Masks a lack of belief in himself and his own judgments with a mask of chirpy happiness and an almost manic need for advice. Because they so want to be liked, the Cerato type will wear a mask of cheerfulness that is similar to the Agrimony and the Centaury. They are our three crying clowns, variations of a theme of a weak sense of self masked by a cheerful demeanor. In the case of the Cerato type, the patient lacks confidence and as a result seeks the advice of others rather relentlessly. The fact that he seldom actually follows their advice never seems to register with him.

**Heather:** Masks a deep loneliness with talkative behavior. Heather's usually overt demand for attention often manages to mask their inner loneliness, and enhances it at the same time by driving away the people who, under most circumstances, would be willing to give them the connection they crave.

**Water Violet:** Like Heather, Water Violet covers their inner loneliness. However, they do so by presenting themselves as blissfully self-sufficient or by seeming to be rather haughty and aloof. Look for the Water Violet to commonly turn to artistic or intellectual pursuits to fill the void left from a lack of human connection.

**Chicory:** With perhaps the most tightly held mask, Chicory presents himself or herself as loving and given to self-sacrifice. Under the mask, Chicory's motives are less noble, as the Chicory tends toward selfishness and greed. Chicorys are commonly rather powerful people, who may be holding a family together single-handedly, while demanding affection, loyalty, and obedience from all.

# The Ultimate (Baker's) Dozen: Healers for Your Home Kit

I certainly agree that, as Bach wrote, each of us will need all thirty-eight Bach remedies at some point or other throughout our lives, but it is also true that some of the remedies are more useful than others. Some remedies speak to specific personality and behavioral types that are not as common as others and some remedies are helpful less often than others. So, in selecting the remedies below, I sought the remedies that, in my opinion, belong in every home and are most useful in the most common situations.

## First, the "Primary Remedies"

**1. Holly: for aggression.** No other Bach Remedy speaks to so many different behavior patterns as Holly. This remedy can be considered for any form of negative aggression, from anger, hatred, jealousy, simple irritability or mistrust to utter paranoia. Holly speaks to the full range of these negative states, and includes most (if not all) of us within the range of its impact in doing so. If any of us were to be honest for a moment, who among us does not experience some level of irritability each and every day? Hopefully, few of us give vent to rage, but all of us know anger, and all of us have felt jealous at one time or another. Along with fear (with which it is intricately entwined), anger is the most pervasive of all negative emotions, which makes Holly one of the most needed of all Bach remedies. Note that because of its universal importance, Holly is often considered among the best remedies of first use in constitutional Bach treatments. It can be useful for any patient displaying anger of any sort, for any reason. Beware, however, that some patients can have a strong response to Holly and can have physical aggravations to the remedy with the first doses. For this reason I often refrain from using it alone as a first remedy and instead blend it with other, "quieter" remedies at the opening of a case.

**2. Wild Oat: for meaninglessness.** The core issue of the remedy Wild Oat reflects what perhaps is the core issue of humanity: man's search for meaning. Patients in the Wild Oat state seek meaning in their lives. They seek a pathway or work challenge that not only offers meaning to their existence, but also guarantees that they will accomplish something rather permanent, which they can, one day, leave behind. It is said that this remedy is for the person who wants to accomplish something good and important with his life, but does not know what that goal actually means. And that's certainly true, as far as it goes. After all, is there anyone who sets out in life not wanting to accomplish something important and be respected for what they have created? And is there anyone who has some sort of inborn map or book that tells them just what they are to do, and how they should go about doing it? Wild Oat is another remedy of universal need in that we are all doing our best, finding our way, and questioning our work—a remedy that can help any of us focus clearly upon our task in life and help us clear-headedly set about meeting that task. Sure, there will be times in life when we may find ourselves confused about our next step, but Wild Oat is always helpful in finding and staying on our path. Because Wild Oat is so commonly needed, it can be very useful as one of Bach's two "primary remedies," to give to a patient to help refine a case when the case has just been taken and a core or "constitutional" remedy is not apparent. In other words, when in doubt, give Wild Oat.

## Then, the Most Used Remedies

**3. Mimulus: for fears of the known.** I believe that there is no emotion that so controls our lives in a negative manner as does fear, simple fear. By this I mean that most of us have a handful of common fears—whether it be poverty, heights, enclosed spaces, darkness, or something else—that color our experience of life and limit our rightful sense of freedom. Some of these fears may seem irrational and even foolish, while others may be well grounded in rational thought, but all are cancers that eat away at our souls. Therefore, I consider Mimulus, the remedy for those who struggle to get through their lives in spite of specific fears, to be extremely valuable. This remedy could bring relief to millions, and allow them to explore their lives with true courage and freedom of movement and thought.

**4. Aspen: for fears of the unknown.** Between them, Mimulus and Aspen cover all aspects of fear. Mimulus is helpful for the fears that we can identify, often for the fears of things that we have already experienced firsthand in our lives, while Aspen is wonderful for fears that are vague, that are often based in conjecture. (For example, no one wants to be poor or very ill, whether they actually have been or not. We have plenty of evidence to let us know these are not pleasant circumstances.) Aspen is for anxiety, for nagging feelings that all is not well, or soon will not be, although we can't exactly put our fingers on what is wrong. Aspen is fear of the dark, the unknown. It is an excellent remedy for young children who are anxious or emotionally very sensitive. In the same way, it is an excellent remedy for animals of all sorts that are "high strung."

**5. Chestnut Bud: for egocentricity and bad habits.** If there is any Bach remedy that is, in my opinion, the most underused, it is Chestnut Bud. It is for all the people, all the time. It should be given to everybody on the morning of their fiftieth birthday, if not before. Chestnut Bud is the remedy of regret, both of the things we have and have not done in our lives. The remedy for our tendency to put our short-term pleasures ahead of our long-term goals. And, more important, it is the remedy for those of us who find ourselves repeating the same mistakes again and again; loving the wrong people, missing deadlines at work, losing and gaining the same ten pounds, and on and on in a manner that is the theme of millions of people's lives. Chestnut Bud is the remedy that can set us free of old patterns that control our lives. It allows us to create new strategies for success and find new paths in life. Each of us holds a cherished pattern or a desperate need, something we clutch that we know in our hearts we would be better off without. Chestnut Bud can help us to let go.

**6. Gorse: for pessimism and doubt.** This remedy speaks to the angry knot of pessimism that exists within each of us. While it is usually written about as the remedy that can reach into the heart of the truly hopeless—those trapped in extreme conditions, life during warfare or life with a deep, chronic, or even life-threatening illness—it can be just as useful (and more widely used) as a remedy for the nagging loss of hope that can cripple us all. Gorse is the remedy for the Doubting Thomas in us all. The Gorse-stricken mind can always find a logical and sensible reason why things will not go as planned, why illness and poverty will remain and good times will never come. Such doubts can be proven on the front page of every paper, so they are easy to rationalize ("I am not being negative, I am being realistic.") and very easy to cling to. What often begins as a "healthy" cynicism warps with time into a loss of hope that can limit life as surely as fear can.

**7. Pine: for guilt.** Since guilt is one of the most basic and all pervasive of all negative emotional states, I think it is important to have this remedy on hand at all times. Many of us are motivated by guilt and will do nearly anything, whether we want to or not, if we are made to feel guilty. For many of us, sensitivity to this emotional state is so profound that a single word or glance is all it takes to motivate us to do whatever it takes to allow us to feel "good enough" once more. The message of guilt is that we can never be good enough, we can never accomplish enough, give enough, *be* enough, no matter how hard we try. When we are controlled by guilt, we find ourselves apologizing for our own needs and wants, often apologizing for our own existence.

**8. Mustard: for depression.** While Mustard is the remedy for depression—for conditions ranging from "bad moods" to clinical depression—in a more complete sense, it should be considered a remedy for negativity. When our thoughts turn dark and our expectations are for the worst, we should turn to Mustard. When the world as we understand it turns strange, or when we feel like an alien in our own clothing, we should turn to Mustard. Mustard is the remedy for melancholia, for sorrow or pessimism that comes on suddenly and without apparent cause. For the times of darkness in our souls when our lives make so little sense. Mustard is also an excellent remedy to remember for those times when things suddenly, in our perception, move very slowly. When we feel sluggish, mentally, physically, or emotionally, the remedy that can help is Mustard.

**9. Crab Apple: for control issues and for physical illness.** Crab Apple relates to the concept of perfection in our lives. As such, it represents a negative mental and emotional pattern in which we put aside our creative desire for excellence and replace it with a destructive desire for perfection. Crab Apple, therefore, also relates to general control issues and to those times in life when we attempt, through an act of sheer will, to make ourselves, our environment, and those around us attain perfection. The Crab Apple state is one in which cleanliness and order are desired above all else. People needing Crab Apple often feel tainted or dirty, often fear germs and illness, and distain any form of chaos. They are rigid in their thoughts and habits. Crab Apple also relates to physical illness, especially to allergies, including food allergies and poisons. It is a natural cleanser that brings balance and order on both the emotional and physical plane. As one of the very few Bach remedies that have applications in physical illness as well as emotional imbalances, it belongs in every home kit.

**10. Vine: for willfulness.** Vine is the remedy for those times in our lives when we set our wills to certain goals without caring about the consequences. In many instances, the Vine state is somewhat infantile, in that it represents the placement of ego above all else. The person needing Vine tries ever harder, using tactics of intimidation, domination, and rigid determination to achieve his goals. Inflexibility is a core trait, emotionally, mentally, and physically. The person needing Vine cannot tolerate disagreement and demands dogmatic compliance from all those around him. He comes into his own at times of crisis, when others turn to him for clear-sighted and determined leadership, but in times of peace, the Vine type can make for a dictatorial teacher, parent, or boss. When we feel like we know it all and are giving others, especially those over whom we have authority, a message that they had better toe the line, we need to reach for Vine.

**11. Walnut: for life's milestones.** The need for Walnut is one that comes and goes throughout all our lives. From a baby's teething process and his first step, through adolescence, career change, midlife crisis and menopause, to change of address, marriage and divorce, birth and death, Walnut is the remedy that can help us move from endings in our lives into new beginnings. Walnut is the remedy of transition and transformation. Further, it is an excellent remedy to be used whenever we need a "kick in the pants" to get us started on a new course. Use Walnut when you are about to begin a new project or a new diet, but lack the ability to get started. Walnut can also be helpful for those times when we sense a relationship or a situation is ending; that it would be better for all concerned if a period was put on one sentence and another begun. Often Walnut is best given to all involved in a given situation rather than to just one person, whether it is a move or a divorce. Also, use Walnut to help integrate new arrivals, human or animal, as they come into an established environment.

**12. Hornbeam: for "modern malaise."** I believe that the Hornbeam state, one of emotional exhaustion when we feel both a bit overwhelmed and a bit bored with our lives, is the one that best describes our modern lives. We are, by nature, animals, who would spend our days struggling for food and habitation in our natural setting, but our lives have become more and more stylized and conceptual over the centuries. We now spend our days in cubicles staring at the blinking cursor on the computer screen. Hornbeam is for those "blue Mondays," when we do not think we can bear to climb our of bed, fight our way through traffic, and go through another week of what is expected or required of us. Hornbeam helps us work our way through the random tedium of our lives and find the creativity and meaning that is hidden within. Hornbeam refreshes the mind and the heart, and gives us an impetus to find new ways of working and new methods of over-coming frustration.

## Finally:

**13. Rescue Remedy:** This is, or course, a bit of a cheat, as Rescue Remedy is not a single remedy, but a combination of five Bach remedies: Cherry Plum, Clematis, Impatiens, Rock Rose and Star of Bethlehem.* But using it here allows me to narrow the other remedies down to an easy dozen. Rescue Remedy is useful for so many different mental, emotional and physical traumas—everything from nightmares, to accidents and injuries, to heart attacks and strokes—that it belongs in every home, and in every suitcase when we travel. It is not, perhaps, the most important remedy overall for our deepest held neg-ative emotional patterns and self-destructive behavior, but it is without a doubt the most important Bach remedy for emergencies. Even emergencies that require a trip to the emergency room or a call to 911 can be helped by a dose or two of Rescue Remedy, not only for the patient, but also for those who are assisting the patient as well.

---

* This mixing of remedies allows me to sort of double cheat, since I have not listed any of the com-ponents of Rescue Remedy as single remedies for the home kit. Some, especially Star of Bethlehem, would be natural candidates for the kit—I actually think it is a good idea to have Star of Bethlehem on hand as a single remedy even if you have Rescue Remedy as well. But since these remedies are available as part of the mix, I leave them out as solos.

# Bach Treatments for Animals

The Bach Flower Remedies have been very helpful to me over the years not only in treating human patients, but also in treating the animals in my household. I cannot recommend them enough to anyone who has an animal that is physically ill or displaying negative emotional patterns of any sort. If they are well selected and well used, they can work wonders.

I included information on their use in the individual remedy listings in this book because I have seen the Bach remedies work wonders over the years for all sorts of animal patients. But I have found that not all the Bach remedies work as well with animals as they do with humans, perhaps because animals do not possess the same emotional states that human do, or because we simply lack the ability to understand animal behavior profoundly enough to be able to fully map the underlying causes for their negative traits. Therefore I wanted to provide a separate list of the remedies I have found over the years to be of particular help for animals. I believe these should be kept on hand at all times if possible for the treatment of animals.

## Remedies for Animals by Mood

The remedies best used in the treatment of animals are listed by mood, as were the remedies for humans.

### Remedies for Animals that Fear

**Mimulus:** Use this remedy for animals that have specific fears: of noises, of storms, of other animals, or of humans.

**Aspen:** Use this remedy for animals that display anxious behavior, who "spook" easily.

### Remedies for Animals that Despair

**Willow:** Use for animals that exhibit extreme or defiant behavior. Also excellent for elderly animals that are irritable and those that have physical aches and pains.

**Star of Bethlehem:** Use this remedy for any animal that has experienced an emotional or physical trauma.

## Remedies for Animals that Doubt

**Hornbeam:** Just as I think that this is the keynote remedy for our human condition, I think it is very useful for our animals as well. Use this remedy for pets that are left alone for long periods of time each day and for any animal that has no "job."

**Scleranthus:** This remedy is great for animals that have sudden changes in behavior. That are calm most of the time, but can suddenly behave aggressively. For any animal that you feel can't be trusted.

**Cerato:** This remedy is great for any animal that has had its spirit crushed, that lacks initiative through over-training.

## Remedies for Animals that Are Overly Sensitive

**Walnut:** This remedy is just as useful for animals as it is for humans. Use it for any of life's milestones, for a change of home, for any time when another human or animal comes into the home. Also use it to help your animals cope with death.

**Holly:** This the best remedy for aggressive behavior in animals when the animal is striking out in anger. For any bullying instinct in animals.

## Remedies for Animals that Are Controlling

**Chicory:** This remedy and Heather can both be used for the treatment of animals that demand attention. Chicory is especially helpful for dogs that are underfoot constantly and that jump into your lap uninvited.

**Vervain:** Excellent for high-strung animals and for animals that are filled with nervous energy. Think of this remedy as well for animals that are destructive, not out of malice, but out of sheer clumsiness. For dogs who bark too much.

**Vine:** This is the best remedy I know of for any animal that is territorial. For the animal that is the boss of the household. It can also be used for animals that are defiant of humans, dogs who will urinate on the carpet while the human watches.

## Remedies for Animals that Are Indifferent

**White Chestnut:** Use this remedy for any animal that exhibits obsessive behaviors, especially when they obsessively bite or scratch.

**Chestnut Bud:** Think of Chestnut Bud whenever you are dealing with any animal that is hard to train. Helps animals to keep from making the same mistakes over and over again.

## Remedies for Animals that Are Lonely

**Impatiens:** Use this remedy for animals that are uncooperative and irritable. It can also, like Hornbeam, be very helpful for animals that are bored because they are left alone too much and don't receive enough exercise.

## Remedies for Physical Symptoms

**Crab Apple:** Use Crab Apple for animals that have chronic skin conditions, like eczema or mange, or that have seasonal allergies.

**Clematis:** Use this remedy whenever an animal slips into unconsciousness in illness. Clematis can also help an animal to recover its interest in life after a long illness.

**Olive:** This remedy is also excellent for animals in recovery. The Olive animal is physically exhausted, either from illness or circumstances, and needs support in recovery. Also helpful to any animal that hibernates to help speed their recovery in the period after waking.

## Combining Remedies for Animals

The Bach Flower Remedies can be combined for animals just as they can for humans. You may use up to five remedies at a time in a combination geared to either an acute or a constitutional treatment. Just like humans, animals have constitutional remedies (remedies that closely mirror the behavior patterns of the patient and may be used over a long period of time in repeated doses). I also find that remedies are often linked to specific periods of life in animals, just as they are in humans.

However, just as I feel animals do not exhibit the same complex emotional states humans do, and thus have no need for certain remedies (for instance, I feel animals do not feel guilt and therefore have no need for Pine, which most humans sorely need), I also feel that it is easier to overload an animal with too many remedies than it is to overload a human patient. So I tend to blend fewer remedies when I am treating an animal and often find that a single remedy is very effective. In most cases, I will not blend more than three remedies at a time, gearing them as precisely as I can to the gender and age of the animals as well as to its specific patterns of negative behavior.

## Dosing Your Animal

Just as I try not to give any animal too many remedies at any one time, I try not to give them too many doses of a needed remedy. It often will take a couple of weeks of treating an animal (the remedies can be added, a couple of drops at a time, right into the animal's food or drink). As most animals are fed once or twice daily, use them when feeding for a couple of weeks, until a change becomes apparent. But once the changes are noticeable, I tend to slow down the treatment and move to an "as needed" basis. In other words, give the animal a chance to make needed changes before adding more remedies or stepping up the dosage. Patience is important when working with animals.

## Books on Animal Treatments

Finally, if you want more information on treating animals of any sort with Bach remedies, there are two good books on the market. They are:

*Bach Flower Remedies for Animals,* by Helen Graham and Gregory Vlamis. Forres, Scotland: Findhorn Press (1999). I really love this book. It is one of only two that I have found that are of real value in treating animals with the Bach remedies. And since I have never been really good at using homeopathics with animals, except for my own, I also need all the help I can get with the Bach remedies. I recommend this volume for its crisp, clear writing and for its very helpful tips on using the remedies on animals of all sorts. (I could do without the little "paw prints" around the page number, however.)

*Bach Flower Remedies for Animals,* by Stefan Ball and Judy Howard. Essex, England: C.W. Daniel Company, Ltd. (1999). Same title, lesser book. Still, it is a good, comprehensive look at the remedies and their uses for animal patients by two of the best authors on the subject. (One gets the feeling, however, that they and their publisher were just looking for another title on the same subject, and thus turned their attention to animal patients to meet this "quota.")

# Other Flower Essences

It should come as no surprise to you that others have followed in Edward Bach's footsteps and have developed their own systems of flower remedies. Just as Bach found the healing virtues in plants that had been cast aside and ignored for centuries, others walked their own fields and glens and used the flowering plants native to their own geographical area to create their own pharmacies of floral essences. All, in my experience, are used either in combination or singly and are mixed and stored in the same way as Bach's remedies. Some have developed their own system of preserving the remedies and keeping them potent, as noted below.

The logic of developing other pharmacies of remedies, each focusing on using the plants native to a specific geographical area, is undeniable. Some may argue that Bach, at the end of his days, felt that he had discovered a complete system of treatment that needs no adjuncts or adjustments. Others might answer that this could be true for those living in Great Britain or even in Europe, but those living in the rest of the world have the same right to use their own native plants in the treatment of their ills as Bach. And surely it must be noted that all native populations across the globe make use of what they have on hand—primarily the plants that grow wild all around them—in the treatment of their ailments.

My experience with other systems of flower remedies has been limited to just three types of essences, all listed below. In each case, I have found that the remedies work quite well. In one instance, I have come to depend upon the remedies almost as much as I do the Bach remedies.

I include this information on other systems of flower essences so the reader can explore them for himself or herself and decide whether or not they are valuable. Certainly, with the development of the Internet, we all have easy access to an entire planet full of flower remedies. One need only enter "flower remedies" or "floral essences" into any Internet search engine to find out what I mean.

## The Flower Essence Society

Patricia Kaminski and Richard Katz, a married couple, founded the Flower Essence

Society (or "FES" as it is known) in California in 1979. They are therapists who practice using a combination of Bach remedies and their own North American essences. Together they authored *The Flower Essence Repertory* in 1984, which lists both their own remedies and Bach's. The book is an excellent reference, with solid information on all the remedies and their applications, physical and emotional. I have used the North American remedies for many years and have found them to be quite trustworthy. They may be used as a separate form of therapy or may be combined with the Bach remedies. You will find the North American essences, notable for their little bottles with purple labels, placed alongside Bach's remedies at many health food stores and whole food markets across the country.

The Flower Essence Society has two excellent websites. Visit fesflowers.com for information on the organization and its resources. Visit the better site of the two, flowersociety.org, for what are perhaps the best and most in-depth listings on the flower remedies—again the North American remedies as well as Bach's—available on the Internet. Note also that Patricia Kaminiski offers free questionnaires on the use of flower remedies for animals and humans on the Healing Waters web page at essencesonline.com.

The Flower Essence Society mailing address is P.O. Box 1769, Nevada City, CA 95959. Its telephone number is (800) 548-0075.

## Green Hope Farm

I first heard about the Green Hope Farm flower remedies when I was traveling in the Berkshires. In a tiny health food store in Williamstown I saw a whole group of remedies with what looked like hand-printed labels. A little booklet describing their uses was tied to the shelf holding the remedies. Since I had come into the store looking for something to help me recover from an illness that was draining my vacation of all enjoyment, I decided to give the remedies a try. The next day, I was feeling so much better that I drove back to that health food store to buy all the remedies (the owner threw in the book for good measure). I have used the Green Hope remedies with great success for many years now. I have always had a great deal of success with these remedies. Perhaps it is because they are taken from plants grown right here in New England, where I live, or perhaps it is because they are really well-made remedies.

Let me note that the Green Hope remedies are not preserved in combination in brandy or any other form of alcohol, unlike the Bach remedies and the FES essences. Instead, Molly Sheehan, the creator of this line of remedies, has developed something called "red shiso" as a preservative. Although I sometimes just use the brandy I have become accustomed to using with other flower remedies, I have also found the red shiso to be just fine. It is available, as are the many different Green Hope remedies, at the website greenhopeessences.com.

There is something very "New Age" (funny how something with the word "new" in it got old so fast) about Green Hope Farm. They do not, for instance, take credit cards for their orders, because their angels told them not to. But those who work at Green Hope are loving and dedicated to their work, especially Molly.

The mailing address is POB 125, Meriden, NH. Their phone number is (603) 469-3662. Note that Green Hope's self-published guide to its remedies is still available free upon request. It is quite good.

## Perelandra, Ltd.

The Perelandra essences are the product of the Perelandra Center for Nature Research, located on forty-five acres of land at the foothills of the Blue Ridge Mountains in Virginia. The center, which, in spite of its name, is a private venture and not any sort of commune, is a joint venture between Machaelle Small Wright and her husband, Clarence, who moved to Virginia in 1973.

The Perelandra flower remedies are of particular interest to me because they come from a mindset entirely different from Bach's. Where Bach's own background was as a doctor and homeopath, Machaelle Small Wright comes to the essences from her ecological work and intense interest in gardening. Therefore, their brochures do not discuss emotional states of spiritual disharmony. Instead, they write, "The human body has within and surrounding it an electrical network. When we experience health, this electrical network is balanced and fully connected. When something in our life or environment threatens that balance, the electrical system responds by either short-circuiting or overloading." The Perelandra essences, therefore, are not sold on the idea that they balance emotional states, but, instead, seek to balance that "electrical system" and the central nervous system.

I know that, ultimately, there is no difference between this perceived electrical system and the vital force, but something about the quasi-science of the Perelandra system sets my teeth on edge.

Still I have used the remedies, some of which have very interesting garden sources like okra, cauliflower, corn, and zucchini, and have found that they, too, work just fine.

Machaelle Small Wright is the author of two Perelandra garden workbooks, an autobiography called *Dancing in the Shadows of the Moon* and a good book that explains her own particular take on flower remedies called *Flower Essences: Reordering Our Understanding and Approach to Illness and Health*.

Perelandra sells a wide range of remedies, all available in kits or individually. They also sell products, like soil-balancing kits, targeted to gardeners, and books by other authors on a variety of subjects.

They have an excellent website at www.perelandra-ltd.com that gives a good deal of information on a wide variety of topics, even pandemics. Their mailing address is Perelandra, Ltd., P.O. Box 3603, Warrenton, VA 20188. Their phone number is (800) 960-8806.

## Other Flower Remedies from Across the Globe

While I cannot vouch for the quality of the remedies sold by the groups below as I can for those above, I have visited all these websites over the years and find myself fascinated by each group's particular take on the concept of flower remedies. Each represents a specific geographic location and a unique set of native plants and flower essences.

### North American Sites

**David's Garden** (www.davidsgarden.com): These remedies have been created by Jack Braunstein, an "FES-certified flower essence practitioner," who named them for his friend and avid gardener David E. Thomas. The essences originated from the flowers in the garden that David left behind when he died and that Jack began to tend as his own. David's Garden is a line of twenty-four remedies with names like "Take It Easy" and "Get Off Your Butt."

**Desert Alchemy** (desert-alchemy.com): Desert Alchemy takes its remedies a bit more seriously. It was founded in 1983 by Cynthia Athina Kemp Scherer in Tucson, Arizona. As with the other systems of flower essences listed here, Desert Alchemy remedies are taken from native plants. Remedy names include "Camphorweed," "Buffalo Gourd," and "Hoptree." The site lists all remedies in alphabetical order and gives information about each.

**Flower Essences from Tree Frog Farm** (treefrogfarm.com): This wins, hands down, for my favorite name of any system of floral essences. Tree Frog Farm is located on two and three-quarters acres of land on Lummi Island in the north Puget Sound in the state of Washington. The farm was purchased in 1976 by John Robinson, who runs the website and business with his partner Diana Pepper. The floral essences, taken from native plants that grow on the farm, are similar in spirit to those grown on Green Hope Farm in New Hampshire. Both types of remedies are preserved in the same way, with red shiso. All remedies are listed on the site and are available for order.

**Pacific Essences** (essencesonline.com/Pacific.html): Pacific Essences is a small company located just north of Tree Frog Farm on the Pacific coast of Canada. They are interesting because they take their essences from sea plants, including brown kelp, and from sea animals, like jellyfish, mussels, and starfish, instead of land plants. I don't know of any other essences like them. The website is quite interesting and very earnest.

**Alaskan Flower Essence Project** (alaskanessences.com): Given how short the summers are in Alaska, I never would have expected to find a line of flower remedies being made there, but here it is. Based in Homer, Alaska, the company offers a kit of seventy-two essences "prepared from wild and domestic flowers growing in the state of Alaska." About their unique remedies, the site says, "Summer here seldom lasts for more than 65 days, however, plants grow at a phenomenal rate during this time due to the constant presence of sunlight." The sunlight, they say, gives their remedies more potency than others possess.

## International Sites

**Findhorn Flower Essences** (www.findhornessences.com): These Scottish essences are perhaps the best known of those coming from the British Isles, with the exception of Bach's own. The plants from which they are taken are well known to us. Remedies include apple, cherry, daisy, and elder. Remedies are available for order from the website, both individually and in combination. The company is based in Moray, Scotland.

**Australian Bush Flower Remedies** (ausflowers.com.au): These remedies are interesting in that they are taken from the plants that were used medicinally by the native Australian Aboriginals. All of the plants are native to the bush. Remedies include Green Spider Orchid, Kangaroo Paw, and Rough Bluebell. There are many remedies in this pharmacy. All are described and for sale at the website. Australian Bush Flower Remedies is based in Terrey Hills, Australia.

**New Millennium Flower Essences of New Zealand** (nmessences.com): is a very comprehensive site*. It not only contains information on each remedy, but it also has a picture and information on the plant from which the remedy is taken. Remedies are divided into groups, including "Body Energy" and "Sexuality and Gender Issues." Peter Archer, the creator of New Millennium Flower Essences, also has an autobiography called *Modern-Day Alchemist—Following in the Footsteps of Dr. Edward Bach*, which is available online at the website. Based in Christchurch, New Zealand.

**South African Essences** (www.essencesonline.com/SouthAfricanflowers1.html or click on the South African Flower Essences link on essencesonline.com): This is the only company I know of that sells essences indigenous to Africa. The company promises that its remedies will balance your masculine and feminine energies and integrate your left-brain with your right. They are said to be especially helpful for those suffering from learning difficulties. Jannet Unite-Penny is the creator of the South African Essences. Remedies include fig, lotus and oreganum. All remedies are taken from plants grown on Table Mountain in South Africa.

* Note that the Healing Waters website (essencesonline.com) is something of a clearinghouse for various small companies that offer their own systems of floral essences. Visit their site and click on the link for flower essences to be given a list of literally dozens of sites based all over the globe.

## ONE FINAL NOTE

If you would like a book that lists the uses of almost all the many different flower remedies available today, get a copy of *The Flower Remedy Book* by Jeffrey Garson Shapiro. It
was published in 1999 by North Atlantic Books, a publisher of books on homeopathy,
based in Berkeley, CA. While this book is a little confusing when you first try to use it
(there are little icons for the various systems of flower remedies that you have to get
to be able to recognize before you can stop glancing up and down from the copy to
the icons at the bottom of the page), but it is a repertory of the uses for more than 700
different remedies. This is the only book I know that lists so many different forms of
flower remedies or is so comprehensive in the individual symptoms listed. It is well
worth the price if you are going to use remedies other than Bach's.

# Index

**A**

Abandonment, 180, 229, 231
Absent-mindedness, 316–317, 318
Abuse, 80, 114, 118, 122, 125, 131, 137, 187, 201, 209, 214, 261, 278–279, 349
  child, 83
  emotional, 64, 214
  physical, 64, 84, 214
  sexual, 64, 187, 300
  verbal, 84, 248
Acceptance, 301–302
Accidents, 131, 137, 148, 194, 245
  automobile, 77, 350
Acid reflux, 320
Acne, 93, 111, 112
Aconite, 76, 287
Acupuncture, 107
Addictions, 60, 64, 70, 134, 178, 194, 209, 320, 340
Adolescence, 111, 112, 117, 174, 184, 209, 217, 260, 272–273, 286, 288
Adrenal disorders, 194
Aging. *See* Elderly.
Agrimony, 60, 173, 186, 188–195, 267, 409, 417
  adults, 193–194
  animals, 194
  children; 193
  homeopathic remedies and, 194

in combination, 192, 234–235, 336–337
AIDS, 162
Alaskan Flower Essence Project, 432–433
*Alchemy of Healing, The*, 137
Alcohol and alcoholism, 184, 190, 191, 215, 294, 306, 334, 337, 340
Alcoholics Anonymous, 301
Alienation, 182
Allergies, 83, 93, 106, 107, 111, 112, 155, 176, 212, 215, 219, 235, 237, 265, 289, 311, 320, 340
Aloofness, 323, 324–332
Ambition, 87, 94, 261
Amblyopia, 166, 169
Amnesia, 194
Anemia, 105, 294
Anger, 53, 71, 82, 84, 188, 201, 210–220, 327, 349, 350
Angina, 57
Animals. *See* Pets.
Ankles, 290
Anorexia. *See* Eating disorders.
Anxiety, 49, 50, 57–64, 69, 77, 92, 99, 176, 284, 306, 420
Apathy, 105, 119, 162, 268, 281, 283, 299
Apis, 245
Appendicitis, 119

Appetite, 70
Argentum Nitricum, 56, 311
Arnica, 76, 134, 136, 194
Arrogance, 325
Arsenicum Album, 56–57, 63–64, 87,
    112, 223, 244–245, 322
Arteriosclerosis, 219
Arthritis, 93, 105, 118, 119, 148, 201,
    254
Artists, 144
Aspen, 49, 50, 57–64, 72, 270, 345, 391,
    420
  adults, 60, 62–63
  animals, 63, 136, 425
  children, 58, 59, 60, 61–62, 82
  homeopathic remedies and, 63–64
  in combination, 58, 63, 74, 82, 92,
    133, 135, 166, 172, 253, 284, 306,
    348
Asthma, 57, 112, 169, 245, 274, 331
Athlete's foot, 93
Attention, need for, 228–229, 249,
    333–334, 336, 337, 338
Attitude, know-it all, 258, 344
Aurum Metallicum, 105, 130–131, 287
Australian Bush Flower Remedies, 433
Avoidance, 52, 55, 134

**B**

Bach, Edward, 2, 3, 4, 14–18, 19–28, 36,
    38–39, 50, 52, 53, 54, 56, 57, 65,
    71, 77, 88, 93, 99, 106, 113, 120,
    121, 131, 137, 143, 150, 156, 162,
    163, 170, 176, 188, 195, 202, 210,
    219, 221, 224, 225, 231, 237,
    245–246, 254, 261, 263, 267, 269,
    275, 281, 283, 286, 289, 294, 302,
    304, 312, 323, 324, 332, 340,
    354–355, 357–358, 364, 379, 381,
    397–398
  books about, 403–404

Bach Centre, 407
Bach Flower Research Programme, 407
*Bach Flower Therapy,* 292
Backaches, 105, 119, 148, 241, 245, 290,
    294, 326
*Bad Seed, The* (movie), 229
Balance, 165, 185, 188, 206, 213,
    366–367
Barnard, Julian, 407
*Be Here Now,* 264–265
Beard, George Miller, 79
Bedwetting, 83
Beech, 231–237, 417
  adults, 236
  animals, 236–237
  children, 236
  homeopathic remedies and, 237
  in combination, 192, 212, 234, 258
Behaviors, 40–41, 390–391, 397–398
  aggressive, 48, 118, 211, 336, 337,
    413–414, 419
  compulsive/obsessive, 83, 106,
    107–108, 110, 121, 264, 267, 278,
    312–320
  destructive, 83, 210
  explosive, 211, 214
  masked, 417–418
Belching, 70
Belladonna, 131, 132, 287
Betrayal, 114, 116, 328
Bible. New Testament, 140–141
Binging, 180, 192
Birds, 287
Birth, 209
Bitterness, 88, 113–120, 227
Blame, 113–114, 115, 117–118
Bleeding, 119
Blindness, 301
Blood sugar, 349
Boils, 219
Bones, 148, 254

Boredom, 178, 179, 274, 347, 422–423
Bossiness, 256
Boundaries, 70, 103, 224
Breakdowns, 254, 346
Breasts, 70
Breath, bad, 219
Breathing, 312, 345, 370
  problems, 176, 245, 320, 331
Broken-heartedness, 131
Bruises, 301
Bullies, 217
Burns, 219
Bursitis, 119

## C

Calcarea Carbonica, 57, 87, 98, 223, 319
Calendula, 112
Cancer, 112, 162, 281
Candidiasis, 320
Cannabis, 175
Capsicum, 281
Carbo Vegetabilis, 155, 265–266
Career. See Work.
Carpal tunnel syndrome, 250, 254, 311
Cats, 230, 319
Causticum, 112, 223, 253
Cell salts, 107, 245
Cellulite, 320
Centaury, 186, 188, 195–202, 204, 281, 409, 415, 417
  adults, 200–201
  animals, 201
  children, 200
  homeopathic remedies and, 201
  in combination, 192, 199, 207, 271–271, 336–337
Cerato, 71, 165, 170–176, 204, 333, 409–410, 415, 418
  adults, 175
  animals, 175, 426

children, 174–175
  homeopathic remedies and, 175–176
  in combination, 123–124, 172, 207, 336
Chamomile, 287
Charisma, 247–249
Cheer, false, 173, 188–195, 197, 417–418
Cherry Plum, 50, 63, 71, 77–84, 391, 414, 423
  adults, 82
  animals, 83
  children, 82
  homeopathic remedies and, 83
  in combination, 79, 80
Chestnut Bud, 36, 66–67, 146, 184, 205, 210, 304, 306, 308, 312–320, 420
  adults, 318–319
  animals, 319
  children, 317–318
  homeopathic remedies and, 319
  in combination, 90, 152, 170, 199, 203, 278, 283, 298–299, 345
Chestnuts, 40, 222, 304
  See also Chestnut Bud; Red Chestnut; Sweet Chestnut; White Chestnut.
Chicory, 224–231, 328, 339, 410
  adults, 229–230
  animals, 230, 426
  children, 228–229
  homeopathic remedies and, 230–231
  in combination, 227, 278, 291, 333, 336
Chinchona, 11–12
Chopra, Deepak, 51
Chronic fatigue syndrome, 99, 125, 155, 162, 201
Circulation, 261, 303
Claustrophobia, 169
Cleaniness and cleansing, 86, 106, 107–108, 109, 309, 325, 422

Clematis, 17, 71, 72, 263, 265, 267–274,
    276, 281, 303, 391, 410, 415, 423
  adults, 273
  animals, 273, 427
  children, 272–273
  homeopathic remedies and, 274
  in combination, 166, 167, 270–271,
    273, 274, 289
Clumsiness, 349
Co-dependence, 99, 124, 209, 231
  See also Dependence.
Colds, 176, 311
Colors, 346
Coma, 57, 301
Complexions, 411–412
Confidence, 248, 256
Confrontations, 189
Conjunctivitis, 219
Consciousness, loss of, 271, 273–274,
    274
Constipation, 105, 169, 261
Control, 65, 221–262, 271, 306, 422
  loss of, 63, 72, 78, 79–80, 81, 111,
    112, 306
  Beech, 223, 231–237
  Chicory, 223, 224–231
  Rock Water, 223, 237–246
  Vervain, 223, 246–254
  Vine, 223, 254–262
Coping, 55, 60, 75, 86
Courage. See Fearlessness.
Crab Apple, 37, 63, 86, 87, 100, 101,
    106–112, 121, 210, 211, 222–223,
    234, 239, 289, 422
  adults, 111
  animals, 112, 427
  children, 110–111
  homeopathic remedies and, 112
  in combination, 57, 106, 107, 110,
    123, 212, 234, 235, 256–257, 258,
    309, 329

Cramps, 194, 349
Crises, 181, 255, 259, 371, 392
  emotional, 127–128
  midlife, 93, 99, 104, 131, 181, 183,
    184, 194, 209, 250, 294
Cullen, William, 11–12
Curing, 354, 360–361
Cynicism, 142, 145
Cystic fibrosis, 320
Cystitis, 119
Cysts, 176

D

David's Garden, 432
Daydreaming, 267, 270
Deafness, 105, 301
Death and dying, 56, 77, 104, 119, 129,
    131, 136, 137, 144, 162, 208, 209,
    271, 287, 288, 291
Dedication, 254
Delirium, 82
Dementia, 274
Denial, 119
Dependence, 135
  See also Co-dependence.
Depression, 85–137, 155, 263, 265, 266,
    278, 281–288, 297, 421
Desert Alchemy, 432
Desertion, fear of, 335
Despair, 85–137, 191, 222
  Crab Apple, 87, 106–112
  Elm, 87, 93–99
  Larch, 87, 88–93
  Oak, 87, 99–106
  Pine, 88, 120–126
  Star of Bethlehem, 88, 131–137
  Sweet Chestnut, 88, 126–131
  Willow, 88, 113–120
Developmental disorders, 209
Diarrhea, 57, 112, 169, 176, 231
Diet, 294

Digestive disorders, 56, 57, 61, 62, 64, 93, 184, 209, 215, 245, 254, 261, 320
Dilution, 10, 12, 21, 26
Dioscorides, Pedanius, 11
Discouragement, 87, 143
Dissatisfaction, 113, 161
Diuretics, 188
Divorce, 119, 144, 281
Dizziness, 57
Dogs, 63, 73, 112, 175, 201, 226, 230, 244, 253, 260, 311, 319, 425–417
Domination, 256, 260
Doubt, 139–184, 221, 265
  Cerato, 143
  Gentian, 143
  Gorse, 143
  Hornbeam, 143
  rational, 139, 144
  Scleranthus, 143
  Wild Oat, 143
  *See also* Self-doubt.
Doubting Thomas," 140–141
Drugs, use of, 63, 178, 184, 190, 273, 304, 311, 337, 340
Duality, 164, 169
Duplicity, 234
Dutch elm disease, 93

**E**

Ear disorders, 165, 169, 219, 261
*Easy Travel to Other Planets*, 152
Eating disorders, 63, 64, 70, 83, 111, 112, 169, 194, 209, 241, 245, 320, 349
Eczema, 331
Eddy, Mary Baker, 22
Egocentricity. *See* Self-centeredness.
Elderly, 56, 57, 105, 118, 119, 130, 135, 136, 147, 148, 162, 230, 231, 236, 237, 244, 273, 274, 275, 281, 287, 288, 300, 311, 339, 340

Electronics. *See* Technology, electronic.
Elm, 87, 93–99, 100, 184, 204, 291
  animals, 98
  adults, 98
  children, 98
  homeopathic remedies and, 98
  in combination, 79, 106, 152, 204, 273, 284, 287, 289, 297, 304
Embarrassment, 191
Emergencies, 112, 131, 137, 254, 255, 423
Emotions, 4, 23–24, 28, 43–45, 50, 189, 211, 213–214, 388
  unavailability of, 190, 326
  *See also* Moods (Bach).
Endive. *See* Chicory.
Energy, 48, 249, 252
Excitability, 223, 246–254
Exercise, 241, 305
Exhaustion, 52, 93–94, 99, 100, 105, 123, 128, 155, 169, 199, 231, 263, 266, 278, 282, 284, 289–294, 297, 307, 311, 346, 349
Extroverts, 221, 233, 246
Eyes, 155, 254, 309, 318

**F**

Failure, 88–89, 90–91, 92, 131, 151
Fainting, 57, 176
False cheer. *See* Cheer, false.
Fantasy, 58–59, 270, 303
Far-sightedness, 70
Fathers, 93, 245, 261
Fatigue. *See* Exhaustion.
Fear, 47–84, 92, 240, 265, 420
  Aspen, 50, 56, 57–64
  Cherry Plum, 50, 77–84
  conceptual, 47–48
  experiential, 47–48, 51, 72
  Mimulus, 50–57
  Red Chestnut, 50, 65–71

Rock Rose, 50, 71–77
    targets of, 48, 66, 67, 69, 71, 78
    use of, 48
Fearlessness, 54, 61
Ferrum Phosphoricum, 331
Fevers, 169, 219
Finances, 293
Findhorn Flower Essences, 433
Fixations, 304–306, 309, 314
Fleas, 112
*Flower Essence Repertory*, 77, 430
Flower Essence Society, 77, 429–430
Flower Essences from Tree Frog Farm,
    432
Flower remedies, vi, 1–2, 17–18, 26–32,
    35–45, 85, 86, 132–133, 359–360,
    363–365, 365–368, 369–384,
    393–399, 429–434
    acute/mood, 30, 36, 62–63, 66, 71,
        74, 78, 85, 106, 113, 116, 120, 126,
        131, 143, 150, 156, 163, 170, 176,
        202, 206, 210, 231, 246, 267, 275,
        285, 289, 291, 295, 313, 323, 333,
        391–392
    administration of, 365–368, 370–376
    blends, 385–392
    books about, 404–407
    case management, 393–396, 397
    case taking, 353–354, 365–368,
        370–372, 377–378
    constitutional/type, 29–30, 36, 62,
        71, 85, 88, 93, 93, 99, 106, 113,
        115, 120, 131, 143, 150, 156, 159,
        163, 170, 176, 188, 191, 195, 210,
        224, 231, 237, 246, 267, 275, 281,
        289, 295, 302, 313, 323, 324, 333,
        340, 343–344, 348, 372, 382,
        388–391, 394
    core constitutional, 389–391
    dosages, 28, 29, 312, 378–383, 392
    home kit, 419–423

    home kit (animals), 425–427
    in combination, 36, 43, 49, 203, 265,
        370–376, 383, 385–392
    individualized rescue, 391–392
    language of, 40–41
    most used, 420–423
    organizations and Internet sites,
        407–408
    potency, 17, 369, 379, 383, 384
    primary, 419–420
    treatment approaches, 377–378
*Flower Remedy Book, The*, 434
Followers, 90, 123, 172, 174–175
Foot disorders, 70, 155, 184
Forgiveness, 124
*Free Thyself*, 17, 27, 50, 359–360
Frustration, 181, 344, 346, 348, 350
Fulfillment, 143, 176–184

## G

Galen, 357
Gall stones, 331
Gas, 57, 184, 320
Gelsemium, 148, 265, 287
Gem elixirs, 245
Gentian, 143–150, 158, 276–277, 281,
    410
    adults, 147–148
    animals, 148
    children, 147
    homeopathic remedies and, 148
    in combination, 145, 146, 148, 152,
        158–159, 284, 297–298
Germany, 259
Glandular disorders, 176, 184
Gorse, 67, 98, 146, 156–162, 291, 296,
    411, 421
    adults, 160–161
    animals, 161
    children, 160
    homeopathic remedies and, 161

in combination, 53, 123, 129, 130, 158–159, 271, 274, 284, 285, 287, 289, 291, 293, 297

Gout, 105, 148

Graphities, 301

Green Hope Farm, 430–432

Grief, 79, 130, 136, 137, 187, 208, 227, 277, 278, 280, 281, 324, 328

Guilt, 88, 120–126, 199, 331, 421
   survivor's, 291, 292

Gums, bleeding, 93, 105, 194

Gypsy (musical), 225

**H**

Habits, 209, 264, 298, 316, 420–421

Hahnemann, Samuel, 9–14, 20, 21–24, 119, 205, 354–356, 357–

Hangovers, 106

Hatred, 188, 210–220

Hay fever, 112, 155, 184, 331, 340

Headaches, 64, 84, 111, 125, 209, 261, 309, 311, 320, 326, 331, 349

Heal Thyself, 19–20, 27–28, 39

Healing, 43–45, 361–364, 366–368, 383, 399
   self-treatment, 25–26, 27, 31, 38, 45, 354, 359, 365, 367, 378

Health, 109, 160–161, 238–239, 242, 284, 358–360, 393–399

Heart and heart disease, 64, 74, 77, 103, 105, 131, 216, 219, 250, 254, 261, 291, 294, 345

Heartburn, 57

Heather, 70, 321, 323, 329, 332–340, 343, 412, 418
   adults, 338–339
   animals, 339
   children, 338
   homeopathic remedies and, 339–340
   in combination, 172, 234, 336

Helplessness, 63

Herpes, 125

Hippocrates, 20, 21, 356

Hips, 301

Hives, 176

Hodgkin's disease, 105

Holly, 37, 71, 107, 117, 133, 149, 177, 186, 188, 209, 210–220, 231, 391, 398, 413, 419
   adults, 218
   animals, 218, 426
   children, 217–218
   homeopathic remedies and, 218
   in combination, 53, 57, 82, 84, 212, 235, 258, 307, 328–329

Homeopathy, 2, 3, 9–14, 15, 21–24, 26, 36–37, 39, 42–43, 49–50, 56–57, 87, 106, 107, 137, 142–143, 187–188, 193–194, 211, 218, 223, 265–266, 322–323, 353–354, 369–370, 378–379

Homes, 326, 328

Homesickness, 279, 281

Honesty, 367–368, 378, 398

Honeysuckle, 101, 263, 270, 275–281, 328, 415
   adults, 280
   animals, 280
   children, 280
   homeopathic remedies and, 280–281
   in combination, 271, 277, 277, 310, 328, 336

Hopelessness, 143, 156–162, 284, 297, 421

Hormone imbalances, 64, 209

Hornbeam, 95, 150–156, 290, 422–423
   adults, 154–155
   animals, 155, 426
   children, 154
   homeopathic remedies and, 155
   in combination, 274, 282–283, 289, 290, 291, 297

Horses, 63

Hospitalization, 209

Humiliation, 191

Humility, 292–293

Hummingbirds, 51

Humor, sense of, 54, 101, 151, 156, 189, 233, 257–258

Hyperactivity, 64, 82, 84, 179, 249, 252, 348

Hypericum, 136–137

Hypertension, 103, 105, 119, 216, 219, 250, 254, 261, 311, 349

Hyperventilation, 64, 176

Hypoglycemia, 105, 201, 274, 281, 301

Hysteria, 50, 62, 64, 77–84

## I

Ignatia Amara, 83, 87, 119, 183, 187, 208, 218, 288, 322

Ileitis, 245

Illnesses, 146, 148, 157–158, 159–160, 162, 285, 288, 289–290, 294, 300, 301, 358–359, 409–412

   psychosomatic, 111, 169, 340

   sudden, 99, 131, 346

Imagination, 58–59, 303

Immune dysfunction, 112, 125, 148, 209, 237, 250, 254, 320, 340

Impatience, 323, 340–350

Impatiens, 17, 58, 60, 71, 72, 192, 257, 270, 276, 321, 323, 340–350, 410, 414, 423

   adults, 348–349

   animals, 349, 426

   children, 347–348

   homeopathic remedies and, 349

   in combination, 82, 179, 212, 218, 250, 253, 307, 308, 345, 348

Impulsiveness, 78

Indecisiveness, 143, 163–170, 271

Independence, 225

Indifference, 263–320

   Chestnut Bud, 267, 312–320

   Clematis, 266, 267–274

   Honeysuckle, 266, 275–281

   Mustard, 266, 281–288

   Olive, 266, 289–294

   Wild Rose, 266, 294–302

   White Chestnut, 267, 302–312

Inertia. See Apathy.

Infantilization, 172, 176

Infections, 219, 254, 261, 311, 349

Inferiority, sense of, 88–89

Inflammation, 109, 118, 254

Influenza, 119

Inhibitions, 191, 192, 334

Injuries, 349

Insecurity, 64, 171

Insomnia, 57, 59, 64, 70, 155, 169, 245, 254, 281, 294, 306–307, 308–309, 311, 345, 349

Intolerance, 223, 231–237, 256

Intrusiveness, 333, 337

Intuition, 58–59

Irritability, 60, 216, 341, 344, 346

Irritable bowel syndrome, 169, 261, 349

Itching, 331, 349

## J

Jaws, 119, 148, 201, 250, 254, 261, 309, 311

Jealousy, 188, 210–220

Jesus, walking on water, 141

Joints, 103, 105, 118, 119, 209, 219, 331

## K

Kali Carbonica, 105

Kent, J. T., 209

Kidney disorders, 105, 231, 294, 331

King of the Hill (TV show), 102

Knees, 290

**L**

Lachesis, 87, 142–143, 322, 349
Larch, 86, 87, 88–93
  adults, 92
  animals, 92
  children, 91–92
  homeopathic remedies and, 92–93
  in combination, 90, 92, 111, 152,
    192, 234
Laryngitis, 219, 254, 311
Lateness. See Tardiness.
Law of Similars, 12, 23
Law of Simplex, 370
Laws of Cure, 12–13
Lazy eye. See Amblyopia.
Learning, 274, 315, 317–318
Legs, 119, 176, 194, 301
Lethargy, 143, 150–156
Lies and lying, 202, 234, 297
Liver disorders, 119
Lockjaw, 219, 261
Loneliness, 291, 321–350
  Heather, 323, 332–340
  Impatiens, 323, 340–350
  Water Violent, 323, 324–332
Love, 65–66, 67–68, 69, 213–214,
  224–227, 229–230
Lung disorders, 274, 281, 331
Lupus, 162
Lycopodium, 87, 92–93, 142–143, 218,
  261, 288, 322, 349
Lymph disorders, 162, 201

**M**

Malaise, modern, 422
Manic depression, 288
Martial issues, 119
Masochism, 197, 415
Materia Medica, 11, 49
Meaninglessness, 181, 419–420

Medea (mythology), 225
Medical Discoveries of Edward Bach,
  Physician, The, 14, 385
Medicine, 353–368, 369
  allopathic, 1–2, 12, 15, 24–25, 36,
    39, 107, 238, 355, 356–357
  "energy," 2, 107
  herbal, 1, 16, 26, 27188, 282, 289,
    295, 303
  See also Homeopathy.
Memories, 275, 277, 281, 304–305,
  316–317, 328, 344
Men, 194, 260, 348
Menopause, 112, 119, 184, 209, 237,
  281
Mental acuity, 87
Mercurius, 169, 187
Miasms, 205, 354
Middle-age, 93, 99, 104, 250, 280
  See also Crises, midlife.
Migraines. See Headaches.
Mimulus, 17, 27, 49, 50–57, 286, 410,
  420
  adults, 55–56
  animals, 56, 73, 136, 218, 425
  children, 55
  homeopathic remedies and, 56–57
  in combination, 57, 74, 92, 135, 136,
    146, 148, 166, 172, 206, 217, 308
Money. See Finances.
Mononucleosis, 119, 148
Moods (Bach), 28, 31–32, 35, 37;
  40–41, 42, 43–44, 370–371,
  377–378, 382–383
  1st (fear), 47–84
  2nd (despair), 85–137
  3rd (doubt), 139–184
  4th (oversensitivity), 186–220
  5th (control), 221–262
  6th (indifference), 263–320
  7th (loneliness), 321–350

Moods swings, 168, 187, 284, 288
Morning sickness, 169
Mortality. *See* Death and dying.
Mother Tinctures, 26
Motherhood, 201, 231, 237
Mothers, 224, 226, 231, 237, 336
Motivation, lack of, 296, 315
Mouth, 254, 261, 294, 309, 311
Multiple sclerosis, 148, 162, 165
Muscles, 209, 241, 249, 309, 345, 349
Muscular dystrophy, 349
Music, 346
Mustard, 36, 263, 265, 281–288, 290,
    421
  adults, 287
  animals, 287
  children, 286
  homeopathic remedies and, 287–288
  in combination, 105, 106, 115, 123,
    133, 278, 282–283, 284–285, 286,
    287, 289, 290, 291, 292, 297
Myopia, 57, 64, 201, 281

## N

Nail biting, 231, 237
Narcolepsy, 274
Natrum Muriatricum, 70, 87, 223, 265,
    280–281, 331
Nausea, 62
Neck, 105, 148, 241, 245, 249–250, 254,
    294, 309, 311
Neediness, 323, 332–340
Negativity, 86, 88, 113–120, 149, 160,
    258–259, 296, 366–367, 398, 421
Neibuhr, Reinhold, 301
Nelson's, 407–408
Nervous conditions, 84
Neurasthenia, 79
Neutering, 208
New Millennium Flower Essences of
    New Zealand, 433

Nightmares, 58, 59, 62, 77, 135, 155,
    254, 311, 348
Nose bleeds, 176, 201
Nosodes, 16, 17
Nostalgia, 266, 275–281
Numbness, 219, 231
Nurture, 225
Nux Vomica, 187, 218, 261

## O

Oak, 44, 86, 87, 95, 96, 98, 99–106,
    121, 149, 184, 204, 243, 291, 412
  adults, 104
  animals, 104
  children, 103
  homeopathic remedies and, 105
  in combination, 55, 57, 80, 100, 105,
    106, 129, 130, 199, 284, 284–285,
    287, 289, 291, 329
Obsessions, 40, 50, 53, 65–71, 79, 115,
    241, 263–264, 267, 278, 302–320
Old age. *See* Elderly.
Olive, 95, 263, 265, 289–294, 412
  adults, 294
  children, 293
  animals, 294, 427
  homeopathic remedies and, 294
  in combination, 57, 105, 106, 128,
    129, 130, 199, 201, 206, 271, 274,
    278, 284, 285, 287, 289, 297
Onosmodium, 184
Opium, 274
Organization, 86, 107, 108
*Organon of Medicine, The*, 13, 14, 354
Oversensitivity. *See* Sensitivity.
Overwhelmedness, 87, 93–99, 156, 284,
    297
Overwork. *See* Work.

## P

Pacific Essences, 432

Pain, 192, 241, 346
  ankle, 290
  chronic, 105, 118, 157–158, 216,
    294, 341
  eye, 155, 309
  hips, 301
  jaw, 119, 148, 201, 250, 254, 261,
    309, 311
  joint, 103, 105, 118, 119, 209, 219,
    331
  knee, 290
  leg, 119, 176, 301
  mouth, 254, 261, 294, 309, 311
  muscle, 209, 241, 249, 309, 345, 349
  neck, 105, 148, 241, 245, 249–250,
    254, 294, 309, 311
  shoulder, 241, 245, 290, 309, 311
  toe, 184
Palpitations, 56, 57, 64
Pancreas disorders, 274
Panic and panic attacks, 50, 63, 77,
    71–77, 92
Paracelsus, 10, 20, 21–22
Paranoia, 64, 80, 216
Parents, 82–83, 111, 118, 135, 200, 257,
    260
  See also Fathers; Mothers.
Passion, 179–180, 222, 326
Passivity, 108, 200, 264, 268, 281, 415
Patients, 15–16, 257, 258, 355–360,
    363–364, 365–368, 372–373,
    380–381, 387–388, 393, 395–397
Perelandra, Ltd., 431–432
Perfectionism, 87, 98, 106–112, 201,
    234, 238, 329, 422
Personality
  archetypes, 18, 31, 390–391
Pessimism, 67–68, 145, 153, 421
Pets, 56, 130, 136, 137, 155, 175, 208,
    226, 230, 231, 250, 253, 272, 280,
    301, 319, 339, 349, 425–428

Phobias, 63, 172, 420
  being alone, 56–57, 64, 127, 172
  commitment, 165, 178
  darkness, 169, 172
  germ, 110
  tests, 74, 147
  water, 169
  See also Claustrophobia.
Phosphoric acid, 161, 294
Phosporus, 63–64, 184, 187, 265, 322
Picricum Acidum, 294
Pine, 88, 120–126, 421, 427
  adults, 125
  animals, 125
  children, 122, 124
  homeopathic remedies and, 125
  in combination, 106, 123–124, 135,
    136, 199, 286, 291, 292
Platinum, 237
Pneumonia, 105
Poisoning, 112, 212
  food, 106, 112
Polio, 219
Polycrests, 35
Possessiveness, 223
Postnasal drip, 176, 194
Power, 258
Pregnancy, 70, 162, 184, 209
Premenstrual syndrome, 184
Pride, 327
Primary Remedies, 177, 210, 210
Procrastination, 93, 153, 201
Proportion, 89
Psora, 205
Psoriasis, 274
Psyche and Substance, 137
Psychic abilities, 59
Public speaking, 74, 90
Pulsatilla, 169, 187, 194, 266, 288, 322,
    339–340
Purging, 180

Purity, 106, 107
Pushiness, 256

**R**

Rabies, 219
Rage. *See* Anger.
Rashes, 237, 349
Reality, 272
    avoidance of, 269, 274
Red Chestnut, 50, 65–71, 304, 308
    adults, 69
    animals, 69
    children, 68–69
    homeopathic remedies and, 70
    in combination, 172
Rejection, 93
Repetition, 150–151
Rescue Remedy, 1, 17, 56, 63; 76, 129,
        133, 268, 286, 345, 371–372, 373,
        423
    components, 71, 78, 131, 267, 341,
        385–392, 423
Resignation, 263, 288, 290, 295–298,
        300, 301–302
Responsibilities, 86, 94, 102, 252
Restlessness, 60, 246–247, 253,
        321–322, 341, 346
Revenge. *See* Vengeance.
Rheumatism, 231, 237, 254, 311
Rhus Tox, 125, 187, 322
Rigidity, 100, 101, 115, 118, 126,
        128–129, 223, 233, 237–247,
        326–327
Ringworm, 237
Road rage, 350
Rock Rose, 36, 50, 71–77, 184, 391,
        410–411, 414, 423
    adults, 76
    animals, 76
    children, 75–76
    homeopathic remedies and, 76

    in combination, 49, 63, 74, 75, 130,
        212, 217, 240, 253
Rock Water, 100, 101, 172, 237–246,
        412
    adults, 243–244
    animals, 244
    children, 243
    homeopathic remedies and, 244–245
    in combination, 110, 111, 234, 241,
        258
Rose hips, 295
Rumex, 187

**S**

Sciatica, 119, 184, 201, 219, 254
*Science of the Mind*, 22
Scleranthus, 143, 163–170, 171, 204,
        411, 415–416
    adults, 168–169
    animals, 169, 426
    children, 168
    homeopathic remedies and, 169
    in combination, 166, 170, 207, 271,
        284, 346
Seasons, 187
Sedatives, 246
Self, sense of, 25–26, 38–39, 88, 89–90,
        121, 141, 164, 173, 175, 190,
        191–192, 196, 197–198, 200, 233,
        340
Self-centeredness, 333, 336, 337, 420
Self-consciousness, 87, 88–93
Self-doubt, 143, 145–146, 164,
        170–176
Selfishness. *See* Self-centeredness.
Self-treatment. *See* Healing, self-
        treatment.
Senility, 281, 301
Sensitivity, 58, 59, 60, 62, 64, 81,
        185–220
    Agrimony, 188–195

Centaury, 188, 195–202
  Holly, 188, 210–220; 188
  Walnut, 202–210
Sepia, 218, 223, 230–231, 288
Serenity Prayer, 301
Seven Helpers, 18, 411–412
Sexual dysfunction, 93, 112, 125, 184,
  331
Sexuality, 93, 122, 286, 331, 334–335
Sexually transmitted diseases, 184
Shame, 121, 199
Shell shock, 74
Shock, 77, 88, 131–137, 212
Shoulders, 241, 245, 290, 309, 311
Shyness, 88, 89, 91, 93, 329
Silicea, 148, 201
Skin, 62, 109, 112, 209, 237, 320, 331,
  340, 349
Sleep, 58, 59, 62, 194, 252, 290, 292,
  294, 306–307, 343
Sleepwalking, 274
Sloth, 153
Snoring, 125, 320
Solar plexus, 56, 76
Sore throats, 261
Sounds, 215
South African Essences, 433
Space, personal, 257, 260, 343
Spaying, 208
Speech disorders, 274
Speed, 349–350
Spinal disorders, 93, 274
Spontaneity, 214, 217, 249, 327
Sprains, 219
Staphysagria, 83, 119, 187, 265
Star of Bethlehem, 56, 71, 74, 85, 88,
  131–137, 210, 211, 391, 398, 423
  adults, 135–136
  animals, 136, 425
  children, 135
  homeopathic remedies and, 136–137

  in combination, 80, 130, 133, 203,
    207, 278, 286, 287, 300, 328
Starvation, 130
Sterility, 70
Stoicism, 101, 238, 302
Storms, 187, 253
Stress, 97, 99, 137, 152, 190, 198, 215,
  250, 254, 274
  post-traumatic, 74
Stroke, 77, 74
Stubbornness, 256, 316, 317
Stuttering, 57
Sulphur, 87, 143, 209, 287, 322
Sulphuric acid, 294
Superiority, 329–330, 342
Sweet Chestnut, 36, 85, 88, 126–131,
  308, 318, 391, 414
  adults, 130
  animals, 130
  children, 130
  homeopathic remedies and,
    130–131
  in combination, 79, 128, 129, 159,
    227, 253, 286, 291, 328, 336
Sympathy, 54–55
Symptoms, suppression of, 24–25,
  193–194, 205

T

Tai chi, 312
Talk, amount of, 173, 191, 247, 248,
  337, 338–339, 340, 344
Tantrums, 348
Tardiness, 201, 270
Tattlers, 252
Technology, electronic, 179, 250, 270
Teenagers. See Adolescence.
Teeth, grinding of, 309
Teething, 209
Terror, 71–77
Therapy, 340

Thoughts, obsessive, 66, 80, 90, 267, 278, 302–312
Thuja, 184
Thyroid disorders, 155
Ticks, 112
Time, 179, 239, 257, 270, 276, 341–342, 348
Timidity, 124
Tinnitus, 237
Toes, 184
Tonsillitis, 57
Toothaches, 82, 201, 219, 345
Transition, 202, 203, 207–208, 209, 422
Travel sickness, 64, 168, 169
*Treatise on Materia Medica, A,* 11–12
Treatment
    left-brained (systematic), 377–378
    right brained (intuitive), 378
Truthfulness, 217
Twelve Healers, 18, 35, 50, 51, 71, 143, 163, 170, 188, 195, 224, 246, 267, 324, 341, 409–411
*Twelve Healers and Seven Helpers, The,* 18, 29, 409
Twitches, 349

**U**

Ulcers, 57, 194, 320
Unemployment, 144, 184, 206, 209
Upheaval, 188, 202–210

**V**

Vagueness, 266, 267–274
Vanity, 336, 337
Veins, varicose, 155, 303
Vengeance, 114, 116, 119–120, 216, 255
Veratrum Album, 87, 261
Verbena. *See* Vervain.
Vertigo, 168, 169
Vervain, 37, 72, 100, 172, 239, 246–254, 256, 345, 346, 391, 411, 414

adults, 252–253
animals, 253, 426
children, 252
homeopathic remedies and, 253–254
in combination, 106, 130, 212, 217, 250, 253, 256, 258, 336, 341, 346, 348
Vine, 100, 117, 172, 239, 254–262, 412, 413, 422
adults, 260
animals, 260, 426
children, 259–260
homeopathic remedies and, 261
in combination, 106, 212, 234, 256, 257, 258, 260, 307, 348
Vital Force, 19, 23, 358
Vithoulkas,George, 362

**W**

Walnut, 63, 133, 186, 188, 196, 202–210, 276, 281, 315, 422
adults, 208
animals, 208, 426
children, 207–208
homeopathic remedies and, 208–209
in combination, 90, 135, 136, 148, 181, 203, 206–207, 273, 280
War, 74, 76
Warts, 237
Water Violet, 81, 277, 321, 323, 324–332, 343, 410, 418
adults, 330–331
animals, 331
children, 330
homeopathic remedies and, 331
in combination, 110, 116, 241, 277, 278, 328–329
Weak will. *See* Will, weak.
Weather, changes in, 61, 64, 187
Weeks, Nora, 14, 15, 385, 386
Weight

over-, 57, 64, 155, 176, 281, 320, 331
under-, 64
White Chestnut, 66, 110, 302–312, 304, 308, 314–315, 345
adults, 310–311
animals, 311, 426
children, 310
homeopathic remedies and, 311
in combination, 53, 57, 58, 80, 90, 115, 116, 212, 250, 271, 274, 278, 307–309, 336, 346
Whitmont, Edward C., 137
Wild Oat, 171, 176–184, 209, 210, 212–213, 220, 276, 281, 315–316, 339, 374, 398, 412, 419
adults,183
animals, 184
children, 182–183
homeopathic remedies and, 184
in combination, 36, 90, 152, 166–167, 181, 206, 241, 273, 285, 298, 316
Wild Rose, 263, 265, 288, 290–291, 294–302
adults, 300
animals, 301
children, 300
homeopathic remedies and, 301
in combination, 159, 181, 199, 289, 293, 297–298, 300
Will, 222
weak, 188, 195–202, 207, 415

Willfulness, 223, 254–262, 422
Willow, 70, 86, 88, 96, 98, 100, 101, 113–120, 149, 210, 211, 215, 227, 236, 258, 288, 290, 296–297, 299, 327, 339, 398
adults, 118
animals, 118–119, 425
children, 117–118
homeopathic remedies and, 119
in combination, 115–116, 145, 161, 258, 260, 307, 328
Withdrawal, 94, 271, 276, 323, 328, 331
Women, 172, 175, 176, 200, 230, 260
Woolf, Virginia, 79
Work, 80, 90, 93, 95–96, 97, 98, 100, 103, 152, 154, 167, 180–181, 182, 196, 206, 209, 239, 240, 250, 257, 284, 291, 305–306, 342, 346
World, post 9/11, 59
Worms, 112
Worry, 145
obsessive, 50, 53, 65–71, 172, 310

**Y**

Yang, 100, 114, 181, 246, 297, 323, 391, 413–415
Ye Suffer from Yourselves, 21–24, 30, 32
Yin, 181, 297, 323, 391, 415–416
Yoga, 312, 345

**Z**

Zeal, 251, 254

# About the Author

Vinton McCabe is the author of six books on the subject of health and healing. Most notably, he is the author of several books on the subject of homeopathy, including *Homeopathy, Healing & You* (1998) and *Practical Homeopathy* (2000), both published by St. Martin's Press. Most recently, he is the author of *Household Homeopathy*, published in January of 2005 by Basic Health Publications. He is also the co-author, with Dr. Marc Grossman, of *Greater Vision*, a book on natural vision improvement, which was published in 2002 by Keats Publishing.

He has studied homeopathy for the past twenty-five years, and served as a homeopathic educator for the past fifteen. He also served as the president of the Connecticut Homeopathic Association from the establishment of that non-profit organization in 1985 until his move to rural Connecticut in the year 2000. As the chief educator for that organization, he has been responsible for training thousands of laypeople and medical professionals alike in the basics of homeopathic philosophy and in the proper uses of homeopathic remedies.

In addition, McCabe has served on the faculty both of the Open Center of Manhattan and the Wainwright House of Rye, New York as a homeopathic educator. He also taught homeopathy at the Learning Annex, the Omega Institute, the New York Botanical Garden, and the Seminar Center in Manhattan. He also served as a member of the Board of Directors for the Hudson Valley School for Classical Homeopathy, for whom he also developed educational materials. He also traveled throughout the United States, teaching courses in homeopathic philosophy and the uses of homeopathic and Bach flower remedies.

Vinton McCabe is presently at work on a series of three new books for Basic Health Publications on the subjects of homeopathy, Bach flower remedies, and cell salts. He is also at work on a book on moderating high blood pressure through natural treatments.

McCabe has worked with medical professionals, including acupuncturists, naturopaths, and chiropractors, as a homeopathic consultant. He also is a trained vision therapist, and practiced vision therapy for seven years (1993–2000) at the Rye Learning Center in Rye, New York.

In addition to his work in vision therapy and homeopathy, Vinton McCabe has won awards for his journalism, as well as for poetry and theatrical writing. He is a published novelist. Recently, he was awarded an individual artist grant by the Connecticut Commission on the Arts for the creation of his first full-length drama, "Appassionata." In 1990, he was given the Dewar's Young Artist award in poetry.

Vinton McCabe has also worked as a producer, a writer, and a host in both television and radio. He was producer and host of the PBS series *Artsweek*, and creator and executive producer of *Healthplan*, an award-winning health-care special produced by Connecticut Public Television. On radio, he has acted as a film and theater critic and hosted his own daily talk show.

As a print journalist, Vinton McCabe has done features work for many weekly and daily papers, as well as monthly publications, including *New England Monthly*, *The Stamford Advocate* and *The New York Times*.

# THE HEALING ENIGMA
## DEMYSTIFYING HOMEOPATHY
Vinton McCabe

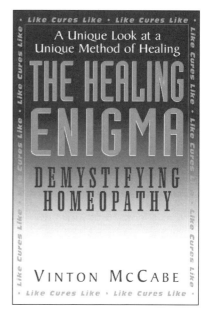

In his twenty-five years as a homeopathic educator, Vinton McCabe has taught thousands of medical professionals and laypersons alike both the philosophy and practice of homeopathic medicine. And through his books on the subject, he has reached many more, giving his readers both the tenets of homeopathy as put forth originally by Samuel Hahnermann more than two hundred years ago and his own unique viewpoint on the subject of homeopathic healing.

In *The Healing Enigma: Demystifying Homeopathy*, McCabe makes use of his full experience in homeopathy to give a fully rounded assessment of the principles of homeopathy and the manner in which it is practiced today. Throughout a text that combines a passionate argument for a mode of healing that is "rapid, gentle, and permanent" in its action, with personal insights and unexpected humor, readers will not only learn what constitutes classical homeopathy and the possibility for healing that it represents for their own lives, but they will also be challenged to consider that the reality of the healing process fundamentally differs from the allopathic concept of curing disease.

Where other books on the subject of homeopathy are limited in their scope to readers who are interested in the mechanics of its practice and the oversimplified selection of remedies, *The Healing Enigma* speaks as much to the practitioners and patients of traditional "allopathic" medicine as it does to those already in the alternative camp. While the "enigma" of the title speaks most directly to the practice of homeopathy, the underlying mystery has to do with the nature of healing itself and the methods that can be used to encourage the healing process.

$17.95 U.S. • 240 pages • 6 x 9 Paperback • ISBN-13: 978-1-59120-071-0

# HOUSEHOLD HOMEOPATHY

## A Safe and Effective Approach to Wellness for the Whole Family

### VINTON McCABE

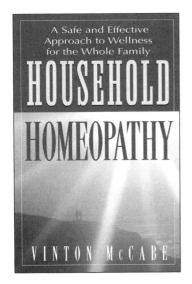

Homeopathy is an alternative medical practice that treats a health condition by administering minute doses of a remedy that would produce symptoms of that condition in a healthy person. Homeopathy is the full expression of holistic medicine, one that sees all people as whole beings in body, mind, and spirit, in whom all symptoms must then be both interconnected and interrelated. As a specific form of medical treatment, homeopathy dates back to just over 200 years ago, but the underlying principles of homeopathy go back to the time of Hippocrates.

Those who wish to gain a practical understanding of homeopathy know that study and dedication are required. This book makes the subject of homeopathy as down to earth and as practical as it can be and provides readers with plenty of food for thought. It discusses the most common homeopathic remedies—such as Arnica, Hypericum, Calendula, Aconite, and many others—and how they can be used safely and effectively. Household Homeopathy teaches readers how to promote healing in themselves and their loved ones—in their own homes. It covers how to handle remedies, how to select them, and how to use them wisely.

From short-term solutions to long-term fixes, the homeopathic approach to wellness can benefit sufferers of virtually every common health condition—from headaches and sore throats to digestive ailments and motion sickness. There will be no need to turn to unnecessary and potentially harmful medications to relieve everyday health complaints. This will also mean fewer trips to the doctor and reduced medical expenses. Armed with the information in this book and the will to fully understand homeopathic treatments, readers will be able to take control of their well-being and that of their loved ones safely and effectively.

$18.95 U.S. • 400 pages • 6 x 9 Paperback • ISBN-13: 978-1-59120-070-3